D0394616

Cardiovascular Diseases and Disorders SOURCEBOOK

Third Edition

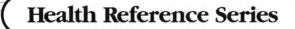

Health Reference Series

Third Edition

Cardiovascular Diseases and Disorders SOURCEBOOK

Basic Consumer Health Information about Heart and Vascular Diseases and Disorders, Such as Angina, Heart Attacks, Arrhythmias, Cardiomyopathy, Valve Disease, Atherosclerosis, and Aneurysms, with Information about Managing Cardiovascular Risk Factors and Maintaining Heart Health, Medications and Procedures Used to Treat Cardiovascular Disorders, and Concerns of Special Significance to Women

Along with Reports on Current Research Initiatives, a Glossary of Related Medical Terms, and a Directory of Sources for Further Help and Information

Edited by
Sandra J. Judd

Omnigraphics

615 Griswold Street • Detroit, MI 48226

Bibliographic Note

Because this page cannot legibly accommodate all the copyright notices, the Bibliographic Note portion of the Preface constitutes an extension of the copyright notice.

Edited by Sandra J. Judd

Health Reference Series

Karen Bellenir, *Managing Editor*
David A. Cooke, M.D., *Medical Consultant*
Elizabeth Barbour, *Permissions and Research Coordinator*
Cherry Stockdale, *Permissions Assistant*
Dawn Matthews, *Verification Assistant*
Laura Pleva Nielsen, *Index Editor*
EdIndex, Services for Publishers, *Indexers*

* * *

Omnigraphics, Inc.

Matthew P. Barbour, *Senior Vice President*
Kay Gill, *Vice President—Directories*
Kevin Hayes, *Operations Manager*
Leif Gruenberg, *Development Manager*
David P. Bianco, *Marketing Director*

* * *

Peter E. Ruffner, *Publisher*

Frederick G. Ruffner, Jr., *Chairman*

Copyright © 2005 Omnigraphics, Inc.

ISBN 0-7808-0739-1

Library of Congress Cataloging-in-Publication Data

Cardiovascular diseases and disorders sourcebook : basic consumer health information about heart and vascular diseases and disorders, such as angina, heart attacks, arrhythmias, cardiomyopathy, valve disease, atherosclerosis, and aneurysms, with information about managing cardiovascular risk factors and maintaining heart health, medications and procedures used to treat cardiovascular disorders, and concerns of special significance to women ; along with reports on current research initiatives, a glossary of related medical terms, and a directory of sources for further help and information / edited by Sandra J. Judd.-- 3rd ed.
    p. cm. -- (Health reference series)
  Includes bibliographical references and index.
  ISBN 0-7808-0739-1 (hardcover : alk. paper)
  1. Heart--Diseases--Popular works. I. Judd, Sandra J. II. Series.
  RC672.C35 2005
  616.1--dc22

                                                                    2004026510

The information in this publication was compiled from the sources cited and from other sources considered reliable. While every possible effort has been made to ensure reliability, the publisher will not assume liability for damages caused by inaccuracies in the data, and makes no warranty, express or implied, on the accuracy of the information contained herein.

∞

This book is printed on acid-free paper meeting the ANSI Z39.48 Standard. The infinity symbol that appears above indicates that the paper in this book meets that standard.

Printed in the United States

Table of Contents

Visit www.healthreferenceseries.com to view *A Contents Guide to the Health Reference Series*, a listing of more than 10,000 topics and the volumes in which they are covered.

Part III: Facts about Heart Diseases and Disorders

Part IV: Facts about Vascular Diseases and Disorders

Part V: Diagnosing Cardiovascular Disorders

Part VI: Medications and Procedures Used to Treat Cardiovascular Disorders

Part VII: Cardiovascular Concerns for Women

Part VIII: Cardiovascular Research

Part IX: Additional Help and Information

Preface

About This Book

Cardiovascular disease is the number-one killer in America today. More than 64 million Americans have some form of cardiovascular disease, including heart disease, high blood pressure, congestive heart failure, congenital heart defects, hardening of the arteries, and other diseases of the circulatory system. As research continues to advance our understanding of cardiovascular disease, the outlook for those suffering from or at risk of developing cardiovascular disease is favorable. Lifestyle changes, along with prompt diagnosis and treatment of existing cardiovascular conditions, can help preserve cardiovascular health for many.

Cardiovascular Disease Sourcebook, Third Edition, provides information about the symptoms, diagnosis, and treatment of cardiovascular diseases and disorders, including heart disease, stroke, and other vascular disorders, along with demographic and statistical data, an overview of the cardiovascular system, a discussion of risk factors and prevention techniques, a look at cardiovascular concerns specific to women, and a report on current research initiatives. A glossary and resources for additional help and information are included.

How to Use This Book

This book is divided into parts and chapters. Parts focus on broad areas of interest. Chapters are devoted to single topics within a part.

Part I: Understanding Cardiovascular Risks looks first at how the cardiovascular system works, then investigates a number of the primary risk factors for cardiovascular disease, including genetic predisposition, aging, stress, smoking, and metabolic syndrome. The part finishes with a description of cardiopulmonary resuscitation (CPR) techniques and a look at automatic external defibrillators.

Part II: Maintaining Heart Health discusses methods of keeping your heart healthy, including healthy diet; controlling blood cholesterol, blood pressure, and diabetes; maintaining a healthy weight; pursuing a regular regimen of physical activity; and daily aspirin therapy. It also includes a discussion of cardiac rehabilitation and information about sexual activity for heart patients.

Part III: Facts about Heart Diseases and Disorders describes the primary types of diseases and disorders affecting the heart, including coronary heart disease, angina, heart attack, and arrhythmias. Each chapter includes a description of symptoms, causes, diagnosis, and treatments.

Part IV: Facts about Vascular Diseases and Disorders focuses on diseases and disorders affecting the vascular system, including, atherosclerosis, stroke, and aneurysms. Each chapter describes symptoms, causes, diagnosis, and treatments.

Part V: Diagnosing Cardiovascular Disorders provides information about the various methods used to diagnose cardiovascular disorders, including blood tests, exercise stress testing, echocardiograms, electrocardiograms, and computer imaging.

Part VI: Medications and Procedures Used to Treat Cardiovascular Disorders describes the primary forms of medical and surgical treatment of cardiovascular diseases and disorders, including cholesterol-lowering drugs, angiotensin converting enzyme (ACE) inhibitors, and other medications and various procedures and devices, such as angioplasty, coronary artery bypass grafting, and cardiac pacemakers.

Part VII: Cardiovascular Concerns for Women discusses concerns about cardiovascular disease that are specific to women, including the effects of heart disease on childbearing, birth control pills and heart disease risk, hormone therapy and cardiovascular risk, and current research on women and heart disease.

Part VIII: Cardiovascular Research describes the latest research in the area of cardiovascular diseases and disorders, including research on homocysteine as a risk factor, C-reactive protein as a predictor of heart disease, vitamin E and garlic as methods of cardiovascular disease prevention, the link between periodontal disease and cardiovascular disease risk, effects of alcohol on heart disease risk, new stroke treatment methods, and chelation and cellular therapies.

Part IX: Additional Help and Information offers a glossary of terms related to cardiovascular disease, a listing of heart-healthy cookbooks, and a directory of organizational resources that can provide further information and help in specific areas.

Bibliographic Note

This volume contains documents and excerpts from publications issued by the following U.S. government agencies: Agency for Healthcare Research and Quality (AHRQ); Centers for Disease Control and Prevention (CDC); National Cancer Institute (NCI); National Center for Complementary and Alternative Medicine (NCCAM); National Heart, Lung, and Blood Institute (NHLBI); National Institute of Dental and Craniofacial Research (NIDCR); National Institute of Diabetes and Digestive and Kidney Disorders (NIDDK); National Institute of Neurological Diseases and Disorders (NINDS); National Institute on Aging; National Institute on Mental Health (NIMH); National Institutes of Health (NIH); National Women's Health Information Center (NWHIC); Office of the Surgeon General; U.S. Department of Agriculture (USDA); U.S. Department of Health and Human Services (HHS); U.S. Food and Drug Administration (FDA); and the Women's Health Initiative (WHI).

In addition, this volume contains copyrighted documents from the following organizations and individuals: A.D.A.M., Inc.; Alliance for Aging Research; American Academy of Family Physicians; American Heart Association; American Society of Echocardiography; American Society of Health-System Pharmacists; American Society of Interventional and Therapeutic Neuroradiology; Cleveland Clinic Department of Rheumatic and Immunologic Diseases; Cleveland Clinic Heart Center; Congenital Heart Information Network; Gale Group; HealthandAge.com; Heart Center Online; Heart Rhythm Society; Howard Gilman Institute for Valvular Heart Disease; Johns Hopkins Bayview Medical Center; Lippincott Williams and Wilkins; March of Dimes Birth Defect Foundation; McKesson Health Solutions LLC; Medical College of Wisconsin's *MCW HealthLink*; *Medical Journal of Australia*; Mount

Sinai School of Medicine; MyDR.com.au; National Coalition for Women with Heart Disease; National Stroke Association; New York State Office for the Aging; Norfolk County Cardiology Associates; St. Jude Medical, Inc.; St. Luke's Regional Medical Center; Thyroid Foundation of Canada; University of Pennsylvania Health System; University of Washington School of Medicine; Vascular Disease Foundation; Washington University School of Medicine, St. Louis-Division of Cardiothoracic Surgery; and WebMD Corporation.

Full citation information is provided on the first page of each chapter. Every effort has been made to secure all necessary rights to reprint the copyrighted material. If any omissions have been made, please contact Omnigraphics to make corrections for future editions.

Acknowledgements

Thanks go to the many organizations, agencies, and individuals who have contributed materials for this *Sourcebook* and to medical consultant Dr. David Cooke, verification assistant Dawn Matthews, and document engineer Bruce Bellenir. Special thanks go to managing editor Karen Bellenir and permissions specialist Liz Barbour for their help and support.

About the Health Reference Series

The *Health Reference Series* is designed to provide basic medical information for patients, families, caregivers, and the general public. Each volume takes a particular topic and provides comprehensive coverage. This is especially important for people who may be dealing with a newly diagnosed disease or a chronic disorder in themselves or in a family member. People looking for preventive guidance, information about disease warning signs, medical statistics, and risk factors for health problems will also find answers to their questions in the *Health Reference Series*. The *Series*, however, is not intended to serve as a tool for diagnosing illness, in prescribing treatments, or as a substitute for the physician/patient relationship. All people concerned about medical symptoms or the possibility of disease are encouraged to seek professional care from an appropriate health care provider.

Locating Information within the Health Reference Series

The *Health Reference Series* contains a wealth of information about a wide variety of medical topics. Ensuring easy access to all the fact sheets, research reports, in-depth discussions, and other material contained within the individual books of the series remains one of our highest priorities. As the *Series* continues to grow in size and scope, however, locating the precise information needed by a reader may become more challenging.

A Contents Guide to the Health Reference Series was developed to direct readers to the specific volumes that address their concerns. It presents an extensive list of diseases, treatments, and other topics of general interest compiled from the Tables of Contents and major index headings. To access *A Contents Guide to the Health Reference Series*, visit www.healthreferenceseries.com.

Medical Consultant

Medical consultation services are provided to the *Health Reference Series* editors by David A. Cooke, M.D. Dr. Cooke is a graduate of Brandeis University, and he received his M.D. degree from the University of Michigan. He completed residency training at the University of Wisconsin Hospital and Clinics. He is board-certified in Internal Medicine. Dr. Cooke currently works as part of the University of Michigan Health System and practices in Brighton, MI. In his free time, he enjoys writing, science fiction, and spending time with his family.

Our Advisory Board

We would like to thank the following board members for providing guidance to the development of this series:

Dr. Lynda Baker, Associate Professor of Library and
Information Science, Wayne State University,
Detroit, MI

Nancy Bulgarelli, William Beaumont Hospital Library,
Royal Oak, MI

Karen Imarisio, Bloomfield Township Public Library,
Bloomfield Township, MI

Karen Morgan, Mardigian Library, University of Michigan-
Dearborn, Dearborn, MI

Rosemary Orlando, St. Clair Shores Public Library,
St. Clair Shores, MI

Health Reference Series *Update Policy*

The inaugural book in the *Health Reference Series* was the first edition of *Cancer Sourcebook* published in 1989. Since then, the *Series* has been enthusiastically received by librarians and in the medical community. In order to maintain the standard of providing high-quality health information for the layperson the editorial staff at Omnigraphics felt it was necessary to implement a policy of updating volumes when warranted.

Medical researchers have been making tremendous strides, and it is the purpose of the *Health Reference Series* to stay current with the most recent advances. Each decision to update a volume is made on an individual basis. Some of the considerations include how much new information is available and the feedback we receive from people who use the books. If there is a topic you would like to see added to the update list, or an area of medical concern you feel has not been adequately addressed, please write to:

Editor
Health Reference Series
Omnigraphics, Inc.
615 Griswold Street
Detroit, MI 48226
E-mail: editorial@omnigraphics.com

Part One

Understanding Cardiovascular Risks

Chapter 1

How the Heart Works

Introduction to the Cardiovascular System

The cardiovascular system is sometimes called the blood-vascular or simply the circulatory system. It consists of the heart, which is a muscular pumping device, and a closed system of vessels called arteries, veins, and capillaries. As the name implies, blood contained in the circulatory system is pumped by the heart around a closed circle or circuit of vessels as it passes again and again through the various "circulations" of the body.

The vital role of the cardiovascular system in maintaining homeostasis depends on the continuous and controlled movement of blood through the thousands of miles of capillaries that permeate every tissue and reach every cell in the body. It is in the microscopic capillaries that blood performs its ultimate transport function. Nutrients and other essential materials pass from capillary blood into fluids surrounding the cells as waste products are removed.

This information is excerpted from "Unit Seven: Cardiovascular System," SEER Web-based Training Modules, 2000. SEER training modules are funded by the U.S. National Cancer Institute's Surveillance, Epidemiology and End Results (SEER) Program, via contract number N01-CN-67006, with Emory University, Atlanta SEER Cancer Registry, Atlanta, Georgia, U.S.A. The complete text of this unit can be accessed through http://training.seer.cancer.gov/module_anatomy/anatomy_map.html.

3

Structure of the Heart

The human heart is a four-chambered muscular organ, shaped and sized roughly like a man's closed fist, with two-thirds of the mass to the left of midline.

The heart is enclosed in a pericardial sac that is lined with the parietal layers of a serous membrane. The visceral layer of the serous membrane forms the epicardium.

Layers of the Heart Wall

Three layers of tissue form the heart wall. The outer layer of the heart wall is the epicardium, the middle layer is the myocardium, and the inner layer is the endocardium.

Chambers of the Heart

The internal cavity of the heart is divided into four chambers:

- Right atrium
- Right ventricle
- Left atrium
- Left ventricle

The two atria are thin-walled chambers that receive blood from the veins. The two ventricles are thick-walled chambers that forcefully pump blood out of the heart. Differences in thickness of the heart chamber walls are due to variations in the amount of myocardium present, which reflects the amount of force each chamber is required to generate.

The right atrium receives deoxygenated blood from systemic veins; the left atrium receives oxygenated blood from the pulmonary veins.

Valves of the Heart

Pumps need a set of valves to keep the fluid flowing in one direction, and the heart is no exception. The heart has two types of valves that keep the blood flowing in the correct direction. The valves between the atria and ventricles are called atrioventricular valves (also called cuspid valves), while those at the bases of the large vessels leaving the ventricles are called semilunar valves.

The right atrioventricular valve is the tricuspid valve. The left atrioventricular valve is the bicuspid, or mitral, valve. The valve between the right ventricle and pulmonary trunk is the pulmonary semilunar valve. The valve between the left ventricle and the aorta is the aortic semilunar valve.

When the ventricles contract, atrioventricular valves close to prevent blood from flowing back into the atria. When the ventricles relax, semilunar valves close to prevent blood from flowing back into the ventricles.

Pathway of Blood through the Heart

While it is convenient to describe the flow of blood through the right side of the heart and then through the left side, it is important to realize that both atria contract at the same time and both ventricles contract at the same time. The heart works as two pumps, one on the right and one on the left, working simultaneously. Blood flows from the right atrium to the right ventricle, and then is pumped to the lungs to receive oxygen. From the lungs, the blood flows to the left atrium, then to the left ventricle. From there it is pumped to the systemic circulation.

Blood Supply to the Myocardium

The myocardium of the heart wall is a working muscle that needs a continuous supply of oxygen and nutrients to function with efficiency. For this reason, cardiac muscle has an extensive network of blood vessels to bring oxygen to the contracting cells and to remove waste products.

The right and left coronary arteries, branches of the ascending aorta, supply blood to the walls of the myocardium. After blood passes through the capillaries in the myocardium, it enters a system of cardiac (coronary) veins. Most of the cardiac veins drain into the coronary sinus, which opens into the right atrium.

Classification and Structure of Blood Vessels

Blood vessels are the channels or conduits through which blood is distributed to body tissues. The vessels make up two closed systems of tubes that begin and end at the heart. One system, the pulmonary vessels, transports blood from the right ventricle to the lungs and back to the left atrium. The other system, the systemic vessels, carries blood from the left ventricle to the tissues in all parts of the body and then returns the blood to the right atrium. Based on their structure and function, blood vessels are classified as either arteries, capillaries, or veins.

5

Arteries

Arteries carry blood away from the heart. Pulmonary arteries transport blood that has a low oxygen content from the right ventricle to the lungs. Systemic arteries transport oxygenated blood from the left ventricle to the body tissues. Blood is pumped from the ventricles into large elastic arteries that branch repeatedly into smaller and smaller arteries until the branching results in microscopic arteries called arterioles. The arterioles play a key role in regulating blood flow into the tissue capillaries. About 10 percent of the total blood volume is in the systemic arterial system at any given time.

The wall of an artery consists of three layers. The innermost layer, the tunica intima (also called tunica interna), is simple squamous epithelium surrounded by a connective tissue basement membrane with elastic fibers. The middle layer, the tunica media, is primarily smooth muscle and is usually the thickest layer. It not only provides support for the vessel but also changes vessel diameter to regulate blood flow and blood pressure. The outermost layer, which attaches the vessel to the surrounding tissue, is the tunica externa or tunica adventitia. This layer is connective tissue with varying amounts of elastic and collagenous fibers. The connective tissue in this layer is quite dense where it is adjacent to the tunica media, but it changes to loose connective tissue near the periphery of the vessel.

Capillaries

Capillaries, the smallest and most numerous of the blood vessels, form the connection between the vessels that carry blood away from the heart (arteries) and the vessels that return blood to the heart (veins). The primary function of capillaries is the exchange of materials between the blood and tissue cells.

Capillary distribution varies with the metabolic activity of body tissues. Tissues such as skeletal muscle, liver, and kidney have extensive capillary networks because they are metabolically active and require an abundant supply of oxygen and nutrients. Other tissues, such as connective tissue, have a less abundant supply of capillaries. The epidermis of the skin and the lens and cornea of the eye completely lack a capillary network. About 5 percent of the total blood volume is in the systemic capillaries at any given time. Another 10 percent is in the lungs.

Smooth muscle cells in the arterioles where they branch to form capillaries regulate blood flow from the arterioles into the capillaries.

Veins

Veins carry blood toward the heart. After blood passes through the capillaries, it enters the smallest veins, called venules. From the venules, it flows into progressively larger and larger veins until it reaches the heart. In the pulmonary circuit, the pulmonary veins transport blood from the lungs to the left atrium of the heart. This blood has a high oxygen content because it has just been oxygenated in the lungs. Systemic veins transport blood from the body tissue to the right atrium of the heart. This blood has a reduced oxygen content because the oxygen has been used for metabolic activities in the tissue cells.

The walls of veins have the same three layers as the arteries. Although all the layers are present, there is less smooth muscle and connective tissue. This makes the walls of veins thinner than those of arteries, which is related to the fact that blood in the veins has less pressure than in the arteries. Because the walls of the veins are thinner and less rigid than arteries, veins can hold more blood. Almost 70 percent of the total blood volume is in the veins at any given time. Medium and large veins have venous valves, similar to the semilunar valves associated with the heart, that help keep the blood flowing toward the heart. Venous valves are especially important in the arms and legs, where they prevent the backflow of blood in response to the pull of gravity.

Physiology of Circulation

Role of the Capillaries

In addition to forming the connection between the arteries and veins, capillaries have a vital role in the exchange of gases, nutrients, and metabolic waste products between the blood and the tissue cells. Substances pass through the capillary wall by diffusion, filtration, and osmosis. Oxygen and carbon dioxide move across the capillary wall by diffusion. Fluid movement across a capillary wall is determined by a combination of hydrostatic and osmotic pressure. The net result of the capillary microcirculation created by hydrostatic and osmotic pressure is that substances leave the blood at one end of the capillary and return at the other end.

Blood Flow

Blood flow refers to the movement of blood through the vessels from arteries to the capillaries and then into the veins. Pressure is a measure of the force that the blood exerts against the vessel walls as it moves the blood through the vessels. Like all fluids, blood flows from a high pressure area to a region with lower pressure. Blood flows in the same direction as the decreasing pressure gradient: arteries to capillaries to veins.

The rate, or velocity, of blood flow varies inversely with the total cross-sectional area of the blood vessels. As the total cross-sectional area of the vessels increases, the velocity of flow decreases. Blood flow is slowest in the capillaries, which allows time for exchange of gases and nutrients.

Resistance is a force that opposes the flow of a fluid. In blood vessels, most of the resistance is due to vessel diameter. As vessel diameter decreases, the resistance increases and blood flow decreases.

Very little pressure remains by the time blood leaves the capillaries and enters the venules. Blood flow through the veins is not the direct result of ventricular contraction. Instead, venous return depends on skeletal muscle action, respiratory movements, and constriction of smooth muscle in venous walls.

Pulse and Blood Pressure

Pulse refers to the rhythmic expansion of an artery that is caused by ejection of blood from the ventricle. It can be felt where an artery is close to the surface and rests on something firm.

In common usage, the term blood pressure refers to arterial blood pressure, the pressure in the aorta and its branches. Systolic pressure is due to ventricular contraction. Diastolic pressure occurs during cardiac relaxation. Pulse pressure is the difference between systolic pressure and diastolic pressure. Blood pressure is measured with a sphygmomanometer and is recorded as the systolic pressure over the diastolic pressure. Four major factors interact to affect blood pressure: cardiac output, blood volume, peripheral resistance, and viscosity. When these factors increase, blood pressure also increases.

Arterial blood pressure is maintained within normal ranges by changes in cardiac output and peripheral resistance. Pressure receptors (baroreceptors), located in the walls of the large arteries in the thorax and neck, are important for short-term blood pressure regulation.

Chapter 2

Heart Disease and Stroke Statistics

Diseases of the Heart

Heart disease is the nation's leading cause of death. Much of the burden of heart disease could be eliminated by reducing the prevalence rates of its major risk factors: high blood pressure, high blood cholesterol, tobacco use, diabetes, physical inactivity, and poor nutrition. Modest reductions in the rates of one or more of these risk factors can have a large public health impact. Heart disease can also be prevented or controlled through governmental policies (such as restricting access to tobacco) and through environmental changes (such as providing better access to healthy foods and opportunities for physical activity).

- Heart disease, which killed more than 700,000 Americans in 2001, accounted for 29 percent of all deaths in the United States.

- In 2001, the rate of death from heart disease was 31 percent higher among blacks than among whites and 49 percent higher among men than among women.

This chapter includes information from the following publications of the Centers for Disease Control: "The Burden of Heart Disease, Stroke, Cancer, and Diabetes, United States: Diseases of the Heart," updated June 10, 2004; "Heart Disease" (FASTATS), updated July 26, 2004; "Hypertension" (FASTATS), updated July 26, 2004; "The Burden of Heart Disease, Stroke, Cancer, and Diabetes, United States: Stroke," updated June 10, 2004; and "Stroke/Cerebrovascular Disease" (FASTATS), updated July 22, 2004.

- In 2001, heart disease cost the nation $193.8 billion.
- About 66 percent of heart attack patients do not make a complete recovery.
- About 42 percent of people who experience a heart attack in a given year will die from it.

Heart Disease Statistics

(Data are for U.S. for year in parentheses)

Morbidity

- Number of noninstitutionalized adults with diagnosed heart disease: 23.0 million (2001)
- Percentage of noninstitutionalized adults with diagnosed heart disease: 11.5 (2001)

Source: Summary Statistics for U.S. Adults, 2001

Health Care Use

Ambulatory Care

- Number of office-based physician visits: 26.2 million (2001)

Source: National Ambulatory Medical Care Survey: 2001 Summary

- Number of hospital outpatient department visits: 1,075,000 (2002)

Source: National Hospital Ambulatory Medical Care Survey: 2002 Outpatient Department Summary

Hospital Inpatient Care

- Number of discharges: 4.4 million (2002)
- Average length of stay: 4.6 days (2002)

Source: 2002 National Hospital Discharge Survey

Home Health Care

- Number of current patients with heart disease as primary diagnosis: 147,600 (2000)

- Percentage of current patients with heart disease as primary diagnosis: 10.9 (2000)

Source: National Home and Hospice Care Survey

Hospice Care

- Number of current patients with heart disease as primary diagnosis: 13,500 (2000)

- Percentage of current patients with heart disease as primary diagnosis: 12.8 (2000)

Source: National Home and Hospice Care Survey

Nursing Home Care

- Number of residents with heart disease as primary diagnosis: 165,100 (1999)

- Percentage of residents with heart disease as primary diagnosis: 10.1 (1999)

Source: National Nursing Home Survey: 1999 Summary

Mortality

- Number of deaths: 700,142 (2001)
- Deaths per 100,000 population: 245.8 (2001)
- Cause of death rank: 1 (2001)

Source: Deaths: Final Data for 2001

- Percentage of hospital inpatient deaths from heart disease: 21.0 (2000)

Source: National Hospital Discharge Survey: 2000 Annual Summary with Detailed Diagnosis and Procedure Data

Hypertension Statistics

(Data are for U.S. for year in parentheses)

Morbidity

- Percentage of noninstitutionalized adults ages twenty and over: 32 (1999–2000)

Source: Health, United States, 2002, table 68

11

Health Care Use

Ambulatory Care

- Number of visits to office-based physicians: 10.4 million (2001)

Source: National Ambulatory Medical Care Survey: 2001 Summary

- Number of hospital outpatient department visits: 1.2 million (2002)

Source: National Hospital Ambulatory Medical Care Survey: 2002 Outpatient Summary

Home Health Care

- Number of current patients with hypertension as primary diagnosis: 41,900 (2000)

- Percentage of current patients with hypertension as primary diagnosis: 3.1

Source: National Home and Hospice Care Survey

Nursing Home Care

- Number of residents with hypertension: 481,800 (1999)

- Percentage of residents with hypertension: 26.4 (1999)

- Average length of stay for discharges with hypertension as primary diagnosis: 494 days

Source: National Nursing Home Survey: 1999 Summary

Mortality

- Number of deaths: 19,250 (2001)

- Deaths per 100,000 population: 8.7 (2001)

Source: Deaths: Final Data for 2001

Stroke

Stroke, or cerebrovascular disease, is the third-leading cause of death and a major cause of disability in the United States. The major risk factors for stroke are high blood pressure, high blood cholesterol, tobacco use, heart disease, diabetes, physical inactivity, and poor nutrition. Preventing stroke and controlling its risk factors are essential to reducing health care costs and improving the quality of life among older Americans. A person's chance of having a stroke more than doubles for each decade of life after age fifty-five.

- Each year, about 700,000 Americans have a stroke. On average, a stroke occurs every forty-five seconds.

- In 2001, stroke accounted for more than 163,500 deaths.

- In 2001, rates of death from stroke were 43 percent higher among blacks than among whites.

- Each year, about 40,000 more women than men have a stroke.

- In a recent study, only 17 percent of the public recognized enough of the major warning signs of stroke to call 911.

- Emergency therapy, if applied within three hours, can drastically reduce disabilities from certain kinds of strokes.

Stroke and Cerebrovascular Disease Statistics

(Data are for U.S. for year in parentheses)

Morbidity

- Number of noninstitutionalized adults who ever had a stroke: 4.8 million (2002)

- Percentage of noninstitutionalized adults who ever had a stroke: 2.4 (2002)

Source: Summary Health Statistics for U.S. Adults, 2002

Health Care Use

Hospital Inpatient Care

- Number of discharges: 942,000 (2002)

- Average length of stay: 5.3 days (2002)

Source: 2002 National Hospital Discharge Survey

Home Health Care

- Number of current patients with stroke as primary diagnosis: 99,400 (2000)

- Percentage of current patients with stroke as primary diagnosis: 7.3 (2000)

Source: National Home and Hospice Care Survey

Mortality

- Number of deaths: 163,538 (2001)
- Deaths per 100,000 population: 57.4 (2001)
- Cause of death rank: 3 (2001)

Source: Deaths: Final Data for 2001

- Percentage of hospital inpatient deaths from stroke/cerebrovascular disease: 7.2 (2001)

Source: National Hospital Discharge Survey, 2001 Annual Summary with Detailed Diagnosis and Procedure Data

Disease

Chapter 3

Risk Factors for Cardiovascular Disease

About Cardiovascular Risk Factors

Risk factors are conditions or behaviors that increase your chance of getting a certain disease. This chapter discusses risk factors for coronary heart disease (also called coronary artery disease).

Some risk factors for coronary heart disease can be treated or controlled and some cannot.

- The more risk factors you have, the greater your risk of developing coronary heart disease.

- The higher your level of each risk factor, the greater your risk of developing coronary heart disease.

The best way to prevent coronary heart disease is to:

- Know your risk factors
- Tell your doctor if you have any risk factors
- Take steps to control your controllable risk factors

Uncontrollable Risk Factors

Increasing Age

- The risk of coronary heart disease increases with age.

Reprinted from "Risk Factors for Cardiovascular Disease," U.S. Food and Drug Administration, updated February 27, 2004.

- Men ages forty-five and older have increased risk.
- Women ages fifty-five and older have increased risk.

Family History

- Children of parents who developed coronary heart disease before age fifty-five are more likely to develop it themselves.

Racial or Ethnic Background

- African Americans, Mexican Americans, American Indians, and other Native Americans have greater risk than Caucasians.

Controllable Risk Factors

Physical Inactivity

- People with inactive lifestyles have increased risk.
- Thirty to sixty minutes of physical activity on most days helps reduce the risk of coronary heart disease.

Smoking

- People who smoke cigarettes have the greatest risk.
- People who smoke cigars or pipes seem to have greater risk, but their risk is not as great as that of cigarette smokers.
- Exposure to other people's smoke increases the risk of cardiovascular disease even for nonsmokers.
- Quitting smoking helps reduce the risk of coronary heart disease.

Overweight or Obesity

- People who have too much body fat, especially around the waist, have increased risk.
  - Women with waist measurements of more than thirty-five inches have increased risk.
  - Men with waist measurements of more than forty inches have increased risk.
- People with Body Mass Index (BMI) values of 25 or greater have increased risk.

- Losing weight helps reduce the risk of coronary heart disease.

High Blood Pressure

- People who have blood pressure of 140/90 mm Hg or higher have increased risk.

- Lowering blood pressure reduces the risk of coronary heart disease.

High Blood Cholesterol

- People with total blood cholesterol levels of 200 mg/dL or higher have increased risk.

- People with heart disease or diabetes, who have low-density lipoprotein (LDL) cholesterol levels of 100 mg/dL or higher, have increased risk.

- People with no other risk factors, who have low-density lipoprotein (LDL) levels of 160 mg/dL or higher, have increased risk.

- People with high-density lipoprotein (HDL) cholesterol levels of less than 40 mg/dL may have increased risk.

- People with triglyceride levels above 150 mm/dL may have increased risk.

Diabetes Mellitus

- People who have type 1 or type 2 diabetes have increased risk.

Other Contributing Factors

Stress

- People who have too much stress or who have unhealthy responses to stress may be at greater risk of having coronary heart disease.

Hormone Replacement Therapy (HRT) for the Treatment of Menopause

- Some women who take hormone replacement therapy for the treatment of menopause may have increased risk of blood clots, heart attack, and stroke.

Chapter 4

Blood Tests Can Help Determine Risk of Coronary Artery Disease

These blood tests help to determine your risk for coronary artery disease and guide your treatment.

Lipoprotein a (Lp(a))

Desirable level for adult: less than 30 mg/dl

Preparation

Blood should be collected after a twelve-hour fast (no food or drink, except water). For the most accurate results, wait at least two months after a heart attack, surgery, infection, injury, or pregnancy to check this blood level.

Lp(a) is LDL (low density lipoprotein) attached to a protein called apo (a). It is not fully known what Lp(a) does, but if Lp(a) is greater than 30 mg/dl, it is related to an increased risk for heart attack and stroke. It is also related to development of fatty matter in vein grafts after bypass surgery, coronary artery narrowing after angioplasty, and increased risk for the development of blood clots. If Lp(a) is high, it is even more important to bring the LDL levels down to an acceptable level. Lp(a) is higher in African Americans. The causes of high Lp(a) are kidney disease and certain family (genetic) lipid disorders.

Apolipoprotein A1 (Apo A1)

Desirable level for adult: more than 123 mg/dl

Preparation

Blood should be collected after a twelve-hour fast (no food or drink, except water). For the most accurate results, wait at least two months after a heart attack, surgery, infection, injury, or pregnancy to check this blood level.

Apo A1 is the major protein of HDL. Low levels of Apo A1 are associated with a diet high in fat and smoking and may lead to early heart and blood vessel disease.

Apolipoprotein B (Apo B)

Desirable level for adult: less than 100 mg/dl

Preparation

Blood should be collected after a twelve-hour fast (no food or drink, except water). For the most accurate results, wait at least two months after a heart attack, surgery, infection, injury, or pregnancy to check this blood level.

Apo B is a major protein found in cholesterol particles. New research suggests Apo B may be a better overall marker of risk than LDL alone.

Homocysteine

Desirable level for adult: less than 10 µmol/ml

Preparation

This test may be measured any time of the day without fasting. For the most accurate results, wait at least two months after a heart attack, surgery, infection, injury, or pregnancy to check this blood level.

Homocysteine is a common amino acid (one of the building blocks that make up proteins) found in the blood. High levels of homocysteine are related to the early development of heart and blood vessel disease. In fact, it is considered an independent risk factor for heart disease. High homocysteine is associated with low levels of vitamin B_6, B_{12}, and folate, and renal disease.

Fibrinogen

Desirable range: less than 300 mg/dl

Preparation

Blood should be collected after a twelve-hour fast (no food or drink, except water). For the most accurate results, wait at least two months after a heart attack, surgery, infection, injury, or pregnancy to check this blood level.

Fibrinogen is a protein found in the blood that is necessary for blood clotting. High levels of fibrinogen may be an independent risk factor for vascular disease, especially fibrinogen levels greater than 350 mg/dl. Higher blood pressure, body weight, LDL and age are related to higher levels of fibrinogen. On the other hand, alcohol use and exercise are related to lower fibrinogen levels. Higher fibrinogen levels are also seen with African Americans, and a rise is seen with menopause.

Ultra Sensitive C-Reactive Protein (US-CRP; also called high sensitivity CRP)

Desirable range:

- Less than 1.0 mg/L = Low Relative Risk for CVD
- 1.0–3.0 mg/L = Average Relative Risk for CVD
- Greater than 3.0 mg/L = High Relative Risk for CVD

Levels above these ranges indicate increased risk for heart and blood vessel disease.

Preparation

This test may be measured any time of the day without fasting.

C-reactive protein measures an inflammatory response in the body. In some cases, inflammation in the arteries may play a role in heart disease. Research is showing promising results for testing CRP (along with other risk factors) to determine heart disease risk in those with undetected heart disease, and risk of complications for those who have already had a heart event (such as a heart attack).

Global Risk Score (GRS)

Desirable range:

- less than 10% = low risk
- 10–20% = intermediate risk
- greater than 20% = high risk

A tool that looks at a person's risk factors, weighs them in importance, and then gives a percentage risk of that patient developing heart disease or having a heart attack within the next ten years.

Source: What you need to know about laboratory tests, Preventive Cardiology & Rehabilitation, 2003; CCF Pathology and Lab Medicine Guide, 2003.

Chapter 5

Genetics of Coronary Artery Disease

This chapter provides an overview of coronary heart disease and its genetics. As with all health conditions, it is important for you to talk with your doctor about health issues regarding yourself or your family.

What Everyone Should Know about Coronary Heart Disease

Your heart is a four-chambered muscular organ that pumps blood throughout your body. A healthy heart is necessary to assure that your tissues receive needed oxygen and nutrients while removing waste products such as carbon dioxide. As we age, the heart can be damaged by a number of processes. The heart's electrical system can wear out, and lead one to require an artificial pacemaker. The contraction and relaxing of the heart's muscular walls can decline, leading to a condition known as congestive heart failure. Additionally, the blood vessels (tubes) that supply blood to the heart itself can become partially or completely clogged. This process is known as coronary artery disease.

Coronary artery disease begins in childhood as the walls of our blood vessels take up cholesterol (a fat). As the disease progresses,

---

small cholesterol-filled blisters (or plaques) can form in our coronary arteries. As the narrowing grows, it increasingly limits the flow of blood through the artery. Chest pains occur when the heart requires more blood than can flow through the narrowing arteries.

The process of coronary blockage can also progress rapidly. If plaques break open, a blood clot can form at the site, leading to a sudden complete or nearly complete blockage of the vessel. This can lead to unstable chest pain (angina), symptoms of heart attack, or death of a portion of the heart muscle due to a lack of oxygen.

Coronary artery disease is a leading cause of death and disability in the United States. When the coronary arteries become clogged they can cause the following problems:

- **Angina:** Chest discomfort or pain; shortness of breath. Angina is usually brought on by mental or physical stress or exercise (increased demands for oxygen), and is relieved with rest (decreasing the heart's work).

- **Heart attack:** A sudden blockage of a coronary vessel with measurable damage to the heart muscle.

- **Sudden death:** Lack of blood supply to the heart can also cause irregular electrical heart rhythms, which can cause immediate stoppage of the heart and death.

- **Heart failure:** Damage to the muscle from heart attacks can also cause the heart to stop effectively pumping blood to vital organs.

Several processes are involved in the development of coronary artery disease.

- Factors that damage the coronary vessel wall:
  - High cholesterol and triglycerides (fats in the blood)
  - Smoking
  - High blood pressure (hypertension)
  - Diabetes mellitus

- The body's response to injury:
  - **Immunologic response:** how much inflammation is caused by damage to the vessel wall
  - **Blood clotting factors:** factors in the blood determine the balance between forming blood clots and dissolving them

- Vessel repair processes:
  - How quickly and completely we produce new cells to repair damage

Coronary Artery Disease and Your Family History

If a member of your immediate family (must be a blood relative) has coronary artery disease, your risk of someday developing it is, on average, about twice as high as that of the rest of the population.

Your risk is higher if your relative developed coronary disease at an early age. "Early age" is before age fifty-five in men and before age sixty-five in women. This follows a general rule in genetics: The earlier in life a disease occurs, the greater is the influence of genes.

An increased risk for coronary disease does not mean you will definitely get it. Just as not having coronary heart disease in your family does not mean you won't get it.

Genetic and environmental differences determine the differences in our appearance and health. Some family members will inherit genes that predispose them to coronary artery disease, and others will not. Some family members will be exposed to environmental agents that trigger disease, and others will not. Likewise, some people will inherit "good genes" that protect them from developing coronary disease.

Environmental Factors and Coronary Artery Disease

While your genetics will determine your baseline likelihood for disease, many factors in life will modify this risk. As in most common diseases, coronary artery disease results from an interaction between genes and environment.

Environmental factors that can lower the risk of coronary disease include:

- Avoiding tobacco;
- Controlling blood pressure (by diet, medication, exercise, weight control);
- Controlling diabetes (by diet, medication, exercise, weight control);
- Controlling cholesterol levels (by diet, medication, exercise, weight control);
- Controlling weight (by diet, exercise, and rarely medication);

- Exercising regularly; and
- Taking aspirin daily.

How Genes Are Involved in Coronary Artery Disease

As one might imagine from the preceding discussion, coronary artery disease is a complex disorder, and many genetic and environmental factors can affect its development and prognosis. While the search for genetic keys for diagnosis and treatment of coronary disease is very active today, there is much that remains to be discovered.

First, it is important to understand that there are a number of different genes that can affect the development of coronary disease. For example, there are certain metabolic disorders of the liver that can lead to high cholesterol and blockages in vessels. Alternatively, certain genetic defects can result in a higher likelihood for blood clotting, raising the risk for heart attacks.

Second, for each involved gene, there can be a wide variety of slight changes in the chemical structure of a gene, known as single-nucleotide polymorphisms, or SNPs. Some of these changes can increase one's risk for coronary disease, while others may be protective against the disease.

Third, beyond gene structure, there are complex factors affecting how many times a particular gene will be copied (transcribed) into a protein. And, after the protein is made in a cell, it, too, can be further modified before it ultimately has any impact on the cell or the person as a whole.

Finally, as noted, environmental factors will affect whether someone susceptible for developing disease actually will. Because of these complexities, there have and will be many "false starts" as scientists attempt to fully understand the process of coronary disease. As we develop larger genetic studies and validate early findings, our knowledge of how to diagnose and treat coronary disease will improve.

There are a large number of genes that can affect coronary disease risk. Table 5.1 provides a partial list.

The Future of Coronary Artery Disease and Genetics

Further discoveries about coronary artery disease genes will allow doctors to develop personalized prevention, diagnosis, treatment, and prognosis based upon the strengths and weaknesses found in a person's genes.

Better Use of Existing Treatments

Several medicines have been approved to treat coronary artery disease. Just as specific genes influence the development and progression of coronary artery disease, specific genes may influence the responses to different treatments. Better genetic information could explain why some drugs work better in some people than others. This will make choosing treatments less hit-and-miss than in the past.

Discovery of New Treatments

Whenever scientists discover a gene involved in coronary artery disease, it's a doorway to developing new treatments.

Prevention, Diagnosis, and Prognosis

Prevention, diagnosis, and prognosis all improve when our ability to understand and calculate risk improves. Researchers believe genes will tell us a lot about the risk of developing coronary artery disease and the progression of coronary artery disease.

Table 5.1. Genes Affecting Risk of Coronary Artery Disease (*continued on next page*).

This listing covers only a small portion of the genes involved in coronary artery disease. It does, however, paint a picture of how each person's genetic risk for coronary artery disease is determined by the combined effects of many genes. Further studies will be needed to discover new genes and to better understand how already-discovered genes interact to produce or lower risk.

Gene Name LDLR (LDL receptor)   **Chromosome** 19

This gene is the blueprint for a protein that removes LDL from the blood. Scientists have found over 350 variants of this gene.[a] About one person in five hundred has a variant that leads to a poorly functioning protein, meaning that LDL is not removed from the blood efficiently. These people have high LDL levels and develop coronary artery disease at a young age. The very few people who carry two copies of such a variant have even higher levels of cholesterol and can have a heart attack in childhood.

Gene Name APOA1 (apo-lipo-protein A1)   **Chromosome** 11

This gene is the blueprint for apo A1—a protein that is packaged with cholesterol into HDL. Certain variants of this gene lead to low levels of apo A1. The result is low levels of HDL, early heart attacks, and early strokes.

Table 5.1. (continued)

Gene Name CETP   **Chromosome** 16

This gene is the blueprint for a protein that helps degrade HDL. With certain variants of the gene, degradation is less efficient, and so HDL levels are high. It's not clear whether this results in less coronary artery disease, however. The search for gene variants that raise HDL continues.

Gene Name APOE (apo-lipo-protein E)   **Chromosome** 19

This gene is also involved in Alzheimer's disease. More than thirty variants are known. The apo E protein is involved in removing LDL from the blood. Some variants (most notably the "e2" variant) lead to elevated levels of serum cholesterol and triglycerides.

Gene Name apo(a)   **Chromosome** 6

The protein made from the apo(a) gene combines with LDL to form a particle called "Lp(a)", pronounced "L.P. little A."[b] High levels of Lp(a) increase the risk of developing coronary disease. The structure of apo(a) is similar to that of plasminogen—a protein that powerfully increases the blood's tendency to clot. Interestingly, Lp(a) also accelerates wound healing.

Gene Name ITGB3 (integrin)   **Chromosome** 17

This gene is the blueprint for a protein that sits on the outer surface of platelets. (Platelets are cell fragments that play a critical role in blood clotting.) A recent study found that a certain variant of this gene was present in half of patients under age sixty who were admitted to a hospital intensive care unit with coronary artery disease.[c]

Gene Name ELN (elastin)   **Chromosome** 7

Elastic fibers are found throughout our bodies. They keep our skin tight and our arteries stretchable. Elastic fibers are made of two major components. The ELN gene is the blueprint for one of them—a protein called elastin. Early experiments have shown that arteries deficient in elastin take a shape (thick wall, narrow center) that obstructs blood flow. We all lose elastin as we age. Further experiments will show whether this age-related loss of elastin is related to the development of coronary artery disease.

Gene Name PTGIS   **Chromosome** 20

Unlike a metal pipe, the inner lining of an artery is active and alive. This is well illustrated by the simple fact that blood does not stick to the interior of a normal artery. One reason for this: The inside surface of an artery makes chemicals that are like Teflon® in the sense that they are "nonstick." The PTGIS gene is the blueprint for a protein that makes a nonstick chemical called prostacyclin. Studies of PTGIS in humans have not yet begun.

28

Table 5.1. (continued)

Gene Name ACE   **Chromosome** 20

This gene is one of the most intensively studied in coronary artery disease.[d] It is the blueprint for a protein that ultimately has effects in the kidney, in the heart muscle, and in the walls of arteries. To date, the results of studies in coronary disease have been conflicting.

[a] M. Higgins, "Epidemiology and Prevention of Coronary Heart Disease in Families," *Am J Med* 108, no. 5 (April 1, 2000): 387–95. [Medline]

[b] R. Ross, "The Pathogenesis of Atherosclerosis," chapter 34 in *Heart Disease*, 5th ed., E. Braunwald, ed. (Philadelphia: Saunders, 1997).

[c] E. J. Weiss, P. F. Bray, M. Tayback, S. P. Schulman, T. S. Kickler, L. C. Becker, J. L. Weiss, G. Gerstenblith, and P. J. Goldschmidt-Clermont, "A Polymorphism of a Platelet Glycoprotein Receptor as an Inherited Risk Factor for Coronary Thrombosis," *N Engl J Med* 334, no. 17 (April 25, 1996): 1090–94. [Medline]

[d] G. Gambaro, F. Anglani, and A. D'Angelo, "Association Studies of Genetic Polymorphisms and Complex Disease," *Lancet* 355, no. 9200 (January 22, 2000): 308–11. [Medline]

Chapter 6

Aging and the Heart

Studies show that the heart changes with age but does not necessarily deteriorate in all ways—and that it can continue to support a physically fit body.

Bert Coleman swims three days a week, eighty-eight laps at a time, or about 1.25 miles—not so unusual these days if it weren't for his age: He is sixty-five. Coleman fits anyone's picture of physical fitness: He looks healthy; his muscles are strong; he has no excess fat. Furthermore, for those who need hard evidence, such as cardiovascular scientists, he scores high on the best tests available of physical fitness.

On one level it's no surprise that someone who exercises is also physically fit; we take it for granted. Yet below the surface of that assumption lie intriguing questions. "We know that older people who exercise regularly can do more aerobic work, meaning they are more physically fit," says Edward Lakatta, who is chief of the Laboratory of Cardiovascular Science at the National Institute on Aging (NIA). "But we want to know what changes in the aging heart and blood vessels allow this to happen. What is the link?"

Coleman is a volunteer in a study that is looking for answers to this question. Yet Lakatta and his colleagues already know that the aging heart is not synonymous with a weakening or declining heart. They have learned this through studies over the last two decades that

Reprinted from "Hearts and Arteries: What Scientists Are Learning about Age and the Cardiovascular System," published in 1994 by the National Institute on Aging. Reviewed by David A. Cooke, M.D., on August 3, 2004.

have put together a picture of what happens during "normal" aging—aging in the absence of disease. Now that they understand the aging process, they can turn to the study of lifestyles—such as Coleman's three-times-a-week swimming schedule—to see whether such habits make a difference to the aging heart.

The Effects of Normal Aging

The NIA's studies of normal aging have revealed a series of fine-tuned adjustments that allow the heart to meet the needs of the aging body. This picture is radically different from the one that prevailed several decades ago, when marked declines in overall heart function were thought to be the norm. The revolution in perspective began in the 1970s when researchers came upon their first surprise: The walls of the heart, as it ages, grow thicker.

Thickening of the Heart Walls

Up until then, the people who study aging—gerontologists—thought that the heart shrank with age. One reason was that early researchers knew about the older heart mainly through chest x-rays and autopsy studies of people who were institutionalized, often with chronic illnesses. These people's hearts, which were affected by disease or extremely sedentary lives, often were smaller than those of younger, healthier people.

Then, in the late 1950s, gerontologists began to study healthy volunteers, such as those who take part in the Baltimore Longitudinal Study of Aging (BLSA). Soon after this came new technologies like echocardiography and radionuclide imaging, exciting because they gave information on wall thickness and cavity size and how they change with time during a given heart beat. Where x-rays provide a static, shadowy silhouette, the newer technologies give thickness, diameter, volume, and in some cases, shape before and during the beat. One of the first soundings of the heart's inner compartments was reported in Finland, where A. J. Sjögren's echocardiograms revealed the thickening of the walls of the left ventricle, the heart's main pumping chamber. Of the heart's four compartments, this one holds the most fascination for cardiovascular scientists; it pumps far harder than the other chambers, starting the blood on its roundabout and many-branched journey through the blood vessels. Even a small alteration in this chamber—like wall thickness—makes a significant difference in heart function.

The thicker walls supplied the first clue that the heart might be adjusting, rather than simply declining, with age. Scientists think that the increased thickness allows the walls to compensate for the extra stress they bear with age (stress imposed by pumping blood into stiffer blood vessels, for instance). When walls thicken, stress is spread out over a larger area.

Other findings about the left side of the heart soon followed. In Baltimore, Gary Gerstenblith and his NIA colleagues studied both the left ventricle and the left atrium, the receiving chamber into which the blood flows before passing into the ventricle. Their echocardiograms with BLSA volunteers showed that in addition to the left ventricular wall growing thicker, the cavities of the left atrium and ventricle increased.

This study also yielded one other finding—a curious one: The mitral valve appeared to close more slowly in older people. The mitral valve is at the gateway between the left atrium and ventricle. As the ventricle fills, its two flaps, like a trap door with two separate panels, float up on the rising pool of blood and come almost together to close the passage. If this valve were closing more slowly in older people, as the echocardiograms indicated, then the ventricle must be filling more slowly.

Between Beats

Why should this be so? And did it make any difference?

Researchers turned their attention to a time period, the fraction of a second between heart beats called diastole. During diastole, the heart relaxes, fills with blood, and readies for the next contraction, or systole.

Heart researchers divide the moments of diastole into even shorter periods. There is the early filling phase when blood from the atrium pushes the mitral valve open, flows rapidly into the ventricle, and floats the valves shut. This early diastolic filling is the phase that takes longer as people grow older, according to the Gerstenblith study. Then comes a late filling phase, when the atrium contracts, forces open the valves a second time, and delivers a last surge of blood to the ventricle, just before it too contracts.

Why should early diastolic filling slow down as people age? Could it be because the ventricle wall was not relaxing between heartbeats as quickly as it once had?

This possibility intrigued the Baltimore scientists because it fit neatly with another stray piece to the puzzle. In animal studies several years earlier, Lakatta had learned that rat hearts studied in the laboratory took longer to relax after a contraction when they were from older rats.

Later imaging studies in humans confirmed the animal studies: Between beats, the aging ventricle fills with blood more slowly because it is relaxing more slowly than it had when young.

Just Before the Beat

Yet now another piece of the diastolic puzzle needed to be filled in. If the left ventricle fills more slowly with blood, does this mean it has less blood pooled at the end of diastole and thus less to send out to the body? The answer is no, and the reason was found in another of the adjustments that the heart makes to age. At the National Heart, Lung, and Blood Institute, scientists showed that the heart compensates for the slower early filling rate by filling more quickly in the late diastolic period.

It happens like this: As the mitral valve slowly closes, incoming blood from the lungs pools in the left atrium, which is now larger and holds more blood than when young. In the last moments of diastole, the heart's pacemaker triggers the first electrical impulse (the action potential), which will lead to contraction. The impulse spreads across the cells of the two atriums. The left atrium, stretched with a greater volume of blood in older hearts, contracts harder, pushing open the valves and propelling the blood to the left ventricle. The late surge from the atrium's contraction occurs at all ages but is stronger in older hearts and delivers a greater volume of blood to the left ventricle. As a result, at the end of diastole, the volume of blood in older hearts is about the same (in women) or slightly greater (in men) than in younger hearts.

Pumping

The next step in this chain of events is contraction or systole, and here the puzzle becomes more complex.

Picture the ventricle at the end of diastole filled with a volume of blood that is equal to or slightly greater than the volume in younger hearts; this is called its end diastolic volume. When the contraction comes, it forces out a certain amount of blood—the stroke volume. Yet not all is pumped out at once. A portion remains in the ventricle, and this is the end systolic volume.

These measurements are important because the links between end diastolic volume, stroke volume, and end systolic volume make up a complex set of dynamics that researchers had to sort out as they attempted to understand what difference aging makes in the heart's pumping ability. The various volumes differ according to age, they may differ according to gender—an area that is just beginning to be explored— and they differ depending on degree of physical activity.

Pumping at Rest

The heart rate slows down with age in both men and women when they are sitting at rest. In men, the heart compensates partly for this decline in two ways. First, the increase in end diastolic volume that comes with age means that there is more blood to pump; and second, the greater volume stretches the ventricular walls and brings into play a peculiar property of muscle cells—the more they are stretched, the more they contract. This phenomenon is called the Frank-Starling mechanism and together with the greater volume to be pumped, it helps to make up for the lower heart rate.

In women, end diastolic volume while sitting does not increase with age, so stroke volume does not increase. The difference between the genders probably reflects their different needs rather than a difference in their hearts' pumping abilities. Women tend to have less lean muscle mass than men, and it's lean muscle that needs the most oxygen. When studies compare oxygen consumption based on amount of lean muscle rather than overall body size, the gender differences disappear. Women, in other words, use the same amount of oxygen per unit of lean muscle as do men.

Pumping during Exercise

During any kind of activity—even moving from a sitting to a standing position—the heart must pump more blood to the working muscles. In younger people it does this by increasing the heart rate and squeezing harder during contractions, sending more blood with each beat. Yet age brings changes. Heart rate still rises during exercise, but it can no longer rise as high. Contractions increase in force, but not by as much; one of the most characteristic changes in the aging heart is the loss of the ability to contract as much as it did when young.

If it cannot beat as fast or squeeze down as hard, then how does the heart respond to the demands of vigorous exercise?

This is the scenario: During exercise, the walls of the older ventricle are stretched by the increased load of blood at end diastole. They cannot pump as efficiently as they once could, but because there is a greater end diastolic volume, they put out about the same amount of blood with each beat. In addition, the increased stretch triggers a series of events that adds calcium ions to the heart muscle cells and increases the calcium's ability to interact with the contractile machinery of the cell—the Frank-Starling mechanism at the molecular level. The result of these adaptations and adjustments is that the heart is able to meet the needs of the exercising older body.

Measuring the Heart

Cardiovascular scientists have several ways to measure heart function. Age, physical activity, and gender all make a difference. The figures given here are in milliliters (ml) per square meter of body surface. They are based on studies with healthy adults, age twenty to eighty, in the Baltimore Longitudinal Study of Aging.

- **End diastolic volume:** The volume of blood in the left ventricle at the end of diastole, just before the next beat. At rest, about 65–75 ml per square meter, increasing with age. During exercise, increases in older people, especially in men after age forty.

- **End systolic volume:** The amount of blood left in the heart at the end of the beat or systole. At rest, about 25 ml per square meter, increasing with age until about age seventy. During exercise, decreases, but not as much in older as in younger people.

- **Ejection fraction:** The fraction of end diastolic volume pumped out with each heartbeat. At rest, about 65 percent, decreasing slightly until about age sixty, then rising slightly. During exercise, increases up to about 90 percent at peak exercise capacity in younger people. The increase is less in older people, reaching about 75 percent at peak exercise capacity.

- **Stroke volume:** The amount of blood pumped with each beat. At rest, about 45–55 ml per square meter; resting stroke volume increases with age in men, not in women. During exercise, increases by about the same amount in both older and younger people, in association with the higher end diastolic volume (Frank-Starling phenomenon).

- **Heart rate:** The number of beats per minute. At rest, between fifty and eighty. During exercise, increases dramatically, but less in older than in younger people.

- **Maximum heart rate:** The number of beats per minute during rigorous exercise; declines 25–30 percent between ages twenty and eighty.

- **Cardiac output:** The amount of blood pumped each minute (heart rate x stroke volume). At rest, about 3–4 ml per minute per square meter; decreases in women with age. During exercise, about 10 ml per minute per square meter in young people; decreases by about 30 percent between ages twenty and eighty due to the decline in maximum heart rate.

The Effect of Lifestyle: Regular Exercise

With this understanding of how the heart adjusts with age, researchers are now turning to people like Coleman who have a regular exercise program. How do their hearts work in comparison with those of sixty- and seventy-year-olds who do not exercise? Scientists know that regular exercise causes certain changes in the hearts of younger people: Resting heart rate is lower, heart mass is higher, and stroke volume is higher than in their sedentary counterparts. Now there is evidence that these changes occur even when exercise training begins later in life, at age sixty or seventy, for instance. In other words, points out Lakatta, "you don't lose the ability to be conditioned."

The evidence continues to mount. For example, as activity levels increase, older male athletes have the same increase as younger men in cardiac output, according to studies at NIA and by Ali Ehsani, John Holloszy, and colleagues at Washington University in St. Louis, Missouri. At maximum exercise capacity, both stroke volume and cardiac output increase in older men. In many ways, at maximum capacity, older athletes' heart function seems to be closer to that of younger men than to that of older men who do not exercise regularly. Other studies are honing in on some of the molecular changes that take place during exercise.

Questions remain about the precise relationships between age and lifestyle, but cardiovascular scientists can begin to make some educated guesses. It looks more and more as though regular physical activity keeps the aging heart working like a younger heart. Regular exercise, moreover, may influence how or when disease develops and with what severity. Going by what is known so far, it seems a good bet that Coleman's exercise program is keeping his heart healthy and his risk of heart disease down.

Physical Fitness and Aging

Many studies have found that physical fitness (measured as maximum oxygen consumption) declines between 5 and 10 percent a decade, but this figure varies widely. Intrigued by the differences, researchers have studied physical fitness in middle-aged and older people who remain competitive in sports. The results: These "master athletes" have twice the physical fitness as sedentary people of the same age.

Other studies have also shown a connection between regular exercise and physical fitness. For instance, sedentary middle-aged men who undertook a six- to eight-month training program had significant increases in fitness, and people who exercise regularly have higher fitness levels as they get older.

Selected Readings

Ehsani, A. A., T. Ogawa, T. R. Miller, R. J. Spina, and S. M. Jilka. "Exercise Training Improves Left Ventricular Systolic Function in Older Men." *Circulation* 83 (1991): 96–103.

Fleg, J. L., and E. G. Lakatta. "Role of Muscle Loss in the Age-Associated Reduction in VO2max." *Journal of Applied Physiology* 65 (1988): 1147–51.

Fleg, J. L., S. P. Schulman, F. C. O'Connor, G. Gerstenblith, L. C. Becker, S. Fortney, A. P. Goldberg, and E. G. Lakatta. "Central and Peripheral Cardiovascular Adaptations in Highly Trained Older Men." *Journal of Applied Physiology* 1994.

Fleg, J. L., S. P. Schulman, F. C. O'Connor, G. Gerstenblith, J. F. Clulow, D. C. Renlund, and E. G. Lakatta. "Effects of Acute Beta Adrenergic Blockade on Age-Associated Changes in Cardiovascular Performance during Dynamic Exercise." *Circulation* 1994.

Gerstenblith, G., J. Frederiksen, F. C. P. Yin, N. J. Fortuin, E. G. Lakatta, and M. L. Weisfeldt. "Echocardiographic Assessment of a Normal Adult Aging Population." *Circulation* 56 (1977): 273–78.

Holloszy, J. O. "Exercise, Health, and Aging: A Need for More Information." *Medicine and Science in Sports and Exercise* 15 (1983): 1–5.

Lakatta, E. G. "Cardiovascular Regulatory Mechanisms in Advanced Age." *Physiological Reviews* 73 (1993): 413–67.

Rodeheffer, R. J., G. Gerstenblith, L. C. Becker, J. L. Fleg, M. L. Weisfeldt, and E. G. Lakatta. "Exercise Cardiac Output Is Maintained with Advancing Age in Healthy Human Subjects: Cardiac Dilatation and Increased Stroke Volume Compensate for a Diminished Heart Rate. *Circulation* 69 (1984): 203–13.

Sjogren, A. L. "Left Ventricular Wall Thickness Determined by Ultrasound in 100 Subjects without Heart Disease." *Chest* 60 (1971): 341–46.

Spirito, P., and B. J. Maron. "Influence of Aging on Doppler Echocardiographic Indices on Left Ventricular Diastolic Function." *British Heart Journal* 59 (1988): 672–79.

The Biology of Physical Fitness

The term "physical fitness" evokes a general picture of health and vitality, but in cardiovascular science it is a measurable entity. The element measured is oxygen (O_2) consumption.

O_2 consumption is the amount of oxygen used by the body.

Scientists calculate oxygen consumption by 1) determining how much oxygen is in the arteries, 2) subtracting from this the oxygen in the veins after the blood passes through the cells, and 3) multiplying the result by the amount of blood the heart pumps each minute (cardiac output).

$$O_2 \text{ consumption} = (O_2 \text{ in arteries} - O_2 \text{ in veins}) \times \text{cardiac output}$$

As oxygen-rich blood leaves the heart, it flows through smaller and smaller arteries, then arterioles, then capillaries, until it reaches individual cells.

The blood diffuses into cells where its oxygen is extracted, then passes back out and into the veins—first the tiny vein capillaries, then larger and larger veins, until it reaches the heart again.

The amount of O_2 consumed at peak exercise (VO_2 max) is considered the best measure of physical fitness.

Both heart and peripheral factors improve with exercise training, boosting physical fitness. Stroke volume is higher in conditioned older men, and oxygen extraction also improves.

Blood Vessels and Aging

Age has a lot to do with stiffening blood vessels, which seem to have a lot to do with heart function.

The exercise physiology laboratory at the National Institute on Aging looks like a den of electronic wizardry. Computer terminals dot the room, one right next to the treadmill, two perched high on a cabinet, one on a rolling cart, one mounted on the wall. Here and there other instruments rest, quiet at the moment or blinking just a little.

So the sound of splashing liquid comes as a surprise. "I keep thinking how noisy the body must be," says Eileen Shields, a marketing director for Carroll County, Maryland, who is here for an echocardiogram. The rhythmic, echoing splashes that fill the room come from a slim, silver-colored tube held gently against the pulse in her carotid artery. The sound is matched by digital waves that dance across the nearby computer terminal, recording the flow and pressure of blood.

Shields is a volunteer in a study that is looking for fresh clues to heart health in a well-known phenomenon: the gradual stiffening of arteries that occurs as people grow older. Arterial stiffening has been known by various names—hardening of the arteries, vascular stiffness, arteriosclerosis—and scientists have long thought that it played a role in diseases like atherosclerosis and high blood pressure. Yet they now have evidence that its impact may reach beyond the blood vessels.

"We suspect that stiffness affects both the heart's structure and its function," says Jerome Fleg, a scientist in the NIA's cardiovascular laboratory, "and we want to know how they match up. Do people with the stiffest arteries have the thickest heart walls? Do their hearts pump out smaller volumes of blood with each beat?"

As they sort out the links between the arteries and the heart, Fleg and his colleagues hope they'll also gain insight into exactly how stiffness relates to disease. Arterial stiffening has long been considered a normal part of aging in industrialized societies. However, in some people, for reasons not yet understood, this common condition turns into a disease process. Stiffening of the arteries is the major cause of high blood pressure in older people, which in turn is a leading risk factor for stroke, coronary artery disease, heart attack, and heart failure. And now stiffening is suspected of making arteries more prone to the cellular processes that underlie atherosclerosis, another key precursor of heart disease and stroke.

Aging is still considered the major risk factor for these diseases. Yet some early evidence from Fleg's studies and those of others suggest that lifestyle may also play a key role. Low-salt diets and regular aerobic exercise may reduce arterial stiffness.

Age and Arteries

What made scientists think there might be a link between blood vessel stiffness and heart function in the first place? It goes back to what they have learned about both over the last few decades, partly through the Baltimore Longitudinal Study of Aging, in which Eileen

Shields is one of about 1,200 participants. The volunteers range in age from twenty through ninety-plus. The scientists, by comparing younger and older volunteers, have been able to put together a picture of what happens in both heart and blood vessels as people age.

The heart, they have learned, adjusts to age in many subtle and interconnecting ways: It develops thicker walls, and it fills with blood and pumps the blood out in a different pattern and even by somewhat different mechanisms than when young.

The large, elastic arteries that are closest to the heart also change in complex ways. Picture an animated computer graphic of the arteries at, say, age twenty-five, when the walls are compliant. The largest artery in the body, the aorta, leads away from the heart, first up toward the neck, where the carotid artery branches off to take blood to the head and brain, and then down toward the rest of the body. When the aortic valve opens, the aorta receives the rushing pulse of blood from the heart. It also receives pressure spreading from the walls of the heart to its own walls. This pressure travels along the aorta's walls in wave after wave until it reaches the walls of the smaller, branching arteries that take the blood to the rest of the body. There the waves of pressure slow and some are sent back through the aorta walls, becoming what are called wave reflections.

Now add, say, fifty years to this picture. The arteries, including the aorta, grow stiffer, their walls thicker, the diameters larger. The stiffer walls no longer expand as much as blood flows through them. Eventually, the resistance of the stiffer aorta walls increases significantly. Commonly it doubles over a lifespan and contributes to the increase in systolic blood pressure that often accompanies aging.

Along the walls of the stiffer aorta, the pressure waves now move more rapidly, and as a result, the wave reflection occurs sooner than it did before. The timing of the wave reflection, in fact, is one of the effects of arterial stiffness that can be measured noninvasively.

As the blood moves on into the smaller arteries, the hydraulics change. The pulse smoothes out, the flow becomes more steady. The opposition to this steady flow is known as peripheral vascular resistance or PVR; so far studies show that among men, resting PVR does not change with normal aging, but that it does rise somewhat in women. In most people with high systolic blood pressure, PVR is elevated.

Next, picture the effects of movement—when a person sits up, stands up, or begins to walk or run. The heart rate increases and blood pressure rises. A group of pressure-sensitive nerves in the aorta respond to the changes in pressure by sending a message to the brain.

The brain, in turn, sends a message back to the heart, which changes its rate and strength of contraction. This aorta/brain/heart message system is called the baroceptor response. Blood vessels also dilate to allow for the extra blood flow. In addition, blood is turned away temporarily from those muscles that don't need it (for instance, the stomach), so that more can be delivered to the working muscles.

In the older picture, the baroceptor response is blunted, perhaps as a result of stiffer arteries; the nerves in the aorta could be affected by increasing stiffness. Also, at maximum exercise, the large arteries do not dilate as much as in the younger picture.

These, in brief outline, are some of the major changes that occur in blood vessel hydraulics with age. One reason these changes intrigue scientists is that they could have a major impact on heart dynamics. Stiffening increases the amount of resistance the heart must overcome to eject blood into the arteries, and any resistance to flow places a load on the heart.

The study in which Eileen Shields is a participant will show the impact of this load.

Exercise and Diet

Perhaps most intriguing of all is the difference that lifestyle may make in arterial stiffness. In one of the tests that study participants routinely take, they walk on a treadmill at increasing speeds until they are exhausted. The test measures physical fitness by gauging oxygen consumption at peak exercise, or VO_2 max.

The individuals who can walk on the treadmill for the longest period—that is, those who are most physically fit—have the least stiff arteries, according to a study by Fleg and his colleagues. The more the volunteers in this study were able to exercise, the less stiff their arteries.

Having learned that physical fitness was linked to less stiff, more compliant arteries, the scientists wondered about cause and effect: Does regular exercise, which increases physical fitness, actually cause less stiff, more compliant arteries?

The answer is a cautious "maybe," according to the next study. In this one, the researchers measured arterial stiffness in a group of endurance-trained men, age fifty-four to seventy-five, and compared them to sedentary men of the same age. The scientists also compared the older group to younger sedentary men. The exercise capacity of the older athletes was similar to that of younger men and greatly surpassed that of the older group. Most striking of all, the arterial stiffening in the older athletes was far less than in their sedentary counterparts. "This demonstrates that endurance training may give us at least some control over the condition of our arteries, a variable we thought controlled us," says the NIA's Edward Lakatta.

Control over the condition of our arteries may also lie in how much salt we consume. In cultures where little sodium (in the form of salt) is consumed, blood pressures do not rise with age as they do in Western countries. Cultural differences have also been found in arterial stiffness. One study compared rural and urban populations in China. The urban population consumed much higher levels of salt than the rural groups, and they had stiffer arteries.

Now a study in Taiwan is following up on this finding by comparing two other rural and urban groups. However, this one is looking not only at arterial stiffness but also at heart structure and function. Early results show that among those with the stiffest arteries, heart walls were thicker, according to Harold Spurgeon, who heads this study at the NIA's Baltimore laboratory.

Some of the next questions facing cardiovascular researchers center on the cells and molecules of the cardiovascular system. How can exercise keep arteries more compliant? It may be that exercise triggers a chain of events within the cells of the arterial walls that ends by reducing collagen and increasing elastin. Ultimately, cardiovascular scientists think, the puzzle of arterial stiffening will come down to the biochemistry and biophysics of the cardiovascular system, a vast territory with many regions still to be explored.

Measuring Stiffness

Over time, changes in arterial stiffness are much more marked than changes in blood pressure and may be a better gauge of cardiovascular health. New, reliable measures of arterial stiffness are currently used only by researchers, but they could someday be a prognostic and clinical tool.

The new tests gauge stiffness by measuring the speed of pulse waves—the waves of pressure that travel down artery walls as blood pulses through them. In one test, researchers monitor pulse waves at two spots, one near the ascending aorta and one on the femoral artery in the thigh, then calculate the time it takes the wave to travel from neck to thigh. The faster the blood flows, the stiffer the arteries.

"It's pure hydraulics," says Amit Nussbacher, a postdoctoral fellow in NIA's Laboratory of Cardiovascular Science, who conducts these tests as part of the laboratory's studies of vascular stiffness. In still-compliant arteries, he explains, waves of pressure travel more slowly; stiffness speeds them up.

The second test monitors wave reflections in the walls of the aorta. Wave reflections occur when the pulse waves encounter the smaller arteries that branch off this large artery. The waves of pressure are bounced or reflected back along the walls of the aorta, augmenting the pressure from the oncoming waves.

This means that if the wave reflection shows up soon after the heart's contraction (as measured by a simultaneous electrocardiogram), then the aorta is relatively stiff. If it occurs later in the cardiac cycle, that is, after the aortic valve closes, there is less stiffness. A computer program translates the timing of the wave reflection into a number known as the augmentation index. The higher the augmentation index, the greater the stiffness of the arteries.

Selected Readings

Avolio, A. P., S. G. Chen, R. P. Wang, C. L. Zhang, M. F. Li, and M. F. O'Rourke. "Effects of Aging on Changing Arterial Compliance and Left Ventricular Load in a Northern Chinese Urban Community." *Circulation* 68 (1983): 50–58.

Avolio, A. P., F. Q. Deng, W. Q. Li, Y. F. Luo, Z. D. Huang, L. F. Xing, and M. F. O'Rourke. "Effects of Aging on Arterial Distensibility in Populations with High and Low Prevalence of Hypertension: Comparison between Urban and Rural Communities in China." *Circulation* 71 (1985): 202–10.

Vaitkevicius, P. V., J. L. Fleg, J. H. Engel, F. C. O'Connor, J. G. Wright, L. E. Lakatta, F. C. P. Yin, and E. G. Lakatta. "Effects of Age and Aerobic Capacity on Arterial Stiffness in Healthy Adults." *Circulation* 88 (1993): 1456–62.

Yin, F. C. P, M. L. Weisfeldt, and W. R. Milnor. "Role of Aortic Input Impedance in the Decreased Cardiovascular Response to Exercise with Aging in Dogs." *Journal of Clinical Investigation* 68 (1981): 28–38.

Chapter 7

Stress and Heart Disease

There is intense public interest in possible links between "stress" and coronary heart disease (CHD). Until recently, organizations such as the National Heart Foundation of Australia have only been able to make judgments based on limited data in this area.

In 1988 the National Heart Foundation of Australia published a report, "Stress and cardiovascular disease," which concluded that, although acute catastrophic events might trigger acute myocardial infarction or sudden death, there was insufficient existing evidence from prospective studies that any form of "stress" consistently predicted the subsequent development of CHD.[1] The report concluded that psychosocial risk factors had effects on conventional risk factors, but no independent effect.

Since then, a considerable number of prospective cohort studies have examined the links between various forms of stress and the development and prognosis of CHD; there have also been a multitude of reviews, both narrative and systematic. However, these reviews have used different methods and at times have come to different conclusions. Because systematic reviews attempt to find, appraise, and summarize the findings of all studies in a systematic and transparent way, these reviews should be the more reliable. Unfortunately, the reported systematic reviews have varied in their quality and come to different conclusions. Recently, methods for critically appraising systematic reviews have been developed, and this position statement is based on a review of the systematic reviews using this methodology.[2, 3]

An Expert Working Group considered all the major suggested psychosocial risk factors ("stressors") to identify evidence of independent associations with CHD.

What is "stress"?

Although the term "stress" is in general use, it is so imprecise that, in agreement with other review groups,[4] the Expert Working Group examined separately those variables that are commonly regarded as components of stress. These include:

- depression, anxiety, panic disorder;
- social isolation and lack of quality social support;
- acute and chronic life events;
- psychosocial work characteristics; and
- Type A behavior, hostility.

Is depression a risk factor for CHD?

There was strong and consistent evidence across all the reviews that depression is an independent risk factor for clinical CHD and its prognosis. The association exists for men and women, subjects living in different countries, and various age groups. Furthermore, the CHD risk is directly related to the severity of depression: a one- to twofold increase in CHD for minor depression and three- to fivefold increase for major depression.[4, 10–13] The strength of the association is of similar magnitude to that of standard risk factors such as smoking or hypercholesterolemia.

Are social isolation or lack of social support risk factors for CHD?

There is strong and consistent evidence across all the reviews that social isolation and lack of quality social support are independent risk factors for CHD onset and prognosis: the risks are increased two- to threefold and three- to fivefold, respectively. The association exists for both men and women, subjects living in different countries, and various age groups. An association was found in studies that examined some aspect of the size and nature of a person's social network and in studies that examined the type of support received.[4, 11, 14, 15]

Can acute life-event "stressors" trigger CHD events?

Acute life event "stressors" can trigger CHD events, although it is very difficult to study and quantify the magnitude of effects. Acute "stressors" include significant common events such as bereavement,[11] as well as catastrophic events such as earthquakes or terrorist attacks.[11, 15, 16] Although the deleterious physiological effects of acute "stressors" as CHD triggers are well documented, the role of chronic "stressors" in CHD onset and prognosis remains unclear.

Are work-related "stressors" risk factors for CHD?

This topic refers specifically to the characteristics of the work environment as distinct from the life-event "stressors" referred to previously. The studies included in one review[4] under psychosocial work characteristics were heterogeneous, with a wide variety of factors being examined individually and collectively. When the results for job control, demands, and strain were recalculated, there was not a preponderance of positive over negative studies. The Expert Working Group found no consistency between this review[4] and the other two reviews of work-related "stressors."[11, 17]

Reasons for the discordance between the reviews of prospective studies in healthy populations were explored by following a set of steps applicable to all types of systematic reviews, including etiological and prognostic studies, developed from an algorithm devised to interpret discordant meta-analyses of intervention studies.[8] Two of the reviews[4, 11] covered the job-strain model, job control, and the effort–reward model, whereas the third review[17] covered only the job-strain model. Of the first two reviews, one[4] included twice as many studies as the other[11] and summarized their findings more fully. Consequently, the Expert Working Group gave more credence to this "negative" review,[4] and concluded that there was neither strong nor consistent evidence of a causal association between work-related "stressors" and CHD.

Is Type A behavior pattern a risk factor for CHD?

Type A behavior pattern refers to a number of personality trait characteristics, including rushed, ambitious, and competitive behavior; impatience; hostility; and intolerance.[18] Early positive studies have now been displaced by a large number of studies concluding that Type A behavior pattern has no effect.[4]

Is hostility a risk factor for CHD?

One review of prospective studies concluded that there was consistent positive evidence of association between hostility and CHD.[13] Two other reviews reported an almost equal number of positive and negative prospective studies in healthy populations.[11, 19] The most recent review concluded that there was no evidence of association.[4]

When the discordance between these reviews was examined, we found that the review that found no clear association between hostility and CHD[4] included two to six times as many large studies as the other reviews, and that the other reviews had only two to four primary studies in common with the most recent review.[4] As well as including several more recent studies, this review included studies with better measures of hostility and more studies of the general population. Its inclusion of studies of Type A behavior patterns[18] did not account for the preponderance of "negative" studies. The Expert Working Group therefore gave greater credence to this better-quality "negative" review and considered that hostility is not a risk factor for CHD.

Are anxiety disorders risk factors for CHD?

A review of primary studies where anxiety was the specific exposure[4] (rather than anxiety associated with depression) found an equal number of positive and null findings among both the etiological and the prognostic studies and concluded there was no association with CHD. Other reviews came to the opposite conclusion or were equivocal.[11, 12]

When the reasons for the discordance between the reviews of etiological studies were explored, it was found that the reviews which had concluded that there was[12] or may be[11] an association between anxiety and CHD had included fewer of the "negative" primary studies than the review which concluded that there was no clear association.[4] This latter review also summarized the primary studies more fully. For those reasons the Expert Working Group gave more credence to that review.[4]

In addition, when the reasons for the discordance between the two reviews of prognostic studies were explored, it was found that the review which had concluded that there was no clear association between anxiety and the prognosis of CHD had included eighteen large primary studies,[4] whereas the review which concluded that there was an association[11] included only four primary studies, two of which were small and one which included patients with cardiopulmonary disease. The Expert Working Group therefore gave greater credence to the negative review.[4]

Patients with panic disorder are subject to episodes of recurring, often inexplicable, psychophysiological arousal. The one review of this area found little evidence to link panic disorder with either CHD development or progression.[20]

What were the outcomes of the expert working group deliberations?

- Depression, social isolation, and lack of social support are significant risk factors for CHD that are independent of conventional risk factors such as smoking, hypercholesterolemia, and hypertension and are of similar magnitude to these conventional risk factors.

- Acute life-event "stressors" can trigger coronary events.

- Absolute risk of CHD depends upon the strength and number of risk factors. However, a substantial proportion of the variation of CHD incidence between populations is not explained by conventional risk factors, and those factors clearly identified in this review—depression, social isolation, and lack of social support— may explain some of the variance in CHD occurrences. These risk factors should be considered in the development of future risk assessment tools.

- Psychosocial risk factors may cluster together in a similar way to conventional risk factors. Psychosocial and conventional risk factors often coexist (e.g., patients with depression are more likely to smoke and be physically inactive).

- Depression is common and is clearly a risk factor for CHD. It can be easily identified and treated. As yet, there are no published studies of whether treatment of depression will reduce CHD morbidity.

- Depression and CHD frequently coexist. Patients with CHD should be assessed for depression and patients with depression should be assessed for CHD risk factors.

- In patients with CHD, the presence of depression is more likely to lead to poorer outcomes. They may need more assertive management of their conventional risk factors and attention to the extent to which depression is affecting their adherence to treatments and lifestyle modifications.

- Social disadvantage is strongly associated with both adverse psychosocial and conventional risk factor status. There is a need for research to investigate the extent to which CHD rates in populations might be influenced by adverse social and cultural factors.

- Until this time, public health approaches to CHD have focused largely on modification of conventional risk factors. We highlight the need to consider the burden imposed by these additional CHD risk factors. Attention to these psychosocial factors may also improve outcomes in CHD patients.

- The term "stress" has proved to be so imprecise as to be unhelpful. It should be replaced in the clinical, public health, and medical and legal environments by more specific terms for which there is evidence, such as the terms used in this review.

References

1. Stress Working Party. Stress and cardiovascular disease: a report from the National Heart Foundation of Australia. *Med J Aust* 1988; 148: 510–13.

2. National Health and Medical Research Council. *A guide to the development, implementation and evaluation of clinical practice guidelines.* Canberra: AGPS, 1995.

3. Oxman AD, Guyatt GH. Validation of an index of the quality of review articles. *J Clin Epidemiol* 1991; 44: 1271–78.

4. Kuper H, Marmot M, Hemingway H. Systematic review of prospective cohort studies of psychosocial factors in the aetiology and prognosis of coronary heart disease. *Semin Vasc Med* 2002; 2: 267–314.

5. Counsell C. Formulating questions and locating primary studies for inclusion in systematic reviews. *Ann Intern Med* 1997; 127: 380–87.

6. Jadad AR, McQuay HJ. Meta-analyses to evaluate analgesic interventions: a systematic qualitative review of their methodology. *J Clin Epidemiol* 1996; 49: 235–43.

7. Hill AB. The environment and disease association or causation. *Proc R Soc Med* 1965; 58: 295–300.

8. Peach H. Reading systematic reviews. *Aust Fam Phys* 2002; 31: 736–40.

9. United States Preventive Services Task Force. *Guide to clinical preventive services*. 2nd ed. Baltimore: Williams and Wilkins, 1996.

10. Musselman DL, Evans DL, Nemeroff CB. The relationship of depression to cardiovascular disease: epidemiology, biology and treatment. *Arch Gen Psychiatry* 1998; 55: 580–92.

11. Rozanski A, Blumenthal JA, Kaplan J. Impact of psychological factors on the pathogenesis of cardiovascular disease and implications for therapy. *Circulation* 1999; 99: 2192–2217.

12. Kubzansky LD, Kawachi I. Going to the heart of the matter. Do negative emotions cause coronary heart disease? *J Psychosom Res* 2000; 48: 323–37.

13. Scheier MF, Bridges MW. Person variables and health: personality predispositions and acute psychological states as shared determinants for disease. *Psychosom Med* 1995; 57: 255–68.

14. Eriksen W. The role of social support in the pathogenesis of coronary heart disease: a literature review. *Fam Pract* 1994; 11: 201–9.

15. Tennant C. Life stress, social support and coronary heart disease. *Aust N Z J Psychiatry* 1999; 33: 636–41.

16. Hemingway H, Malik M, Marmot M. Social and psychosocial influences on sudden cardiac death, ventricular arrhythmia and cardiac autonomic function. *Eur Heart J* 2001; 22: 1082–1101.

17. Schnall PL, Landsbergis PA, Baker D. Job strain and cardiovascular disease. *Annu Rev Public Health* 1994; 15: 381–411.

18. Friedman M, Roseman RH. *Type A behaviour and your heart*. New York: Knopf, 1974.

19. Miller TQ, Smith TW, Turner CW, et al. A meta-analytic review of research on hostility and physical health. *Psychol Bull* 1996; 119: 322–48.

20. Fleet RP, Lavoi K, Beitman B. Is panic disorder associated with coronary artery disease? A critical review of the literature. *J Psychosom Res* 2000; 48: 347–56.

21. Easterbrook PJ, Berlin JA, Gopalan R, Matthews DR. Publication bias in clinical research. *Lancet* 1991; 337: 867–72.

Chapter 8

Smoking and Cardiovascular Diseases

Cardiovascular Consequences of Smoking

Heart disease and stroke are cardiovascular (heart and blood vessel) diseases caused by smoking. Heart disease and stroke are also the first and third leading causes of death in the United States.

More than 61 million people in the United States suffer from some form of heart and blood vessel disease. This includes high blood pressure, coronary heart disease, stroke, and congestive heart failure. Nearly 2,600 Americans die every day as a result of cardiovascular diseases. This is about one death every thirty-three seconds. You are up to four times more likely to die from heart disease if you smoke. In 2003, heart disease and stroke cost the United States an estimated $351 billion in health care costs and lost productivity from death and disability.

The link between smoking and heart disease was noted in the first Surgeon General's report in 1964. Later reports revealed a much stronger connection. Researchers found that smoking is a major cause

This chapter begins with excerpts from "The Health Consequences of Smoking: What It Means to You," prepared by the Centers for Disease Control and Prevention (CDC), May 2004, and also includes excerpts from "Chapter 3: Cardiovascular Diseases," *The Health Consequences of Smoking: A Report of the Surgeon General*. U.S. Department of Health and Human Services, Centers for Disease Control and Prevention, National Center for Chronic Disease Prevention and Health Promotion, Office on Smoking and Health, 2004. The full text of these reports is available online through the U.S. Surgeon General's website at www.surgeongeneral.gov.

of diseases of blood vessels inside and outside the heart. Most cases of these diseases are caused by atherosclerosis, a hardening and narrowing of the arteries. Damage to your arteries and blood clots that block blood flow can cause heart attacks or strokes.

Cigarette smoking speeds up this process even in smokers in their twenties. Cigarette smoke damages the cells lining the blood vessels and heart. The damaged tissue swells. This makes it hard for blood vessels to get enough oxygen to cells and tissues. Your heart and all parts of your body must have oxygen. Perhaps most important, cigarette smoking can increase your risk of dangerous blood clots, both because of swelling and redness and by causing blood platelets to clump together. Cigarettes aren't the only dangerous kind of tobacco. Even smokeless tobacco can lead to heart and blood vessel disease.

Facts You Should Know about Cardiovascular Disease and Smoking

- Coronary heart disease is the leading cause of death in the United States.

- You are up to four times more likely to die from coronary heart disease if you smoke.

- In 2000, about 1.1 million Americans had heart attacks.

- Even with treatment, 25 percent of men and 38 percent of women die within one year of a heart attack.

- Smoking causes atherosclerosis, or hardening and narrowing of your arteries.

- Smoking causes coronary heart disease.

- Smoking low-tar or low-nicotine cigarettes rather than regular cigarettes does not reduce the risk of coronary heart disease.

- Smoking causes strokes.

- Smoking causes abdominal aortic aneurysm, a dangerous weakening and ballooning of the major artery near your stomach.

Conclusions from the Surgeon General's Report, 2004

Smoking and Subclinical Atherosclerosis

Recently developed techniques can measure markers of subclinical atherosclerosis in healthy persons in community settings. These techniques have now been applied in a number of different kinds of studies with repeated findings of a higher frequency of abnormalities in smokers. Consistently, studies measuring carotid artery wall thickness or the ankle-arm index (AAI) have demonstrated strong, dose-response associations between smoking and the presence and progression of subclinical atherosclerosis. Results from earlier and other studies also suggest that smoking affects the progression of intermediate to advanced atherosclerotic lesions at early ages. Knowledge of the underlying mechanisms by which smoking causes atherosclerosis adds plausibility to these observations. Smoking has immediate adverse effects on the homeostatic balance of the cardiovascular system.

Conclusion: The evidence is sufficient to infer a causal relationship between smoking and subclinical atherosclerosis.

Implications: Cigarette smoking has a causal relationship with the full natural history of atherosclerosis from the time that it can be detected by sensitive, subclinical markers to its late and often fatal stages. The new findings on subclinical disease indicate the potential for preventing more advanced and clinically symptomatic disease through quitting smoking and maintained cessation.

Smoking, Coronary Heart Disease, and Sudden Death

New data reaffirm the already well-documented causal association of smoking with the risk for CHD (coronary heart disease). Compared with lifetime nonsmokers, the relative risk in smokers rises with the number of cigarettes smoked and falls after cessation. The type of cigarette smoked has little influence on CHD risk. The association cannot be explained by confounding.

Conclusions: 1. The evidence is sufficient to infer a causal relationship between smoking and coronary heart disease. 2. The evidence suggests only a weak relationship between the type of cigarette smoked and coronary heart disease risk.

Implications: Because of its prevalence, smoking is a major cause of CHD, particularly among younger smokers. While CHD mortality rates have continued to fall, a substantial proportion of the population's burden of CHD could be avoided with smoking prevention and cessation. Products with lower yields of tar and nicotine, as measured by a smoking machine, have not been found to reduce CHD risk substantially and they are not a lower-risk alternative for smokers who cannot quit. By causing CHD and MI (myocardial infarction), smoking may also contribute to the development of CHF (congestive heart failure), an increasingly frequent disease that is disabling and has a poor prognosis.

Smoking and Cerebrovascular Disease

Recent evidence remains fully consistent with a causal effect of smoking on risk for cerebrovascular disease. The recent evidence extends the range of populations in which an association with smoking has been demonstrated and shows consistent associations of smoking with all major types of stroke.

Conclusion: The evidence is sufficient to infer a causal relationship between smoking and stroke.

Implication: Cigarette smoking remains a major cause of stroke in the United States.

Smoking and Abdominal Aortic Aneurysm

Smoking causes atherosclerosis in arteries, including the abdominal aorta. Autopsy studies show that even young adults who smoke have more plaque in their aortas than do lifetime nonsmokers. Other mechanisms by which smoking might injure the abdominal aorta include inflammation and damage to elastin.

The epidemiologic evidence, coming from multiple studies of differing design and location, shows a strong association of smoking with risk for abdominal aortic aneurysm. Dose-response relationships with the amount and duration of smoking have been reported and risks are lower in former than in current smokers.

Conclusion: The evidence is sufficient to infer a causal relationship between smoking and abdominal aortic aneurysm.

Implication: Smoking is one of the few currently avoidable causes of this frequently fatal disease.

Summary

Research during the past decade has produced further evidence that tobacco smoking is causally related to all of the major clinical cardiovascular diseases. A large body of evidence coming from multiple populations, age groups, and both genders outlined in Surgeon General's reports prior to 2004 indicates that tobacco smoking causes atherosclerosis and associated clinical syndromes. A dose-response relationship has been repeatedly demonstrated with higher levels of cigarette smoking and a longer duration of smoking. Evidence now suggests that light smokers (fewer than ten cigarettes per day) have moderate but measurable increases in the risks for CVD (cardiovascular disease), and passive smoking has been causally associated with CHD. New evidence also documents that tobacco smoking is associated with subclinical or very early atherosclerosis.

Chapter 9

Metabolic Syndrome and Cardiovascular Risks

What is metabolic syndrome?

Metabolic syndrome is a collection of health risks that increase your chance of developing heart disease, stroke, and diabetes. The condition is also known by other names, including syndrome X, insulin resistance syndrome, and dysmetabolic syndrome. According to a national health survey, more than one in five Americans has metabolic syndrome. The number of people with metabolic syndrome increases with age, affecting more than 40 percent of people in their sixties and seventies.

What are these health risks?

You are diagnosed with metabolic syndrome if you have three or more of the following:

- A waistline of forty inches or more for men and thirty-five inches or more for women (measured across the belly)
- A blood pressure of 130/85 mm Hg or higher
- A triglyceride level above 150 mg/dl

"Metabolic Syndrome," © 2004 The Cleveland Clinic Foundation, 9500 Euclid Avenue, Cleveland, OH 44195. Additional information is available from the Cleveland Clinic Health Information Center, 216-444-3771, toll-free at 800-223-2273 est. 43771, or www.clevelandclinic.org/health.

- A fasting blood glucose (sugar) level greater than 100 mg/dl

- A high density lipoprotein level (HDL) less than 40 mg/dl (men) or under 50 mg/dl (women)

Who typically has metabolic syndrome?

According to the American Heart Association, three groups of people often have metabolic syndrome:

- People with diabetes who cannot maintain a proper level of glucose (glucose intolerance)

- People without diabetes who have high blood pressure and who also secrete large amounts of insulin (hyperinsulinemia) to maintain blood glucose levels

- Heart attack survivors who have hyperinsulinemia without glucose intolerance

What are the symptoms of metabolic syndrome?

Usually, there are no immediate physical symptoms; the syndrome's associated medical problems develop over time. If you are unsure if you have metabolic syndrome, see your health care provider. He or she will be able to make the diagnosis by ordering the necessary tests.

What causes metabolic syndrome?

The exact cause of metabolic syndrome is not known. Most researchers believe it is caused by a combination of your genetic makeup and lifestyle choices—including the types of food you eat and your level of physical activity.

If you have metabolic syndrome, your body experiences a series of biochemical changes. Over time, these changes lead to the development of one or more associated medical conditions. The sequence begins when insulin, a hormone excreted from your pancreas, loses its ability to make your body's cells absorb glucose from the blood—your body uses glucose for energy. When this happens, glucose levels remain high after you eat. Your pancreas, sensing a high glucose level in your blood, continues to excrete insulin. Loss of insulin production may be genetic or secondary to high fat levels with fatty deposits in the pancreas.

If I have metabolic syndrome, what health problems might develop?

Consistently high levels of insulin and glucose are linked to many harmful changes to the body, including:

1. Damage to the lining of coronary and other arteries, a key step toward the development of heart disease or stroke

2. Changes in the kidneys' ability to remove salt, leading to high blood pressure, heart disease, and stroke

3. An increase in triglyceride levels, resulting in an increased risk of developing cardiovascular disease

4. An increased risk of blood clot formation, which can block arteries and cause heart attacks and strokes

5. A slowing of insulin production, which can signal the start of type 2 diabetes, a disease that can increase your risk for a heart attack or stroke and may damage your eyes, nerves, or kidneys

How do I prevent or reverse metabolic syndrome?

Since physical inactivity and excess weight are the main underlying contributors to the development of metabolic syndrome, getting more exercise and losing weight can help reduce or prevent the complications associated with this condition. Your doctor may also prescribe medications to manage some of your underlying problems. Some of the ways you can reduce your risk include:

-   **Lose weight:** Moderate weight loss, in the range of 5 percent to 10 percent of body weight, can help restore your body's ability to recognize insulin and greatly reduce the chance that the syndrome will evolve into a more serious illness.

-   **Exercise:** Increased activity alone can improve your insulin levels. A brisk thirty-minute walk a day can result in a weight loss, improved blood pressure, improved cholesterol levels, and a reduced risk of developing diabetes.

-   **Consider dietary changes:** Maintain a diet that keeps carbohydrates to no more than 50 percent of total calories. Eat foods defined as complex carbohydrates, such as whole grain bread (instead of white), brown rice (instead of white), and sugars that are unrefined (instead of refined; for example, cookies, crackers). Increase your fiber consumption by eating legumes (for example, beans), whole grains, fruits, and vegetables. Reduce your intake of red meats and poultry. As much as 30 percent to 45 percent of your daily calories can come from fat, but consume healthy fats, such as those in canola oil, olive oil, flaxseed oil, and nuts.

• **Limit alcohol intake:** Consume no more than one drink a day for women or two drinks for men.

Chapter 10

The Heart and
the Thyroid Gland

Diseases of the thyroid gland can directly alter the normal function of the heart, causing symptoms and resulting in significant complications. To understand how the heart is affected it is first necessary to appreciate how the heart works.

The heart contains muscular chambers that contract and cause blood to circulate around the body. Because of valves within the heart, blood normally circulates in one direction only. Blood is returned to the heart through the veins, and the right atrium and right ventricle of the heart pump blood into the lungs. From the lungs blood is returned to the left atrium and left ventricle, from which it is ejected into the arteries, which distribute blood to the different organs in the body.

With respect to thyroid disease it is important to understand two principles. One, as the heart itself is called a muscle it requires oxygen to work and receives oxygen through special arteries called coronary arteries. If there is disease in these coronary arteries causing a blockage within the lumen and reduction in coronary artery blood flow, the heart muscle then works with an inadequate oxygen supply and heart pain or "angina" can be produced. Two, in order for the heart to beat in a coordinated fashion and expel blood smoothly and efficiently, the heart muscle is stimulated to contract in a synchronized fashion

Reprinted from "The Heart and the Thyroid Gland," by J. Malcolm O. Arnold, M.D., © 2000. Reprinted with permission from the author and the Thyroid Foundation of Canada, http://www.thyroid.ca.

by specialized tissues within the heart that conduct electrical impulses. The impulse normally starts at the top of the right atrium and spreads down through the heart.

Hyperthyroidism

Symptoms and Signs

Increased levels of thyroxine released from the thyroid gland stimulate the heart to beat more quickly and more strongly. Initially this may produce a fast heart rate, which is called a tachycardia. This is observed by a nurse or physician but is usually not noticed by the patient. However, if the fast heart rate becomes severe, then palpitations may be observed by the patient. This is an awareness of the heart beating within the chest. Occasionally it can be noticed by normal individuals and may be caused by excessive exercise or drinking too much caffeine. However, if it occurs at rest and is a fast prolonged heart rate, then it may be abnormal. Palpitations may occur in other types of heart disease, but, if caused by an overactive thyroid gland, they do not necessarily mean that a more serious underlying heart disease is present. In some patients, prolonged stimulation of the heart with thyroxine may cause an incoordination of the conduction of electrical impulses within the heart and atrial fibrillation may ensue. This is where the impulses arising in the right atrium, rather than being conducted normally into the ventricles, form a short circuit within atria and rapidly go around in circles, causing incoordinated atrial contraction and loss of regular stimulation of the ventricle with an irregular heartbeat.

Prolonged stimulation of heart contraction can cause some increase in blood pressure, which is called systolic hypertension. The diastolic blood pressure, that is, the lower of the two blood pressure numbers, is not normally increased. The increased contraction of the heart with increased cardiac output causes a pulse that is easily felt at the wrist and contributes to warm sweaty hands.

Complications

If there is prolonged untreated stimulation of heart rate and heart contraction this can cause the two complications of angina and heart failure. Angina occurs when heart muscle does not get enough oxygen supply and causes a discomfort in the center of the chest that may also be felt in the throat, in the neck or jaw, and in the arms (often the left arm). If severe it may be described as an actual pain and not just a discomfort. If such pain is left untreated an actual heart attack or myocardial infarction can occur, where an area of heart muscle is irreversibly damaged.

Heart failure may occur when the increased demands on the heart from the fast heart rate and increased contraction cause a weakening of the heart muscle and it is no longer able to pump blood efficiently out of the lungs into the rest of the body. The usual symptom is therefore shortness of breath due to congestion of blood in the lungs. Ankle swelling may also occur.

Angina and heart failure do not normally occur in hyperthyroidism in young healthy hearts. However, in older patients with underlying heart disease, the presence of an overactive thyroid gland may be sufficient to unmask the underlying heart disease or aggravate symptoms that are already present.

Treatment

The first essential is to correct the hyperthyroidism. The decision whether to use drugs, radioactive iodine therapy, or thyroid surgery depends on the nature of the thyroid problem. At the same time as treating the hyperthyroidism, specific treatment for angina may be commenced with a drug that slows the heart rate such as a "beta blocker", for example, propranolol. There is a wide variety of drugs similar to propranolol and all are equally effective. These drugs are also useful to decrease other symptoms of hyperthyroidism, such as finger tremor and anxiety. Heart failure is usually treated in the standard way, with heart medications to improve heart function, such as digoxin, and drugs to increase excretion of water by the kidneys, diuretics, for example, furosemide. We do not fully understand the direct actions of thyroxine on the heart, but it appears that some patients may be relatively resistant to normal doses of digoxin and it may be necessary to measure blood digoxin levels and increase the dose to obtain a desired effect.

Hypothyroidism

Symptoms and Signs

These tend to be the opposite to those mentioned previously for an overactive thyroid gland and consist of slow heart rate and low blood pressure. Neither of these signs usually produce symptoms in patients. Prolonged hypothyroidism causes metabolic changes in the body and may produce elevated levels of cholesterol. We are aware that some types of elevated cholesterol levels may produce or aggravate narrowing of the coronary arteries. However, as heart rate and blood pressure are also lowered, the complications of angina or heart attack are relatively uncommon.

Complications

In severe prolonged hypothyroidism the heart muscle fibers may become diseased, with the development of a weak heart, producing heart failure. There is often a collection of fluid around the heart and this is called a pericardia effusion but rarely produces any symptoms. As discussed previously, there may be an increased risk for coronary artery disease, but the importance of this is not fully understood. As with hyperthyroidism, the occurrence of heart complications is more likely to occur in patients who have underlying heart disease caused by factors other than their thyroid problem.

Treatment

If heart disease is present, then hypothyroidism needs to be corrected slowly. If thyroxine replacement is commenced at doses given to otherwise healthy people, then the demands on the heart may be quickly increased with resultant symptoms of angina or heart failure. Thus it is often necessary to begin thyroid replacement at half or even one quarter of the normal replacement dose. Depending on the patient's response and the lack of heart symptoms, this dose may be increased over a period of weeks or months to the normal thyroid replacement dose.

Summary

Thyroid disease may directly affect the heart, especially whenever the thyroid gland is overactive. This may produce symptoms of palpitations, heart pain, or heart failure. Similar symptoms may occur with an underactive thyroid if it is treated too rapidly with thyroid replacement therapy. Symptoms of heart disease are much more likely to occur in patients who have underlying heart disease from another cause. Permanent changes in the heart are unusual in patients with normal healthy hearts, unless the thyroid disease is particularly severe and left untreated for very long periods of time.

Chapter 11

Depression and Heart Disease

Symptoms of Depression

- Persistent sad, anxious, or "empty" mood
- Feelings of hopelessness, pessimism
- Feelings of guilt, worthlessness, helplessness
- Loss of interest or pleasure in hobbies and activities that were once enjoyed, including sex
- Decreased energy, fatigue, being "slowed down"
- Difficulty concentrating, remembering, making decisions
- Insomnia, early-morning awakening, or oversleeping
- Appetite or weight changes
- Thoughts of death or suicide, or suicide attempts
- Restlessness, irritability

If five or more of these symptoms are present every day for at least two weeks and interfere with routine daily activities such as work, self-care, and childcare or social life, seek an evaluation for depression.

Introduction

Depression can strike anyone. However, research over the past two decades has shown that people with heart disease are more likely to

Reprinted from "Depression and Heart Disease," National Institute of Mental Health, NIH publication no. 02-5004, May 2002.

suffer from depression than otherwise healthy people, and conversely, that people with depression are at greater risk for developing heart disease.[1] Furthermore, people with heart disease who are depressed have an increased risk of death after a heart attack, compared to those who are not depressed.[2] Depression may make it harder to take the medications needed and to carry out the treatment for heart disease. Treatment for depression helps people manage both diseases, thus enhancing survival and quality of life.

Heart disease affects an estimated 12.2 million American women and men and is the leading cause of death in the United States.[3] While about 1 in 20 American adults experiences major depression in a given year, the number goes to about 1 in 3 for people who have survived a heart attack.[4,5]

Depression and anxiety disorders may affect heart rhythms, increase blood pressure, and alter blood clotting. They can also lead to elevated insulin and cholesterol levels. These risk factors, with obesity, form a group of signs and symptoms that often serve as both a predictor of and a response to heart disease. Furthermore, depression or anxiety may result in chronically elevated levels of stress hormones, such as cortisol and adrenaline. As high levels of stress hormones are signaling a "fight or flight" reaction, the body's metabolism is diverted away from the type of tissue repair needed in heart disease.

Despite the enormous advances in brain research in the past twenty years, depression often goes undiagnosed and untreated. Persons with heart disease, their families and friends, and even their physicians and cardiologists (physicians specializing in heart disease treatment) may misinterpret depression's warning signs, mistaking them for inevitable accompaniments to heart disease. Symptoms of depression may overlap with those of heart disease and other physical illnesses. However, skilled health professionals will recognize the symptoms of depression and inquire about their duration and severity, diagnose the disorder, and suggest appropriate treatment.

Depression Facts

Depression is a serious medical condition that affects thoughts, feelings, and the ability to function in everyday life. Depression can occur at any age. NIMH-sponsored studies estimate that almost 10 percent of American adults, or about 19 million people age eighteen and older, experience some form of depression every year.[4] Although available therapies alleviate symptoms in over 80 percent of those treated, less than half of people with depression get the help they need.[4,6]

Depression results from abnormal functioning of the brain. The causes of depression are currently a matter of intense research. An interaction between genetic predisposition and life history appear to determine a person's level of risk. Episodes of depression may then be triggered by stress, difficult life events, side effects of medications, or other environmental factors. Whatever its origins, depression can limit the energy needed to keep focused on treatment for other disorders, such as heart disease.

Heart Disease Facts

Heart disease includes two conditions called angina pectoris and acute myocardial infarction ("heart attack"). Like any muscle, the heart needs a constant supply of oxygen and nutrients that are carried to it by the blood in the coronary arteries. When the coronary arteries become narrowed or clogged and cannot supply enough blood to the heart, the result is coronary heart disease. If not enough oxygen-carrying blood reaches the heart, the heart may respond with pain called angina. The pain is usually felt in the chest or sometimes in the left arm and shoulder. (However, the same inadequate blood supply may cause no symptoms, a condition called silent angina.) When the blood supply is cut off completely, the result is a heart attack. The part of the heart that does not receive oxygen begins to die, and some of the heart muscle may be permanently damaged.

Chest pain (angina) or shortness of breath may be the earliest signs of heart disease. A person may feel heaviness, tightness, pain, burning, pressure, or squeezing, usually behind the breastbone but sometimes also in the arms, neck, or jaws. These signs usually bring the person to a doctor for the first time. Nevertheless, some people have heart attacks without ever having any of these symptoms.

Risk factors for heart disease other than depression include high levels of cholesterol (a fat-like substance) in the blood, high blood pressure, and smoking. On the average, each of these doubles the chance of developing heart disease. Obesity and physical inactivity are other factors that can lead to heart disease. Regular exercise, good nutrition, and smoking cessation are key to controlling the risk factors for heart disease.

Heart disease is treated in a number of ways, depending on how serious it is. For many people, heart disease is managed with lifestyle changes and medications, including beta-blockers, calcium-channel blockers, nitrates, and other classes of drugs. Others with severe heart disease may need surgery. In any case, once heart disease develops, it requires lifelong management.

Get Treatment for Depression

Effective treatment for depression is extremely important, as the combination of depression and heart disease is associated with increased sickness and death. Prescription antidepressant medications, particularly the selective serotonin reuptake inhibitors, are generally well-tolerated and safe for people with heart disease. There are, however, possible interactions among certain medications and side effects that require careful monitoring. Therefore, people being treated for heart disease who develop depression, as well as people in treatment for depression who subsequently develop heart disease, should make sure to tell any physician they visit about the full range of medications they are taking.

Specific types of psychotherapy, or "talk" therapy, also can relieve depression. Ongoing research is investigating whether these treatments also reduce the associated risk of a second heart attack. Preventive interventions based on cognitive-behavior theories of depression also merit attention as approaches for avoiding adverse outcomes associated with both disorders. These interventions may help promote adherence and behavior change that may increase the impact of available pharmacological and behavioral approaches to both diseases.

Exercise is another potential pathway to reducing both depression and risk of heart disease. A recent study found that participation in an exercise training program was comparable to treatment with an antidepressant medication (a selective serotonin reuptake inhibitor) for improving depressive symptoms in older adults diagnosed with major depression.[7] Exercise, of course, is a major protective factor against heart disease as well.

Use of herbal supplements of any kind should be discussed with a physician before they are tried. Recently, scientists have discovered that St. John's wort, an herbal remedy sold over the counter and promoted as a treatment for mild depression, can have harmful interactions with some other medications.

Treatment for depression in the context of heart disease should be managed by a mental health professional—for example, a psychiatrist, psychologist, or clinical social worker—who is in close communication with the physician providing the heart disease treatment. This is especially important when antidepressant medication is needed or prescribed, so that potentially harmful drug interactions can be avoided. In some cases, a mental health professional that specializes in treating individuals with depression and co-occurring physical illnesses such as heart disease may be available.

While there are many different treatments for depression, they must be carefully chosen by a trained professional based on the circumstances of the person and family. Recovery from depression takes time. Medications for depression can take several weeks to work and may need to be combined with ongoing psychotherapy. Not everyone responds to treatment in the same way. Prescriptions and dosing may need to be adjusted. No matter how advanced the heart disease, however, the person does not have to suffer from depression. Treatment can be effective.

Other mental disorders, such as bipolar disorder (manic-depressive illness) and anxiety disorders, may occur in people with heart disease, and they, too, can be effectively treated.

Remember, depression is a treatable disorder of the brain. Depression can be treated in addition to whatever other illnesses a person might have, including heart disease. If you think you may be depressed, or know someone who is, don't lose hope. Seek help for depression.

References

1. C. B. Nemeroff, D. L. Musselman, and D. L. Evans, "Depression and Cardiac Disease," *Depression and Anxiety* 8, Suppl 1 (1998): 71–79.

2. N. Frasure-Smith, F. Lesperance, and M. Talajic, "Depression and Eighteen-Month Prognosis after Myocardial Infarction," *Circulation* 91, no. 4 (1995): 999–1005.

3. "Morbidity and Mortality: 2000 Chart Book on Cardiovascular, Lung, and Blood Diseases," National Heart, Lung, and Blood Institute, 2000. http://www.nhlbi.nih.gov/resources/docs/00chtbk.pdf

4. D. A. Regier, W. E. Narrow, D. S. Rae, et al. "The De Facto Mental and Addictive Disorders Service System. Epidemiologic Catchment Area Prospective One-Year Prevalence Rates of Disorders and Services." *Archives of General Psychiatry* 50, no. 2 (1993): 85–94.

5. F. Lesperance, N. Frasure-Smith, and M. Talajic, "Major Depression Before and After Myocardial Infarction: Its Nature and Consequences," *Psychosomatic Medicine* 58, no. 2 (1996): 99–110.

6. National Advisory Mental Health Council, "Health Care Reform for Americans with Severe Mental Illnesses," *American Journal of Psychiatry* 150, no. 10 (1993): 1447–65.

7. J. A. Blumenthal, M. A. Babyak, K. A. Moore, et al. "Effects of Exercise Training on Older Patients with Major Depression," *Archives of Internal Medicine* 159, no. 19 (1999): 2349–56.

Chapter 12

Cardiopulmonary Resuscitation (CPR): You Can Do It

CPR in Three Simple Steps

(Please try to attend a CPR training course.)

1. **Call:** Check the victim for unresponsiveness. If there is no response, call 911 and return to the victim. In most locations the emergency dispatcher can assist you with CPR instructions.

2. **Blow:** Tilt the head back and listen for breathing. If not breathing normally, pinch nose and cover the mouth with yours and blow until you see the chest rise. Give 2 breaths. Each breath should take 2 seconds.

3. **Pump:** If the victim is still not breathing normally, coughing, or moving, begin chest compressions. Push down on the chest 1-1/2 to 2 inches 15 times right between the nipples. Pump at the rate of 100/minute, faster than once per second.

Continue with 2 breaths and 15 pumps until help arrives.

Note: This ratio is the same for one-person and two-person CPR. In two-person CPR the person pumping the chest stops while the other gives mouth-to-mouth breathing.

This chapter includes information reprinted from "Learn CPR: You Can Do It!" "Learn CPR: CPR for Infants (Age <1)," and "Learn CPR: CPR for Children (Ages 1–8)" prepared by the University of Washington School of Medicine, reviewed October 16, 2003. © 2003 www.learncpr.org. These articles may be accessed at www.learncpr.org.

Unresponsiveness

During cardiac arrest, the heart stops pumping blood, the blood pressure falls to zero, and the pulse disappears. Within ten seconds of cardiac arrest the person loses consciousness and becomes unresponsive. If you shake or shout at the victim, there will be no response.

Sometimes a person in cardiac arrest may make grunting, gasping, or snoring-type breathing sounds for a couple of minutes. Do not be confused by this abnormal type of breathing.

If a person is unresponsive (doesn't respond to shouts or shakes) and not breathing (or breathing abnormally) then call 911 and begin CPR.

Abnormal Breathing

Remember, a person in cardiac arrest may have abnormal breathing for a couple of minutes. This abnormal breathing is called "agonal respiration" and is the result of the brain's breathing center sending out signals even though circulation has ceased. The key point is that the abnormal breathing may sound like grunting, gasping, or snoring. It disappears in two to three minutes. If you see this type of breathing **do not delay CPR**. The person desperately needs air, and only you can provide it.

CPR for Children (Ages 1–8)

CPR for children is similar to performing Quick CPR for adults. There are, however, four differences.

1. If you are alone with the child, give one minute of CPR before calling 911

2. Use the heel of one hand for chest compressions

3. Press the sternum down 1 to 1.5 inches

4. Give 1 full breath followed by 5 chest compressions

CPR for Infants (Age <1)

Shout and Tap

Shout and gently tap the child on the shoulder. If there is no response, position the infant on his or her back.

Open the Airway

Open the airway using a head tilt lifting of chin. Do not tilt the head too far back.

Give Two Gentle Breaths

If the baby is not breathing, give 2 small, gentle breaths. Cover the baby's mouth and nose with your mouth. Each breath should be 1.5 to 2 seconds long. You should see the baby's chest rise with each breath.

Give Five Compressions

Give 5 gentle chest compressions at the rate of 100 per minute. Position your third and fourth fingers in the center of the chest, half an inch below the nipples. Press down only 1/2 to 1 inches.

Repeat

Repeat with 1 breath and 5 compressions. After one minute of re-peated cycles call 911 and continue giving breaths and compressions.

Chapter 13

Automated External Defibrillators (AEDs)

What is an automated external defibrillator?

An automated external defibrillator (AED) is a portable automatic device used to restore normal heart rhythm to patients in cardiac arrest.

An AED is applied outside the body. It automatically analyzes the patient's heart rhythm and advises the rescuer whether or not a shock is needed to restore a normal heart beat. If the patient's heart resumes beating normally, the heart has been defibrillated.

When is it used?

An AED is used to treat cardiac arrest. It is a life-saving device because cardiac arrest is a sudden condition that is fatal if not treated within a few minutes.

Heart attacks and other conditions can cause ventricular fibrillation. In ventricular fibrillation, the electrical signals in the lower part of the heart are uncoordinated and ineffective. Very little blood is pumped from the heart to the body or the lungs. If ventricular fibrillation is not treated, it will result in cardiac arrest.

You can find AEDs in public places, such as airports and office buildings (public access AEDs). Doctors sometimes recommend home defibrillators for patients with heart disease.

Reprinted from "Automated External Defibrillator (AED)," U.S. Food and Drug Administration, updated February 27, 2004.

How does it work?

An AED consists of a small computer (microprocessor), electrodes, and electrical circuitry. The electrodes collect information about the heart's rhythm. The microprocessor interprets the rhythm.

If the heart is in ventricular fibrillation, the microprocessor recommends a defibrillating shock. The shock is delivered by adhesive electrode pads, through the victim's chest wall, and into the heart.

There are special low-power electrode pads for use on children.

What will it accomplish?

The AED delivers an electric shock that stuns the heart momentarily, stopping all activity. This gives the heart a chance to restart normal electrical activity and resume beating effectively.

What are the risks?

Most trained users can operate AEDs safely. There is some risk of electric shock to the operator and others if the operator has not been trained to avoid touching the patient. Other risks include skin burns from the electrodes, abnormal heart rhythms, and blood clots.

When should it not be used?

The device should not be used in a patient who has a pulse. It should also be avoided under conditions where the patient cannot be isolated from other people (for example, in the standing water of a rowboat that is filled with passengers who are either touching the patient or the water).

Part Two

Maintaining Heart Health

Chapter 14

How to Keep Your
Heart Healthy

Sixty-two-year-old Jack Andre says having a heart attack in March 2003 was like getting hit in the head with a baseball bat. "It brought a lot of things to my attention that I never thought about before," he says. He was overweight, didn't exercise, and often ate high-fat foods. Yet he never connected his lifestyle to his heart.

"Six months before the heart attack, my doctor told me I had borderline high cholesterol and high blood pressure," says Andre, of Rockville, Maryland. "But I didn't think much of it."

That all changed after he experienced heart attack symptoms—extreme fatigue, dizziness, and back pain. Tests revealed that Andre had three clogged coronary arteries. "Now I walk every day at lunch, eat smaller portions, and I'm a food label reader," he says.

Bonnie Brown, fifty, of Baltimore, says she also didn't change her life until she had a heart attack in 1997. "I used to smoke, ate cold-cut subs for breakfast, and had lots of fried foods, all the time, any time," Brown says. But her heart attack—which she initially mistook for a bad case of indigestion—led her to give up cigarettes, improve her diet, and sign up for weekly water aerobics and line dancing classes.

"There's nothing that motivates people like having a heart attack or bypass surgery," says Christopher Cates, M.D., director of vascular intervention at the Emory Heart Center in Atlanta. "I've found that people think that heart disease always happens to someone else, until

Reprinted from "How to Keep Your Heart Healthy," by Michelle Meadows, *FDA Consumer*, U.S. Food and Drug Administration, November–December 2003; contains revisions made in February 2004 and May 2004.

it happens to them." Experts say that until Americans change their way of thinking from a viewpoint of damage control to one of proactive prevention, heart disease will remain the number one killer of men and women in the United States.

"In many ways, I think we've become insulated by high-tech care," Cates says. "As physicians, we are partners in the health care of our patients, which means we need to educate them about their risk factors for heart disease. And they need to have some sense of ownership about what they can control. They can't simply look to their doctors or to the FDA [U.S. Food and Drug Administration] or to medicine, and say, 'Cure me, but I'm going to eat fatty foods, smoke, and be sedentary.'"

One of the reasons that some people may shrug off the possibility of developing heart disease is that it's a gradual, lifelong process that people can't see or feel. About the size of a fist, the heart muscle relies on oxygen and nutrients to continually pump blood through the circulatory system. In coronary artery disease, the most common type of heart disease, plaque builds up in the coronary arteries, the vessels that bring oxygen and nutrients to the heart muscle. As the walls of the arteries get clogged, the space through which blood flows narrows. This decreases or cuts off the supply of oxygen and nutrients, which can result in chest pain or a heart attack. Damage can result when the supply is cut off for more than a few minutes. It's called a heart attack when prolonged chest pain or symptoms (twenty minutes or more) are associated with permanent damage to the heart muscle.

Every year, more than one million people have heart attacks, according to the National Heart, Lung, and Blood Institute (NHLBI). About thirteen million Americans have coronary heart disease, and about half a million people die from it each year.

What's Your Risk Profile?

Risk factors for heart disease are typically labeled "uncontrollable" or "controllable." The main uncontrollable risk factors are age, gender, and a family history of heart disease, especially at an early age.

The risk of heart disease rises as people age, and men tend to develop it earlier. Specifically, men ages forty-five and older are at increased risk of heart disease, while women fifty-five and older are at increased risk. A woman's natural hormones give some level of protection from heart disease before menopause.

"Heart disease presents in women an average of seven to ten years later than in men," says Patrice Desvigne-Nickens, M.D., leader of cardiovascular medicine at the National Heart, Lung, and Blood Institute

(NHLBI). "But after menopause, women develop heart disease as often as men, and women who have a heart attack don't fare as well as men." Women are more likely than men to die from a heart attack.

Though heart disease is the leading cause of death for both men and women in this country, surveys have shown that many women don't know it, and that they are more worried about cancer, especially breast cancer. "We want women to know that heart disease is not a man's disease. Rather, heart disease is the leading cause of death for women, and heart disease is preventable and treatable," says Desvigne-Nickens.

The NHLBI defines having a family history of early heart disease this way: A father or brother who had heart disease before age fifty-five, or a mother or sister who had heart disease before age sixty-five. Be sure to tell your doctor if any of your family members have had heart disease. Andre says it was only after he had a heart attack that he learned that he had four uncles who had been diagnosed with coronary artery disease.

Even if you have uncontrollable risk factors for heart disease, it doesn't mean that you can't take steps to limit your risk. Researchers say that controllable risk factors—physical inactivity, smoking, overweight or obesity, high blood pressure, high blood cholesterol, and diabetes—are all major influences on the development and severity of heart disease.

According to Cynthia Tracy, M.D., chief of cardiology at Georgetown University Hospital in Washington, D.C., the best way to combat heart disease is to know the risk factors, "own" the risk factors that apply to you, and address the ones that are controllable. "I think many people can rattle off risk factors, but then they don't internalize them to say: 'That's a risk factor for me. I am at risk for heart disease. And now I'm going to do something about it,'" Tracy says.

Taking Charge of Your Health

Because of advances in medicine and technology, people with heart disease are living longer, more productive lives than ever before. Yet prevention is still the best weapon in the fight against heart disease. As with anything in life, there are no guarantees. You could do all the right things and still develop heart disease because there are so many factors involved. Yet by living a healthier life, you could delay heart disease for years or minimize its damage. Whether you are already healthy, are at high risk for heart disease, or have survived a heart attack, the advice to protect your heart is the same.

Get Moving and Maintain a Healthy Weight

Exercise improves heart function, lowers blood pressure and blood cholesterol, and boosts energy. Being overweight forces the heart to work harder. Yet about one in four U.S. adults are sedentary.

The general recommendation from the NHLBI is to get at least thirty minutes of moderate physical activity on most, and preferably all, days of the week. And you don't need to run a marathon or buy an expensive gym club membership to do it. The thirty minutes also don't have to be done all at once, but can be broken up into ten-minute intervals throughout your day.

"Exercising is like taking the pennies from under the couch cushions and putting them into your piggybank," says Ann Bolger, M.D., a spokeswoman for the American Heart Association (AHA) and a cardiologist in San Francisco. "Every little bit counts."

Vigorous exercise like running or doing aerobics brings more health benefits than lighter-intensity activities, but walking is a great form of exercise. Brisk walking can get your heart rate up and give you a solid workout. Walking at a comfortable pace can work well for many people, too. "The best exercise is the one you feel good about and can do over and over again," Bolger says. And it's easier to work exercise into your everyday routine than you might think.

For example, Bolger suggests parking farther away when you go to the grocery store or to your office to create a longer walk, taking the stairs, walking all the way around a mall the next time you go shopping, and walking around your neighborhood. Getting support from a walking buddy or a walking group can be a good way to keep you motivated.

Talk with your doctor about what form of exercise is best for you. Those with severe heart disease, for example, are advised against strenuous exercise.

Desvigne-Nickens suggests that you teach your children early that exercise is fun and good for them. Families can walk together, ride bikes, and chase after balls in a park. "But we have to show them," she says. "Our children are exercising their thumbs with computers and video games, and obesity in childhood is epidemic."

Stick to a Nutritious, Well-Balanced Diet

This advice might make you groan if your usual lunch consists of cheeseburgers with French fries or pizza slices topped with sausage. Yet the good news is that diet isn't an all-or-nothing affair.

A heart-healthy diet means a diet that's low in fat, cholesterol, and salt, and high in fruits, vegetables, grains, and fiber. "But it doesn't mean that you can never have pizza or ice cream again," Bolger says. You could start by telling yourself that you will eat a big leafy green salad first, and then you will have one slice of cheese pizza, not three slices with sausage. "Or if you must have a burger, don't get your usual order of French fries," Bolger suggests. "That alone cuts hundreds of calories."

Experts point out that a heart-healthy diet should be the routine. That way, when you have high-fat food every now and then, you're still on track. Making a high-fat diet the routine is asking for trouble.

Bolger teaches people about the AHA's Simple Solutions program, which helps women—often the ones who do the cooking and grocery shopping—adopt simple ways to improve eating habits for the whole family. For example, it's wise to make a grocery list so that you can carefully plan your meals. "You have to make a conscious decision to make your snack a bag of grapes instead of a candy bar or cookies," Bolger says.

Bolger also asks her patients to tell her the food or food group that gets them into trouble. If you pin that down you can start to make healthy substitutions. Tell Bolger that overloading on ice cream is your downfall and she'll tell you about her recipe for a berry dessert: Use nonfat yogurt, sweeten it up as much as you want with a sugar substitute, add a drop of vanilla extract, microwave frozen strawberries briefly to soften them up, add the berries, stir it all around, and enjoy.

Like exercise, good eating habits need to start early. "Teaching your children to eat well is one of the most loving things you can do for them," Bolger says. Your children tend to follow your lead, eat what you eat, and eat what you put in front of them. It's up to you how often you put a banana in front of them instead of high-fat cookies.

Look at the Nutrition Facts label on the foods you buy for guidance. The general rule of thumb is that foods that provide 5 percent of the daily value (DV) of fat or less are low in fat, and foods that are labeled as providing 20 percent or more of the daily value are high in fat.

Control Your Blood Pressure

About fifty million American adults have high blood pressure, also called hypertension. The top number of a blood pressure reading, called the systolic pressure, represents the force of blood in the arteries as the heart beats. The bottom number, called diastolic pressure, is the force of blood in the arteries as the heart relaxes between beats. High blood pressure makes the heart work extra hard and hardens artery walls, increasing the risk of heart disease and stroke.

A blood pressure level of 140 over 90 mm Hg (millimeters of mercury) or higher is considered high. The NHLBI recently set a new "prehypertension" level of any reading above 120 over 80 mm Hg.

Poor eating habits and physical inactivity both contribute to high blood pressure. According to the NHLBI, table salt increases average levels of blood pressure, and this effect is greater in some people than in others.

The National Institutes of Health's DASH diet (Dietary Approaches to Stop Hypertension) is rich in fruits, vegetables, and low-fat dairy foods, and low in total and saturated fat. The DASH diet also reduces red meat, sweets, and sugary drinks, and it's rich in potassium, calcium, magnesium, fiber, and protein.

It's important to keep on top of your blood pressure levels through regular doctor visits. High blood pressure disproportionately affects racial and ethnic minority groups, including blacks, Hispanics, and American Indians/Alaska Natives. The condition is known as a silent killer because there are no symptoms. If lifestyle changes alone don't bring your blood pressure within the normal range, medications may also be needed.

Recent NHLBI research has shown that older, less costly diuretics work better than newer medicines to treat high blood pressure. These findings, part of the Antihypertensive and Lipid-Lowering Treatment to Prevent Heart Attack Trial (ALLHAT), were published in the December 18, 2002, issue of the *Journal of the American Medical Association.*

Control Blood Cholesterol

Cholesterol is a fat-like substance in the blood. High levels of triglycerides, another form of fat in the blood, can also indicate heart disease risk.

As with blood pressure, eating a low-fat, low-cholesterol diet and engaging in physical activity can lower cholesterol levels. Your body turns saturated fats into cholesterol. The higher your cholesterol level, the more likely it is that the substance will build up and stick to artery walls.

The only way to find out your cholesterol levels is to go to a doctor and have a blood test after fasting for nine to twelve hours. A lipoprotein profile will reveal your total cholesterol, which is measured in milligrams (mg) of cholesterol per deciliter (dL) of blood. Total cholesterol less than 200 mg/dL is desirable, 200–239 mg/dL is borderline high, and 240 mg/dL or more is high.

Low-density lipoprotein (LDL), also known as "bad" cholesterol, should be less than 100 mg/dL. A level of 100–129 mg/dL is near optimal/above optimal, 130–159 mg/dL is borderline high, 160–189 mg/dL is high, and 190 mg/dL and above is very high.

High-density lipoprotein (HDL), also known as "good" cholesterol, protects the arteries from bad cholesterol buildup, so the higher the HDL, the better. HDL levels of 60 mg/dL or more help lower heart disease risk, and an HDL level of less than 40 mg/dL is considered low.

People ages twenty and older should have cholesterol measured at least once every five years. If lifestyle changes alone don't adequately control cholesterol levels, medications may be needed.

Experts say the drug class known as "statins" marks a significant advance in preventing heart disease. These drugs work by partially blocking the synthesis of cholesterol in the liver, which helps remove cholesterol from the blood. Along with lowering cholesterol, statins help stabilize blood vessel membranes. Examples include Lescol (fluvastatin),

Table 14.1. Heart-Smart Substitutions

Instead of:	Do This:
whole or 2 percent milk and cream	use 1 percent or skim milk
fried foods	eat baked, steamed, boiled, broiled, or microwaved foods
lard, butter, palm, and coconut oils	cook with unsaturated vegetable oils such as corn, olive, canola, safflower, sesame, soybean, sunflower, or peanut
fatty cuts of meat	eat lean cuts of meat or cut off the fatty parts
one whole egg in recipes	use two egg whites
sauces, butter, and salt	season vegetables with herbs and spices
regular hard and processed cheeses	eat low-fat, low-sodium cheeses
salted potato chips	choose low-fat, unsalted tortilla and potato chips and unsalted pretzels and popcorn
sour cream and mayonnaise	use plain low-fat yogurt, low-fat cottage cheese, or low-fat or "light" sour cream

Pravachol (pravastatin), Zocor (simvastatin), and Lipitor (atorvastatin). The most recent addition to this class, AstraZeneca Pharmaceuticals' Crestor (rosuvastatin), was approved by the Food and Drug Administration in August 2003. Even with drug treatment, a cholesterol-lowering diet and exercise are still recommended.

Prevent and Manage Diabetes

About seventeen million people in the United States have diabetes, and heart disease is the leading cause of death of those with the disease. According to the American Diabetes Association (ADA), two out of three people with diabetes die from heart disease or stroke.

Diabetes is a disease in which the body does not properly produce or use insulin. Insulin is a hormone needed to convert sugar, starches, and other nutrients into energy. Another sixteen million Americans have pre-diabetes, a condition in which blood glucose levels are higher than normal, but not high enough to be diagnosed as diabetes. Genetics and lifestyle factors such as obesity and physical inactivity can lead to diabetes.

One in three people who have diabetes don't know they have it. See a doctor if you have any diabetes symptoms, which include frequent urination, excessive thirst, extreme hunger, unusual weight loss, increased fatigue, irritability, and blurry vision.

Quit Smoking

Ditch the cigarettes and you'll dramatically lower your heart attack risk. If you don't smoke, don't start. Along with raising your risk of lung cancer and other diseases, the mixture of tar, nicotine, and carbon monoxide in tobacco smoke increases the risk that your arteries will harden, which restricts blood flow to the heart.

Smokers have more than twice the risk of having a heart attack as nonsmokers. According to the AHA, smoking is the biggest risk factor for sudden cardiac death, and smokers who have a heart attack are more likely to die than nonsmokers who have a heart attack.

In the first year that you stop smoking, your risk of coronary heart disease drops sharply, according to the NHLBI. Over time, your risk will gradually return to that of someone who has never smoked.

Minimize Stress

After having a heart attack in 1987, Dennis Everett, sixty-one, retired early from a high-stress job and moved with his wife, Joyce, from Vienna, Virginia, to Berkeley Springs, West Virginia—a rural resort town that gives Everett a relaxing life.

Stress management was a major part of Everett's recovery, which also included improving his diet, going for daily walks, and giving up smoking. "I couldn't have done it without the support of my wife," he says. "Spouses also have a big adjustment."

The link between stress and heart disease isn't completely clear, but what's known for sure is that stress speeds up the heart rate. People with heart disease are more likely to have a heart attack during times of stress.

Everett was serving as coach for a girls' softball team when the pain he had been experiencing in his left arm for a few days became unbearable. "It hurt so bad that I had to hold my left arm up with my right one," he says. He happened to mention his symptoms to a player's father, a dentist. "He told me, 'I hate to tell you this, but those are the signs of a heart attack,'" Everett says. "That's when we called 911."

Heart Attack Symptoms

Research has shown that people typically wait two hours or more before seeking emergency care for heart attack symptoms. It could be because they are uncertain about their symptoms or concerned that it might be a false alarm. Yet clot-busting medications and other effective treatments that restore blood flow and save heart muscle are most effective in the first hour following a heart attack.

Symptoms of heart attack include chest discomfort or pain; discomfort in the arm(s), back, neck, jaw, or stomach; shortness of breath; breaking out in a cold sweat; nausea; and lightheadedness. Most heart attacks don't involve someone clutching the chest and dropping to the floor like you might see on TV. It's also important to know that heart attack symptoms for men can be different than symptoms for women.

"The classic sign is when someone comes into the emergency room, puts their fist on their chest, and says it feels like a squeezing pressure," says Cynthia Tracy, M.D., chief of cardiology at Georgetown University Hospital in Washington, D.C. "But it's not always like that. For women, it may present as back pain, flu-like symptoms, or a sense of impending doom."

"We need women to be aware of their symptoms, and we need doctors to put the pieces together and say, 'This woman is postmenopausal and her mother died of a heart attack at forty-seven. So even though her symptoms don't sound classic, I need to investigate her for coronary disease.'"

When Bonnie Brown, fifty, of Baltimore, felt a sharp pain in the middle of her chest in 1997, she thought it was indigestion and assumed the feeling would pass. Yet something made her tell her sister, Joan Hamilton, fifty-three, who lived with her at the time. Joan noticed how pale Bonnie looked and insisted they call an ambulance. Soon after, doctors confirmed that she was having a heart attack.

Then, amazingly enough, Joan also had a heart attack—two weeks after Bonnie did. For Joan, her main symptom was persistent pain in the left arm. "I thought it was from lifting boxes," Joan says, "but I don't tolerate pain too well so I checked it out."

Both Bonnie and Joan used to think heart disease was only for men. Both women are part of the Red Dress Project, the centerpiece of the Heart Truth campaign, sponsored by the National Institutes of Health, to educate women about heart disease. The Red Dress Project features a collection of nineteen red dresses from America's most prestigious designers, with the dresses symbolizing the fact that heart disease is a women's issue too.

Treating Heart Disease

Once doctors determine that you have clogged coronary arteries, the treatment plan typically involves a combination of drugs, lifestyle changes, and procedures that open up the arteries.

Drugs

Thrombolytic drugs, also referred to as "clot-busting drugs," are given during a heart attack to dissolve blood clots in coronary arteries and restore blood flow to the heart.

Because of its anti-clotting abilities, aspirin is recognized by the Food and Drug Administration as safe and effective to help lower the risk of having a second heart attack.

Other drugs commonly used to treat people with heart disease include drugs that lower blood pressure, angiotensin-converting enzyme (ACE) inhibitors, which help the heart pump blood better, and beta blockers, which slow the heart down. Nitrates and calcium channel blockers relax blood vessels and relieve chest pain. Diuretics decrease fluid in the body. Blood cholesterol–lowering drugs reduce levels of low-density lipoproteins (LDL), the "bad" cholesterol, in the blood and increase high-density lipoproteins (HDL), the "good" cholesterol.

Catheter-Based Treatments

Angioplasty is a procedure in which a thin tube called a catheter is put into an artery in the groin and threaded up to the narrowed artery in the heart. The catheter, which has a balloon at the tip, is used to widen the artery. Routinely, tiny mesh wire tubes called stents are then inserted into the artery to hold it open permanently. Yet a major challenge is restenosis, which is the reclogging or renarrowing of an artery after angioplasty or stenting.

Maureen Magoon, sixty-seven, of Blairsville, Georgia, who was diagnosed with heart disease in 1999, has experienced problems with restenosis since receiving angioplasty. So when her doctors at the Emory Heart Center in Atlanta recently discovered that another one of her arteries was clogged, they determined that she was a good candidate to receive the Cypher Stent from Cordis Corporation, the first drug-eluting stent. The new stent, approved by the FDA in May 2003, releases the drug sirolimus, which reduces the risk that the artery will reclog.

A process called intravascular radiation therapy, which uses radiation to kill cells that are clogging an artery, is sometimes used during angioplasty procedures. Also known as brachytherapy, this treatment is not approved for use with the placement of a stent for a vessel that has never been treated, says Jonette Foy, Ph.D., a biomedical engineer in the FDA's Center for Devices and Radiological Health. "Brachytherapy is approved for vessels that have been previously stented, but reoccluded over time."

Coronary Bypass Surgery

In cases of severe blockages or when someone is unresponsive to medications or not a candidate for angioplasty, doctors may perform coronary bypass surgery. This involves taking a blood vessel from the leg or chest and grafting it onto the blocked artery to bypass the blockage.

In the last few years, the FDA has approved several devices that improve heart disease diagnosis and treatment. For example, after a person has received coronary bypass surgery, devices are used to catch loose particles that could potentially float downstream and clog another artery. This process is known as embolic protection.

C-Reactive Protein: A New Risk Factor

Among the new risk factors that may be linked to increased risk of cardiovascular disease is C-reactive protein (CRP). It's produced by the liver as a response to injury or infection and is a sign of inflammation in the body. Research correlates high levels of CRP with an increased risk of heart attack and stroke. Though the evidence is conflicting, some researchers believe that CRP itself is not a risk factor, but elevated levels of CRP could mean that some part of the cardiovascular system is inflamed, which can lead to stroke or heart attack. Information about CRP and other new risk factors is still emerging.

Chapter 15

Eating for a Healthy Heart

Why do I need to be concerned about heart healthy eating?

Diet is one of the things that can affect your heart health, and your risk for getting heart disease. Everyone needs to be concerned about heart disease. It is the number-one killer of American men and women. The good news is that diet is one of the things you can control to improve your heart health and lower your risk for heart disease. Making relatively simple changes in your daily eating habits will pay off quickly—not only will you feel better, your overall health will improve as well!

How do I get started with planning a heart healthy diet?

We all know that too much fat and salt are not good for us. Yet it can be hard to change your diet, particularly when you are busy and often don't have time for three healthy, home-cooked meals a day. While the thought of changing your diet might be daunting, there are diets out there to help you! It can be very confusing knowing what to eat, how much to eat, what type of fat to eat, what type of fat to avoid, and how much salt to use. We will describe three easy-to-follow diets, to help you reduce your risk for getting heart disease.

Reprinted from "Heart Healthy Eating," National Women's Health Information Center (www.4woman.gov), December 2002.

What is cholesterol and what diets can help me lower or maintain healthy levels of cholesterol?

Our bodies need cholesterol to function normally. Yet if you have too much cholesterol in your blood, it can build up (called plaque) in your arteries (blood vessels that carry oxygen- and nutrient-rich blood from the heart and lungs to all parts of the body). High cholesterol adds to the narrowing and blockages in arteries, which cause heart disease. We all have "good" cholesterol, called HDL, which helps remove cholesterol from the blood. We also all have "bad" cholesterol, or LDL, which causes cholesterol to build up in the blood.

There are two diets that focus on lowering or maintaining levels of cholesterol—a natural, waxy substance found in all parts of the body, including the blood—to reduce risk for heart disease.

- The **Heart Healthy Diet** helps you keep your blood cholesterol low, decreasing your chances of getting heart disease.

- The **Therapeutic Lifestyles Changes (TLC) Diet** focuses on helping people lower their blood cholesterol. Sometimes a person may also need medicine prescribed by a health care provider to help lower his or her blood cholesterol.

It's important to note that diet isn't the only thing that can affect cholesterol levels. Your genes affect how fast cholesterol is made and removed from the blood, being overweight tends to increase your LDL ("bad" cholesterol), and physical activity (for thirty minutes most days of the week) helps lower your LDL. Before menopause, women usually have cholesterol levels that are lower than those of men the same age. As women and men age, their cholesterol levels rise, up until about age sixty to sixty-five. However, after the age of about fifty (when menopause begins), women often have higher cholesterol levels than men of the same age.

How do the Heart Healthy and TLC Diets work?

Both of these diets help you to develop a personal eating plan. Be sure to talk with your health care provider first, before starting any type of eating plan. You might want to ask your provider for a referral to a registered dietitian (RD) who can help you choose foods and plan menus, monitor your progress, and encourage you to stay on the diet. You might also want to enlist the help of a family member or friend, to give you support and help you stay on track. Finding a "buddy" to go on one of these diets with you can also provide support. Try to stay focused on your ultimate goal—to prevent heart disease and protect your health—and have some fun learning new recipes and different ways to cook!

Here are some general guidelines to follow, for both the Heart Healthy and TLC diets. Check Table 15.1 to determine, for each diet, the daily amounts of saturated fat, total fat, cholesterol, and sodium that you should have.

- **Choose foods low in saturated fat.** Saturated fat raises your LDL ("bad" cholesterol) level more than anything else you eat. It's found the most in animal foods like fatty cuts of meat, poultry with the skin, and whole-milk dairy products, and in tropical oils like coconut, palm kernel, and palm oils. Most other vegetable oils are low in saturated fats. Foods low in saturated fat include fruits, vegetables, whole-grain foods, and low-fat or nonfat dairy products. Some processed foods (such as frozen dinners and canned foods) can be quite high in saturated fat—it' s best to check package labels before purchasing these types of foods.

- **Choose a diet moderate in total fat.** The good news is that you don't have to eliminate all fat from your diet! A diet moderate in fat will give you enough calories to satisfy your hunger, which can help you to eat fewer calories, stay at a healthy weight, and lower your blood cholesterol level. Keep in mind, though, that it's important to keep your total fat level within the levels on Table 15.1, depending on which diet you follow. You should substitute unsaturated fat for saturated fat, in order not to go over these levels.

- **Choose foods low in cholesterol.** Dietary cholesterol found in animal foods can also raise your blood cholesterol level; many of these foods also are high in saturated fat. To reduce dietary cholesterol, eat fruit, vegetables, whole grains, low-fat or nonfat dairy products, and moderate amounts of lean meats, skinless poultry, and fish.

- **Cut down on sodium.** If you have high blood pressure (see next question) as well as high blood cholesterol—and many people do—your health care provider may tell you to cut down on sodium or salt. Even if you don't have high blood pressure or cholesterol, try to have no more than 2,400 milligrams of sodium a day. You can choose low-sodium foods, which will also help lower your cholesterol, such as fruits, vegetables, whole grains, low-fat or nonfat dairy products, and moderate amounts of lean meat. To flavor your food, reach for herbs and spices rather than high-sodium table salt. There are many types of seasoning mixes in salt shaker-like containers you can find in grocery stores, but some do contain salt. Be sure to read the labels of these products before purchasing.

- **Watch your body weight.** It is not uncommon for overweight people to have higher blood cholesterol than people who are not overweight. When you reduce the fat in your diet, you cut down not only on cholesterol and saturated fat, but on calories as well. This will help you to lose weight and improve your blood cholesterol, both of which will reduce your risk for heart disease. If you are overweight, talk with your health care provider about the best ways to lose weight, including having a regular exercise program. Regular exercise is important, even if you are not overweight. It will help lower your blood cholesterol and blood pressure and improve your overall health.

What diets can help me maintain a healthy blood pressure level?

Research has shown that diet affects the development of high blood pressure (hypertension). As blood is pumped from your heart through

Table 15.1. Heart Healthy and TLC Diet Guidelines

Heart Healthy Diet Every Day You Should Have:	TLC Diet Every Day You Should Have:
8 to 10 percent of total calories from saturated fat	less than 7 percent of total calories from saturated fat
30 percent or less of total calories from fat	25–35 percent or less of total calories from fat
less than 300 milligrams (mg) of dietary cholesterol	less than 300 milligrams (mg) of dietary cholesterol
no more than 2,400 milligrams (mg) of sodium	no more than 2,400 milligrams (mg) of sodium
just enough calories to achieve or maintain a healthy weight and reduce your blood cholesterol level[a]	just enough calories to achieve or maintain a healthy weight and reduce your blood cholesterol level[a]

[a] Ask your health care provider or RD what a reasonable daily calorie level is for you.

your body, the blood puts force or pressure against the blood vessel (or artery) walls. Your blood pressure is a reading, or measure, of this pressure. When that pressure goes above a certain point, it is called high blood pressure, another name for hypertension. High blood pressure is called the "silent killer" because it most often has no signs or symptoms. It makes the heart work too hard and if not controlled over time, it can lead to heart and kidney disease, and stroke.

Studies have shown that following the Dietary Approaches to Stop Hypertension (DASH) Diet and reducing sodium lowers blood pressure. If you do not have high blood pressure, following the DASH diet and reducing your sodium intake may help prevent the development of high blood pressure.

How does the DASH Diet work?

The DASH diet is similar to the Heart Healthy and TLC diets. Like these diets, the DASH diet recommends no more than 2,400 mg of sodium a day. However, the DASH diet also recommends a lower level of 1,500 mg sodium a day. Talk with your health care provider before making any type of change in your diet. If you choose the DASH diet, ask your provider what amount of sodium (2,400 or 1,500 mg) you should not exceed on a daily basis. You can ask your provider for a referral to a RD, who can help you choose foods and plan menus, monitor your progress, and encourage you to stay on the diet. You might also want to enlist the help of a family member or friend, to give you support and help you stay on track. Finding a "buddy" to go on one of these diets with you can also provide support.

The DASH diet is made up of foods that are low in saturated fat, cholesterol, and total fat, such as fruits, vegetables, and low-fat dairy products. It also includes whole-grain products, fish, poultry and nuts, and reduced amounts of red meat, sweets, and sugar-containing beverages. It is rich in magnesium, potassium, and calcium, as well as protein and fiber. Eating foods rich in potassium is especially important, since potassium seems to prevent high blood pressure. Try to have more than 3,500 mg of potassium per day. There are different amounts, or servings, of specific food groups recommended for different daily calorie levels, described in Tables 15.2 and 15.3.

Know that the DASH diet has more daily servings of fruits, vegetables, and whole-grain foods than you may be used to eating. This increases the fiber in your diet, which can cause bloating and diarrhea in some persons. To avoid these problems, gradually increase your intake of fruit, vegetables, and whole-grain foods. Also know that only a small amount of sodium occurs naturally in foods. Because most of the sodium we consume is in processed foods, be sure to carefully check the label of these types of foods before purchasing. While some processed foods do have low or reduced sodium levels, some are loaded with it!

Here are some other helpful tips to reduce sodium and salt in your diet:

- Aim for no more than 2,400 milligrams of sodium per day.
- Use reduced-sodium or no-salt-added products.
- Buy fresh, frozen, or canned with no-salt-added vegetables.
- Use fresh poultry, fish, and lean meat, rather than canned, smoked, or processed types.

Table 15.2. DASH Eating Plan for a 2000 Calorie/day (Average) Diet (*continued on next page*)

Food Group: Grains and grain products   **Daily Servings:** 7 to 8
Serving Sizes: 1 slice bread, 1 oz. dry cereal, ½ cup cooked rice, pasta, or cereal
Examples and Notes: whole wheat bread, English muffin, pita bread, bagel, cereal, grits, oatmeal, crackers, unsalted pretzels and popcorn—these are major sources of energy and fiber

Food Group: Vegetables   **Daily Servings:**4 to 5
Serving Sizes: 1 cup raw leafy vegetable, ½ cup cooked vegetable, 6 oz. vegetable juice
Examples and Notes: tomatoes, potatoes, carrots, green peas, squash, broccoli, turnips, greens, collards, kale, spinach, artichokes, green beans, lima beans, sweet potatoes—these are rich sources of potassium, magnesium, and fiber

Food Group: Fruits   **Daily Servings:** 4 to 5
Serving Sizes: 6 oz. fruit juice, 1 medium fruit, ¼ cup dried fruit, ½ cup fresh, frozen, or canned fruit
Examples and Notes: apricots, bananas, dates, grapes, oranges, orange juice, mangoes, melons, peaches, pineapples, prunes, raisins, strawberries, tangerines—these are important sources of potassium, magnesium, and fiber

Food Group: Low-fat of nonfat dairy foods   **Daily Servings:** 2 to 3
Serving Sizes: 8 oz. Milk, 1 cup yogurt, 1.5 oz. Cheese
Examples and Notes: fat-free or low-fat milk, fat-free or low-fat buttermilk, fat-free or low-fat regular or frozen yogurt, low-fat and fat-free cheeses—these are major sources of calcium and protein

- Choose ready-to-eat breakfast cereals that are low in sodium.

- Limit cured foods (like bacon and ham), foods packed in brine (like pickles, olives, and sauerkraut), and condiments (like MSG, mustard, horseradish, catsup, and barbecue sauce). Limit even lower-sodium versions of soy and teriyaki sauce.

- Be spicy instead of salty! Flavor foods with herbs, spices, lemon, lime, vinegar, or salt-free seasoning blends. Start by cutting salt in half.

- Cook rice, pasta, and hot cereals without salt. Cut back on instant or flavored rice, pasta, and cereal mixes, which often contain added salt.

Table 15.2. DASH Eating Plan for a 2000 Calorie/day (Average) Diet (*continued*)

Food Group: Meats, poultry, and fish   **Daily Servings:** 2 or less
Serving Sizes: 3 oz. cooked meats, poultry, or fish

Examples and Notes: select only lean; trim away visible fats; broil, roast, or boil instead of frying; remove skin from poultry—these are rich sources of protein and magnesium

Food Group: Nuts, seeds, and dry beans   **Daily Servings:** 4 to 5 per week
Serving Sizes: 1/3 cup or 1.5 oz nuts. 2 Tbsp or ½ oz. Seeds, ½ cup cooked dry beans

Examples and Notes: almonds, filberts, mixed nuts, peanuts, walnuts, sunflower seeds, kidney beans, lentils, peas—these are rich sources of energy, magnesium, potassium, protein, and fiber

Food Group: Fats and oils   **Daily Servings:** 2 to 3
Serving Sizes: 1 tsp soft margarine, 1 Tbsp low-fat mayonnaise, 2 Tbsp light salad dressing, 1 tsp vegetable oil

Examples and Notes: soft margarine, low-fat mayonnaise, light salad dressing, vegetable oil (such as olive, corn, canola, or safflower)—DASH has 27 percent of calories as fat, including that in or added to foods

Food Group: Sweets   **Daily Servings:** 5 per week
Serving Sizes: 1 Tbsp sugar, 1 Tbsp jelly or jam, ½ oz. jelly beans, 8 oz. lemonade

Examples and Notes: maple syrup, sugar, jelly, jam, fruit-flavored gelatin, jelly beans, hard candy, fruit punch, sorbet, ices—these are sweets that should be low in fat

Note: Ask your health care provider or RD what a reasonable daily calorie level is for you.

- Choose convenience foods that are lower in sodium. Cut back on frozen dinners, pizza, packaged mixes, canned soups or broths, and salad dressings—these often have a lot of sodium.

- Rinse canned foods like tuna to remove some sodium.

What else can I do, besides diet, to keep my heart healthy?

Regular physical activity can help you reduce your risk of heart disease. Being active helps you take off extra pounds, helps to control blood pressure, and boosts your level of "good" cholesterol. Some studies show that being inactive increases the risk of a heart attack. To reduce your risk for heart disease:

- Quit smoking. Talk with your health care provider if you need help quitting.

- Exercise at least thirty minutes a day on most (if not all) days of the week.

- Lose weight if you are overweight and maintain a healthy weight.

- Check blood pressure, cholesterol, and blood sugar levels and keep them under control.

Table 15.3. DASH Eating Plan Number of Servings for Other Calorie Levels

Food Group	1,600 calories/day	3,100 calories/day
Grains and grain products	6 servings/day	12 to 13 servings/day
Vegetables	3 to 4 servings/day	6 servings/day
Fruits	4 servings/day	6 servings/day
Low-fat or nonfat dairy foods	2 to 3 servings/day	3 to 4 servings/day
Meats, poultry, and fish	1 to 2 servings/day	2 to 3 servings/day
Nuts, seeds, and dry beans	3 servings/week	1 serving/day
Fats and oils	2 servings/day	4 servings/day
Sweets	0	2 servings

Ask your health care provider or RD what a reasonable daily calorie level is for you.

Chapter 16

High Blood Cholesterol: What You Need to Know

Why is cholesterol important?

Your blood cholesterol level has a lot to do with your chances of getting heart disease. High blood cholesterol is one of the major risk factors for heart disease. A risk factor is a condition that increases your chance of getting a disease. In fact, the higher your blood cholesterol level, the greater your risk for developing heart disease or having a heart attack. Heart disease is the number one killer of women and men in the United States. Each year, more than a million Americans have heart attacks, and about a half million people die from heart disease.

How does cholesterol cause heart disease?

When there is too much cholesterol (a fat-like substance) in your blood, it builds up in the walls of your arteries. Over time, this buildup causes "hardening of the arteries" so that arteries become narrowed and blood flow to the heart is slowed down or blocked. The blood carries oxygen to the heart, and if enough blood and oxygen cannot reach your heart, you may suffer chest pain. If the blood supply to a portion of the heart is completely cut off by a blockage, the result is a heart attack.

Reprinted from "High Blood Cholesterol: What You Need to Know," National Heart, Lung, and Blood Institute (NHLBI), NIH publication no. 01-3290, May 2001.

High blood cholesterol itself does not cause symptoms, so many people are unaware that their cholesterol level is too high. It is important to find out what your cholesterol numbers are, because lowering cholesterol levels that are too high lessens the risk for developing heart disease and reduces the chance of a heart attack or dying of heart disease, even if you already have it. Cholesterol lowering is important for everyone—younger, middle age, and older adults; women and men; and people with or without heart disease.

What do your cholesterol numbers mean?

Everyone age twenty and older should have their cholesterol measured at least once every five years. It is best to have a blood test called a "lipoprotein profile" to find out your cholesterol numbers. This blood test is done after a nine- to twelve-hour fast and gives information about your:

- Total cholesterol

- LDL (bad) cholesterol—the main source of cholesterol buildup and blockage in the arteries

- HDL (good) cholesterol—helps keep cholesterol from building up in the arteries

- Triglycerides—another form of fat in your blood

If it is not possible to get a lipoprotein profile done, knowing your total cholesterol and HDL cholesterol can give you a general idea about your cholesterol levels. If your total cholesterol is 200 mg/dL or more or if your HDL is less than 40 mg/dL, you will need to have a lipoprotein profile done. See how your cholesterol numbers compare to Tables 16.1 and 16.2.

Table 16.1. Evaluating Total Cholesterol Level

Total Cholesterol Level	Category
Less than 200 mg/dL	Desirable
200–239 mg/dL	Borderline High
240 mg/dL and above	High

Note: Cholesterol levels are measured in milligrams (mg) of cholesterol per deciliter (dL) of blood.

Table 16.2. Evaluating LDL Cholesterol Level

LDL Cholesterol Level	LDL-Cholesterol Category
Less than 100 mg/dL	Optimal
100–129 mg/dL	Near optimal/above optimal
130–59 mg/dL	Borderline high
160–89 mg/dL	High
190 mg/dL and above	Very high

HDL (good) cholesterol protects against heart disease, so for HDL, higher numbers are better. A level less than 40 mg/dL is low and is considered a major risk factor because it increases your risk for developing heart disease. HDL levels of 60 mg/dL or more help to lower your risk for heart disease.

Triglycerides can also raise heart disease risk. Levels that are borderline high (150–99 mg/dL) or high (200 mg/dL or more) may need treatment in some people.

What affects cholesterol levels?

A variety of things can affect cholesterol levels. These are things you can do something about:

- **Diet.** Saturated fat and cholesterol in the food you eat make your blood cholesterol level go up. Saturated fat is the main culprit, but cholesterol in foods also matters. Reducing the amount of saturated fat and cholesterol in your diet helps lower your blood cholesterol level.

- **Weight.** Being overweight is a risk factor for heart disease. It also tends to increase your cholesterol. Losing weight can help lower your LDL and total cholesterol levels, as well as raise your HDL and lower your triglyceride levels.

- **Physical Activity.** Not being physically active is a risk factor for heart disease. Regular physical activity can help lower LDL (bad) cholesterol and raise HDL (good) cholesterol levels. It also helps you lose weight. You should try to be physically active for thirty minutes on most, if not all, days.

103

Things you cannot do anything about also can affect cholesterol levels. These include:

- **Age and Gender.** As women and men get older, their cholesterol levels rise. Before the age of menopause, women have lower total cholesterol levels than men of the same age. After the age of menopause, women's LDL levels tend to rise.

- **Heredity.** Your genes partly determine how much cholesterol your body makes. High blood cholesterol can run in families.

What is your risk of developing heart disease or having a heart attack?

In general, the higher your LDL level and the more risk factors you have (other than LDL), the greater your chances of developing heart disease or having a heart attack. Some people are at high risk for a heart attack because they already have heart disease. Other people at high risk for developing heart disease because they have diabetes (which is a strong risk factor) or a combination of risk factors for heart disease. Follow these steps to find out your risk for developing heart disease.

Step 1: Check the table below to see how many of the listed risk factors you have; these are the risk factors that affect your LDL goal.

Major Risk Factors That Affect Your LDL Goal

- Cigarette smoking
- High Blood Pressure (140/90 mmHg or higher or on blood pressure medication)
- Low HDL cholesterol (less than 40 mg/dL) [If your HDL cholesterol is 60 mg/dL or higher, subtract 1 from your total count.]
- Family history of early heart disease (heart disease in father or brother before age fifty-five; heart disease in mother or sister before age sixty-five)
- Age (men forty-five years or older; women fifty-five years or older)

Even though obesity and physical inactivity are not counted in this list, they are conditions that need to be corrected.

Step 2: Determine how many major risk factors do you have? If you have two or more of the risk factors in the preceding list, use the attached risk scoring tables (which include your cholesterol levels) to find your risk score. Risk score refers to the chance of having a heart attack in the next ten years, given as a percentage.

Step 3: Use your medical history, number of risk factors, and risk score to find your risk of developing heart disease or having a heart attack in Table 16.3.

Table 16.3. Risk of Having a Heart Attack

If You Have	You Are in Category
Heart disease, diabetes, or risk score more than 20%[a]	I. Highest Risk
2 or more risk factors and risk score 10–20%	II. Next Highest Risk
2 or more risk factors and risk score less than 10%	III. Moderate Risk
0 or 1 risk factor	IV. Low-to-Moderate Risk

[a] Means that more than twenty out of one hundred people in this category will have a heart attack within ten years.

How is high cholesterol treated?

The main goal of cholesterol-lowering treatment is to lower your LDL level enough to reduce your risk of developing heart disease or having a heart attack. The higher your risk, the lower your LDL goal will be. To find your LDL goal, see the following list for your risk category. There are two main ways to lower your cholesterol:

- Therapeutic Lifestyle Changes (TLC)—includes a cholesterol-lowering diet (called the TLC diet), physical activity, and weight management. TLC is for anyone whose LDL is above goal.

- Drug Treatment—if cholesterol-lowering drugs are needed, they are used together with TLC treatment to help lower your LDL.

LDL Goals

If you are in:

- Category I, Highest Risk, your LDL goal is less than 100 mg/dL. If your LDL is 100 or above, you will need to begin the TLC diet. If your LDL is 130 or higher, you will need to start drug treatment at the same time as the TLC diet. If your LDL is 100 to 129, you may also need to start drug treatment together with the TLC diet. Even if your LDL is below 100, you should follow the TLC diet on your own to keep your LDL as low as possible.

- Category II, Next Highest Risk, your LDL goal is less than 130 mg/dL. If your LDL is 130 mg/dL or above, you will need to begin treatment with the TLC diet. If your LDL is 130 mg/dL or more after three months on the TLC diet, you may need drug treatment along with the TLC diet. If your LDL is less than 130 mg/dL, you will need to follow the heart-healthy diet for all Americans, which allows a little more saturated fat and cholesterol than the TLC diet.

- Category III, Moderate Risk, your LDL goal is less than 130 mg/dL. If your LDL is 130 mg/dL or above, you will need to begin the TLC diet. If your LDL is 160 mg/dL or more after you have tried the TLC diet for three months, you may need drug treatment along with the TLC diet. If your LDL is less than 130 mg/dL, you will need to follow the heart-healthy diet for all Americans.

- Category IV, Low-to-Moderate Risk, your LDL goal is less than 160 mg/dL. If your LDL is 160 mg/dL or above, you will need to begin the TLC diet. If your LDL is still 160 mg/dL or more after three months on the TLC diet, you may need drug treatment along with the TLC diet to lower your LDL, especially if your LDL is 190 mg/dL or more. If your LDL is less than 160 mg/dL, you will need to follow the heart-healthy diet for all Americans.

To reduce your risk for heart disease or keep it low, it is very important to control any other risk factors you may have, such as high blood pressure and smoking.

What are Therapeutic Lifestyle Changes (TLC), and how do they lower cholesterol?

TLC is a set of things you can do to help lower your LDL cholesterol. The main parts of TLC are:

- **The TLC Diet.** This is a low-saturated-fat, low-cholesterol eating plan that calls for less than 7 percent of calories from saturated fat and less than 200 mg of dietary cholesterol per day. The TLC diet recommends only enough calories to maintain a desirable weight and avoid weight gain. If your LDL is not lowered enough by reducing your saturated fat and cholesterol intakes, the amount of soluble fiber in your diet can be increased. Certain food products that contain plant stanols or plant sterols (for example, cholesterol-lowering margarines and salad dressings) can also be added to the TLC diet to boost its LDL-lowering power.

- **Weight Management.** Losing weight if you are overweight can help lower LDL and is especially important for those with a cluster of risk factors that includes high triglyceride and low HDL levels and being overweight with a large waist measurement (more than forty inches for men and more than thirty-five inches for women).

- **Physical Activity.** Regular physical activity (thirty minutes on most, if not all, days) is recommended for everyone. It can help raise HDL and lower LDL and is especially important for those with high triglyceride or low HDL levels who are overweight with a large waist measurement.

Foods low in saturated fat include fat-free or 1 percent dairy products, lean meats, fish, skinless poultry, whole-grain foods, and fruits and vegetables. Look for soft margarines (liquid or tub varieties) that are low in saturated fat and contain little or no trans fat (another type of dietary fat that can raise your cholesterol level). Limit foods high in cholesterol, such as liver and other organ meats, egg yolks, and full-fat dairy products.

Good sources of soluble fiber include oats, certain fruits (such as oranges and pears), and vegetables (such as Brussels sprouts and carrots), and dried peas and beans.

What if drug treatment is necessary?

Even if you begin drug treatment to lower your cholesterol, you will need to continue your treatment with lifestyle changes. This will keep the dose of medicine as low as possible, and lower your risk in other ways as well. There are several types of drugs available for lowering cholesterol, including statins, bile acid sequestrants, nicotinic acid, and fibric acids. Your doctor can help decide which type of drug is best for you. The statin drugs are very effective in lowering LDL levels and are safe for most people. Bile acid sequestrants also lower LDL and can be used alone or in combination with statin drugs. Nicotinic acid lowers LDL and triglycerides and raises HDL. Fibric acids lower LDL somewhat but are used mainly to treat high triglyceride and low HDL levels.

Once your LDL goal has been reached, your doctor may prescribe treatment for high triglycerides or a low HDL level, if these conditions are present. The treatment includes losing weight, if needed, increasing physical activity, quitting smoking, and possibly drug treatment.

Chapter 17

Understanding Cholesterol and Fat

Cholesterol and Fat: Sorting It Out

Sorting through dietary advice today is not easy, especially when it comes to understanding "fat words" and cholesterol terms. Here is basic information from the National Institute on Health (NIH) and the Food and Drug Administration (FDA) to help you better understand these terms.

The Relationship between Cholesterol and Fat

Cholesterol and fat—let's call them cousins—belong to the lipid family, a family of chemical compounds. The body needs both cholesterol and fat to stay healthy.

Cholesterol is a waxy substance used to build cell membranes and brain and nerve cells and helps the body make steroid hormones and bile acids. All the cholesterol the body needs is made by the liver, so people don't need to consume dietary cholesterol. Yet most American diets include foods that contain dietary cholesterol, found in foods of animal origin: egg yolks, meat, some shellfish, and whole-milk dairy products.

Reprinted from "Cholesterol and Fat: Sorting It Out," Copyright © 2004 New York State Office for the Aging. Reprinted with permission. For additional information, visit http://www.agingwell.state.ny.us. Additional excerpts from "Trans Fat Now Listed with Saturated Fat and Cholesterol on the Nutrition Facts Label," Center for Food Safety and Applied Nutrition, U.S. Food and Drug Administration, updated March 3, 2004.

Fats are chemical compounds that contain fatty acids. Fat is not produced by the body itself but is provided through diet. It is needed for growth and to store energy for the body. There are three main types of fatty acids: saturated, monounsaturated, and polyunsaturated.

Saturated fats are mostly found in foods of animal origin. Monounsaturated fats and polyunsaturated fats are mostly found in plant foods and some seafoods.

Triglyceride, the major form in which fat occurs in nature, appears to be related to heart health. Most of the body's fat is stored in the form of triglyceride. It comes from food and is also made in your body. Triglyceride levels should be below 200 milligrams per deciliter (mg/dl) to be considered normal. However, people with diabetes or kidney disease—conditions that increase the risk of heart disease—are also prone to high triglycerides. The NIH recommends that individuals with high total cholesterol or other risk factors for coronary heart disease have their triglyceride levels checked when the blood cholesterol level is checked.

Cultural Dietary Patterns

Eating less saturated fat has the effect of lowering blood cholesterol levels. High rates of heart disease are commonly found in countries where the diet is heavy with meat and dairy products containing a lot of saturated fats.

Other countries, in which diets are traditionally high in monounsaturated and polyunsaturated fats, may be relatively free of heart disease. It appears, then, that the type of fat one consumes is important when it comes to heart health.

For example, people living on the Greek Island of Crete consume a high dietary fat diet, largely from olive oil, a monounsaturated fat. Yet, they are relatively free of heart disease, as are the Inuit people of Alaska who have a staple food in their diet of fish rich in polyunsaturated fatty acids.

From these patterns and those in other cultures, we see that we should be removing as much saturated fat from our diet as we can. That means eating fewer foods of animal origin, such as meat and whole-milk dairy products, and more plant foods, such as vegetables and grains.

At the same time, people should limit their consumption of calories from all fats to 30 percent of their total calories per day since foods high in fats are usually high in calories as well and may affect body weight.

Build a Healthy Diet Based on Your "Fat" Knowledge

- Choose oils high in unsaturated fats.

- Buy margarine made with unsaturated liquid vegetable oils as the first ingredient.

- Limit butter, lard, fatback, and solid shortenings.

- Buy light or nonfat mayonnaise instead of the regular kinds that are high in fat.

Trans *Fat Now Listed with Saturated Fat and Cholesterol on the Nutrition Facts Label*

Trans *Fat Coming to a Label Near You!*

The Food and Drug Administration (FDA) now requires food manufacturers to list *trans* fat (i.e., *trans* fatty acids) on Nutrition Facts and some Supplement Facts panels. Scientific evidence shows that consumption of saturated fat, *trans* fat, and dietary cholesterol raises low-density lipoprotein (LDL or "bad") cholesterol levels that increase the risk of coronary heart disease (CHD). According to the National Heart, Lung, and Blood Institute of the National Institutes of Health, over 12.5 million Americans suffer from CHD, and more than 500,000 die each year. This makes CHD one of the leading causes of death in the United States today.

The FDA has required that saturated fat and dietary cholesterol be listed on the food label since 1993. By adding *trans* fat on the Nutrition Facts panel (required by January 1, 2006), consumers now know for the first time how much of all three—saturated fat, *trans* fat, and cholesterol—are in the foods they choose. Identifying saturated fat, *trans* fat, and cholesterol on the food label gives consumers information to make heart-healthy food choices that help them reduce their risk of CHD. This revised label, which includes information on *trans* fat as well as saturated fat and cholesterol, will be of particular interest to people concerned about high blood cholesterol and heart disease. However, all Americans should be aware of the risk posed by consuming too much saturated fat, *trans* fat, and cholesterol. But what is *trans* fat, and how can you limit the amount of this fat in your diet?

What Is Trans *Fat?*

Unlike other fats, the majority of *trans* fat is formed when liquid oils are made into solid fats like shortening and hard margarine.

111

However, a small amount of *trans* fat is found naturally, primarily in some animal-based foods. Essentially, *trans* fat is made when hydrogen is added to vegetable oil—a process called hydrogenation. Hydrogenation increases the shelf life and flavor stability of foods containing these fats.

Trans fat, like saturated fat and dietary cholesterol, raises the LDL (or "bad") cholesterol that increases your risk for CHD. On average, Americans consume four to five times as much saturated fat as *trans* fat in their diet.

Although saturated fat is the main dietary culprit that raises LDL, *trans* fat and dietary cholesterol also contribute significantly. *Trans* fat can often be found in processed foods made with partially hydrogenated vegetable oils such as vegetable shortenings, some margarines (especially margarines that are harder), crackers, candies, cookies, snack foods, fried foods, and baked goods.

Are All Fats the Same?

Simply put: no. Fat is a major source of energy for the body and aids in the absorption of vitamins A, D, E, and K, and carotenoids. Both animal and plant-derived food products contain fat, and when eaten in moderation, fat is important for proper growth, development, and maintenance of good health. As a food ingredient, fat provides taste, consistency, and stability and helps us feel full. In addition, parents should be aware that fats are an especially important source of calories and nutrients for infants and toddlers (up to two years of age), who have the highest energy needs per unit of body weight of any age group.

Saturated and *trans* fats raise LDL (or "bad") cholesterol levels in the blood, thereby increasing the risk of heart disease. Dietary cholesterol also contributes to heart disease. Unsaturated fats, such as monounsaturated and polyunsaturated, do not raise LDL cholesterol and are beneficial when consumed in moderation. Therefore, it is advisable to choose foods low in saturated fat, *trans* fat, and cholesterol as part of a healthful diet.

What Can I Do About Saturated Fat, Trans Fat, and Cholesterol?

When comparing foods, look at the Nutrition Facts panel, and choose the food with the lower amounts of saturated fat, *trans* fat, and cholesterol. Health experts recommend that you keep your intake of these nutrients as low as possible while consuming a nutritionally adequate diet. However, these experts recognize that eliminating these three components entirely from your diet is not practical because they are unavoidable in ordinary diets.

Where Can I Find Trans *Fat on the Food Label?*

Consumers can find *trans* fat listed on the Nutrition Facts panel directly under the line for saturated fat. Although some food products already have *trans* fat on the label, food manufacturers have until January 2006 to list it on all their products.

How Do Your Choices Stack Up?

With the addition of *trans* fat to the Nutrition Facts panel, you can review your food choices and see how they stack up.

Don't assume similar products are the same. Be sure to check the Nutrition Facts panel (NFP) when comparing products because even similar foods can vary in calories, ingredients, nutrients, and the size and number of servings in the package. When buying the same brand product, also check the NFP frequently because ingredients can change at any time and any change could affect the NFP information.

How Can I Use the Label to Make Heart-Healthy Food Choices?

The Nutrition Facts panel can help you choose foods lower in saturated fat, *trans* fat, and cholesterol. To lower your intake of saturated fat, *trans* fat, and cholesterol, compare similar foods and choose the food with the lower combined saturated and *trans* fats and the lower amount of cholesterol.

Although the updated Nutrition Facts panel will now list the amount of *trans* fat in a product, it will not show a %Daily Value (%DV). While scientific reports have confirmed the relationship between *trans* fat and an increased risk of CHD, none has provided a reference value for *trans* fat or any other information that FDA believes is sufficient to establish a Daily Reference Value or a %DV.

Saturated fat and cholesterol, however, do have a %DV. To choose foods low in saturated fat and cholesterol, use the Quick Guide to %DV. The general rule of thumb is: 5%DV or less is low and 20%DV or more is high.

You can also use the %DV to make dietary trade-offs with other foods throughout the day. You don't have to give up a favorite food to eat a healthy diet. When a food you like is high in saturated fat or cholesterol, balance it with foods that are low in saturated fat and cholesterol at other times of the day.

Do Dietary Supplements Contain Trans Fat?

Would it surprise you to know that some dietary supplements contain *trans* fat from partially hydrogenated vegetable oil as well as saturated fat or cholesterol? It's true. As a result of FDA's new label requirement, if a dietary supplement contains a reportable amount of *trans* or saturated fat, which is 0.5 grams or more, dietary supplement manufacturers must list the amounts on the Supplement Facts panel. Some dietary supplements that may contain saturated fat, *trans* fat, and cholesterol include energy and nutrition bars.

Practical Tips for Consumers

Here are some practical tips you can use every day to keep your consumption of saturated fat, *trans* fat, and cholesterol low while consuming a nutritionally adequate diet.

- **Check the Nutrition Facts panel** to compare foods because the serving sizes are generally consistent in similar types of foods. Choose foods lower in saturated fat, *trans* fat, and cholesterol. For saturated fat and cholesterol, use the Quick Guide to %DV: 5%DV or less is low and 20%DV or more is high. (Remember, there is no %DV for *trans* fat.)

- **Choose alternative fats.** Replace saturated and *trans* fats in your diet with mono- and polyunsaturated fats. These fats do not raise LDL (or "bad") cholesterol levels, and have health benefits when eaten in moderation. Sources of monounsaturated fats include olive and canola oils. Sources of polyunsaturated fats include soybean oil, corn oil, sunflower oil, and foods like nuts and fish.

- **Choose vegetable oils (except coconut and palm kernel oils) and soft margarines (liquid, tub, or spray)** more often because the amounts of saturated fat, *trans* fat, and cholesterol are lower than the amounts in solid shortenings, hard margarines, and animal fats, including butter.

- **Consider fish.** Most fish are lower in saturated fat than meat. Some fish, such as mackerel, sardines, and salmon, contain omega-3 fatty acids that are being studied to determine if they offer protection against heart disease.

- **Choose lean meats,** such as poultry (without skin, not fried), lean beef, and pork (trim visible fat, not fried).

- **Ask before you order when eating out.** A good tip to remember is to ask which fats are being used in the preparation of your food when eating or ordering out.

- **Watch calories.** Don't be fooled! Fats are high in calories. All sources of fat contain nine calories per gram, making fat the most concentrated source of calories. By comparison, carbohydrates and protein have only four calories per gram.

Here are two actions consumers can take to keep their intake of saturated fat, *trans* fat, and cholesterol "low":

- Look at the Nutrition Facts panel when comparing products. Choose foods low in the combined amount of saturated fat and *trans* fat and low in cholesterol as part of a nutritionally adequate diet.

- When possible, substitute alternative fats that are higher in mono- and polyunsaturated fats, like olive oil, canola oil, soybean oil, sunflower oil, and corn oil.

Chapter 18

Fish Oil and Heart Health

Fish oil can help reduce deaths from heart disease, according to new evidence reports announced today by the Agency for Healthcare Research and Quality (AHRQ). The systematic reviews of the available literature found evidence that long chain omega-3 fatty acids, the beneficial component ingested by eating fish or taking a fish oil supplement, reduce heart attack and other problems related to heart and blood vessel disease in persons who already have these conditions, as well as their overall risk of death. Although omega-3 fatty acids do not alter total cholesterol, HDL cholesterol, or LDL cholesterol, evidence suggests that they can reduce levels of triglycerides—a fat in the blood that may contribute to heart disease.

The review also found other evidence indicating that fish oil can help lower high blood pressure slightly, may reduce risk of coronary artery re-blockage after angioplasty, may increase exercise capability among patients with clogged arteries, and may possibly reduce the risk of irregular heart beats—particularly in individuals with a recent heart attack.

"These findings will help health care professionals and the public understand which benefits of omega-3 fatty acids have been scientifically proven and pinpoint areas where additional evidence is needed," said Carolyn M. Clancy, M.D., AHRQ's director. "Translating scientific evidence into information that can be used to improve health and heath care is key to AHRQ's mission."

Reprinted from "AHRQ Evidence Reports Confirm that Fish Oil Helps Fight Heart Disease," press release, April 22, 2004. Agency for Healthcare Research and Quality (AHRQ), Rockville, MD.

The evidence reports of the health effects of omega-3 fatty acids are part of a series conducted by AHRQ-supported Evidence-based Practice Centers at the request of the National Institutes of Health [NIH]'s Office of Dietary Supplements, which plans to use the findings to develop research agendas on the issues. Five reports are currently being issued, and an additional six reports will be issued next year.

Paul M. Coates, Ph.D., director of NIH's Office of Dietary Supplements, said, "The reports describe some positive findings as well as a number of areas where data are insufficient to draw conclusions about the efficacy and safety of omega-3 fatty acids. The Office of Dietary Supplements, in collaboration with other NIH institutes, will use these reports to develop appropriate research agendas for omega-3 fatty acids that will fill these gaps in knowledge."

Findings from the three other AHRQ evidence reviews indicate that:

- Omega-3 fatty acids do not affect fasting blood sugar or glycosylated hemoglobin in people with type II diabetes, nor do they appear to affect plasma insulin levels or insulin resistance.

- Alpha-linolenic acid (ALA), a type of omega-3 fatty acid from plants such as flaxseed, soybeans, and walnuts, may help reduce deaths from heart disease, but to a much lesser extent than fish oil.

- Based on the evidence to date, it is not possible to conclude whether omega-3 fatty acids help improve respiratory outcomes in children and adults who have asthma.

- Omega-3 fatty acids appear to have mixed effects on people with inflammatory bowel disease, kidney disease, and osteoporosis, and no discernible effect on rheumatoid arthritis.

The evidence reports and Evidence-based Practice Centers (EPCs) that produced them are: *Effects of Omega-3 Fatty Acids on Cardiovascular Disease, Effects of Omega-3 Fatty Acids on Cardiovascular Risk Factors and Intermediate Markers for Cardiovascular Disease,* and *Effects of Omega-3 Fatty Acids on Arrhythmogenic Mechanisms in Animal and Isolated Organ/Culture Studies* (Tufts-New England Medical Center EPC, Boston); *Health Effects of Omega-3 Fatty Acids on Asthma* (University of Ottawa EPC, Ottawa, Ontario); *Health Effects of Omega-3 Fatty Acids on Lipids and Glycemic Control in Type II Diabetes and the Metabolic Syndrome, and on Inflammatory Bowel Disease, Rheumatoid Arthritis, Renal Disease, Systemic Lupus Erythematosus, and Osteoporosis* (Southern California-RAND EPC, Santa Monica).

Chapter 19

If You Have
High Blood Pressure

What Are High Blood Pressure and Prehypertension?

Blood pressure is the force of blood against the walls of arteries. Blood pressure rises and falls throughout the day. When blood pressure stays elevated over time, it's called *high blood pressure.*

The medical term for high blood pressure is *hypertension.* High blood pressure is dangerous because it makes the heart work too hard and contributes to atherosclerosis (hardening of the arteries). It increases the risk of heart disease and stroke, which are the first- and third-leading causes of death among Americans. High blood pressure also can result in other conditions, such as congestive heart failure, kidney disease, and blindness.

Risk Factors for Heart Disease

Risk factors are conditions or behaviors that increase your chances of developing a disease. When you have more than one risk factor for heart disease, your risk of developing heart disease greatly multiplies. So if you have high blood pressure, you need to take action. Fortunately, you can control most heart disease risk factors.

Reprinted from "Your Guide to Lowering Blood Pressure," National Heart, Lung, and Blood Institute (NHLBI), National Institutes of Health (NIH), NIH Publication No. 03-5232, October 2003.

Risk Factors You Can Control

- High blood pressure
- Abnormal cholesterol
- Tobacco use
- Diabetes
- Overweight
- Physical inactivity

Risk Factors Beyond Your Control

- Age (55 or older for men; 65 or older for women)
- Family history of early heart disease (having a father or brother diagnosed with heart disease before age 55 or having a mother or sister diagnosed before age 65)

Defining High Blood Pressure and Prehypertension

A blood pressure level of 140/90 mmHg or higher is considered high. About two-thirds of people over age sixty-five have high blood pressure. If your blood pressure is between 120/80 mmHg and 139/89 mmHg, then you have prehypertension. This means that you don't have high blood pressure now but are likely to develop it in the future unless you adopt the healthy lifestyle changes described in this chapter. (See Table 19.1.)

People who do not have high blood pressure at age fifty-five face a 90 percent chance of developing it during their lifetimes. So high blood pressure is a condition that most people will have at some point in their lives.

Both numbers in a blood pressure test are important, but for people who are age fifty or older, systolic pressure gives the most accurate diagnosis of high blood pressure. Systolic pressure is the top number in a blood pressure reading. It is high if it is 140 mmHg or above.

How Can You Prevent or Control High Blood Pressure?

If you have high blood pressure, you and your health care provider need to work together as a team to reduce it. The two of you need to agree on your blood pressure goal. Together, you should come up with a plan and timetable for reaching your goal.

Blood pressure is usually measured in millimeters of mercury (mmHg) and is recorded as two numbers—systolic pressure (as the

Table 19.1. Blood Pressure Levels for Adults

Category	Systolic (mmHg)[a]		Diastolic (mmHg)[a]	Result
Normal	less than 120	and	less than 80	Good for you!
Prehypertension	120–139	or	80–89	Your blood pressure could be a problem. Make changes in what you eat and drink, be physically active, and lose extra weight. If you also have diabetes, see your doctor.
Hypertension	140 or higher	or	90 or higher	You have high blood pressure.Ask your doctor or nurse how to control it.

Source: The Seventh Report of the Joint National Committee on Prevention, Detection, Evaluation, and Treatment of High Blood Pressure; NIH Publication No. 03-5230, National High Blood Pressure Education Program, May 2003.

Note: Ranges given here are for adults ages eighteen and older who are not on medicine for high blood pressure and do not have a short-term serious illness.

[a] If systolic and diastolic pressures fall into different categories, overall status is in the higher category. mmHg is millimeters of mercury.

heart beats) "over" diastolic pressure (as the heart relaxes between beats)—for example, 130/80 mmHg. Ask your doctor to write down for you your blood pressure numbers and your blood pressure goal level.

Monitoring your blood pressure at home between visits to your doctor can be helpful. You also may want to bring a family member with you when you visit your doctor. Having a family member who knows that you have high blood pressure and who understands what you need to do to lower your blood pressure often makes it easier to make the changes that will help you reach your goal.

The following steps will help lower your blood pressure. If you have normal blood pressure or prehypertension, following these steps will help prevent you from developing high blood pressure. If you have high blood pressure, following these steps will help you control your blood pressure.

This chapter is designed to help you adopt a healthier lifestyle and remember to take prescribed blood pressure-lowering drugs. Following the steps described will help you prevent and control high blood pressure. While you read them, think to yourself . . . "I Can Do It!"

Hypertension can almost always be prevented, so these steps are very important even if you do not have high blood pressure.

- Maintain a healthy weight.
- Be physically active.
- Follow a healthy eating plan.
- Eat foods with less sodium (salt).
- Drink alcohol only in moderation.
- Take prescribed drugs as directed.

Lower Your Blood Pressure by Aiming for a Healthy Weight

Being overweight or obese increases your risk of developing high blood pressure. In fact, your blood pressure rises as your body weight increases. Losing even ten pounds can lower your blood pressure—and losing weight has the biggest effect on those who are overweight and already have hypertension.

Overweight and obesity are also risk factors for heart disease. Furthermore, being overweight or obese increases your chances of developing high blood cholesterol and diabetes—two more risk factors for heart disease.

Finding Your Target Weight

Two key measures are used to determine if someone is overweight or obese. These are body mass index, or BMI, and waist circumference.

BMI is a measure of your weight relative to your height. It gives an approximation of total body fat—and that's what increases the risk of diseases that are related to being overweight.

Yet BMI alone does not determine risk. For example, in someone who is very muscular or who has swelling from fluid retention (called edema), BMI may overestimate body fat. BMI may underestimate body fat in older persons or those losing muscle.

That's why waist measurement is often checked as well. Another reason is that too much body fat in the stomach area also increases disease risk. A waist measurement of more than thirty-five inches in women and more than forty inches in men is considered high.

Check Table 19.2 for your approximate BMI value. Check Table 19.3 to see if you are at a normal weight, overweight, or obese. Overweight is defined as a BMI of 25 to 29.9; obesity is defined as a BMI equal to or greater than 30.

If you fall in the obese range according to the guidelines in Table 19.3, you are at increased risk for heart disease and need to lose weight. You also should lose weight if you are overweight and have two or more heart disease risk factors, as listed previously. If you fall in the normal weight range or are overweight but do not need to lose pounds, you still should be careful not to gain weight.

Table 19.2 gives BMI for men and women of various heights and weights (as measured with underwear but no shoes). To use the table, find your height in the left-hand column labeled Height. Move across to your body weight. The number at the top of the column is the BMI for your height and weight.

If you need to lose weight, it's important to do so slowly. Lose no more than one-half pound to two pounds a week. Begin with a goal of losing 10 percent of your current weight. This is the healthiest way to lose weight and offers the best chance of long-term success.

There's no magic formula for weight loss. You have to eat fewer calories than you use up in daily activities. Just how many calories you burn daily depends on factors such as your body size and how physically active you are. (See Table 19.4.)

One pound equals 3,500 calories. So, to lose one pound a week, you need to eat 500 calories a day less or burn 500 calories a day more than you usually do. It's best to work out some combination of both eating less and being more physically active.

Remember to be aware of serving sizes. It's not only what you eat that adds calories, but also how much.

As you lose weight, be sure to follow a healthy eating plan that includes a variety of foods. A good plan to follow is the DASH eating plan, which is outlined in Table 19.5. Some tips to make the plan lower in calories appear in the section "How to Lose Weight on the DASH Eating Plan."

Lower Your Blood Pressure by Being Active

Being physically active is one of the most important things you can do to prevent or control high blood pressure. It also helps to reduce your risk of heart disease.

Table 19.2. Body Mass Index

BMI	21	22	23	24	25	26	27	28	29	30	31
Height (feet and inches)	**Body Weight (pounds)**										
4'10"	100	105	110	115	119	124	129	134	138	143	148
5'0"	107	112	118	123	128	133	138	143	148	153	158
5'2"	115	120	126	131	136	142	147	153	158	164	169
5'4"	122	128	134	140	145	151	157	163	169	174	180
5'6"	130	136	142	148	155	161	167	173	179	186	192
5'8"	138	144	151	158	164	171	177	184	190	197	203
5'10"	146	153	160	167	174	181	188	195	202	209	216
6'0"	154	162	169	177	184	191	199	206	213	221	228
6'2"	163	171	179	186	194	202	210	218	225	233	241
6'4"	172	180	189	197	205	213	221	230	238	246	254

Table 19.3. What Your BMI Means

Category	BMI	Result
Normal Weight	18.5–24.9	Good for you! Try not to gain weight.
Overweight	25–29.9	Do not gain any weight, especially if your waist measurement is high. You need to lose weight if you have two or more risk factors for heart disease.
Obese	30 or greater	You need to lose weight. Lose weight slowly— about 1/2 pound to 2 pounds a week. See your doctor or a registered dietitian if you need help.

Source: Clinical Guidelines on the Identification, Evaluation, and Treatment of Overweight and Obesity in Adults: The Evidence Report, NIH Publication No. 98-4083, National Heart, Lung, and Blood Institute, in cooperation with the National Institute of Diabetes and Digestive and Kidney Diseases, National Institutes of Health, June 1998.

It doesn't take a lot of effort to become physically active. All you need is thirty minutes of moderate-level physical activity on most days of the week. Examples of such activities are brisk walking, bicycling, raking leaves, and gardening. For more examples, see Table 19.4.

You can even divide the thirty minutes into shorter periods of at least ten minutes each. For instance: Use stairs instead of an elevator, get off a bus one or two stops early, or park your car at the far end of the lot at work. If you already engage in thirty minutes of moderate-level physical activity a day, you can get added benefits by doing more. Engage in a moderate-level activity for a longer period each day or engage in a more vigorous activity.

Most people don't need to see a doctor before they start a moderate-level physical activity. You should check first with your doctor if you have heart trouble or have had a heart attack, if you're over age fifty and are not used to moderate-level physical activity, if you have a family history of heart disease at an early age, or if you have any other serious health problem.

Lower Your Blood Pressure by Eating Right

What you eat affects your chances of getting high blood pressure. A healthy eating plan can both reduce the risk of developing high blood pressure and lower a blood pressure that is already too high.

Table 19.4. Examples of Moderate-Level Physical Activities

Common Chores	Sporting Activities
Washing and waxing a car for 45–60 minutes	Playing volleyball for 45–60 minutes
	Playing touch football for 45 minutes
Washing windows or floors for 45–60 minutes	Walking 2 miles in 30 minutes (1 mile in 15 minutes)
Gardening for 30–45 minutes	Shooting baskets for 30 minutes
Wheeling self in wheelchair for 30–40 minutes	Bicycling 5 miles in 30 minutes
Pushing a stroller 1½ miles in 30 minutes	Dancing fast (social) for 30 minutes
Raking leaves for 30 minutes	Performing water aerobics for 30 minutes
Shoveling snow for 15 minutes	Swimming laps for 20 minutes
Stair walking for 15 minutes	Playing basketball for 15–20 minutes
	Jumping rope for 15 minutes
	Running 1½ miles in 15 minutes (1 mile in 10 minutes)

For an overall eating plan, consider DASH, which stands for "Dietary Approaches to Stop Hypertension." You can reduce your blood pressure by eating foods that are low in saturated fat, total fat, and cholesterol, and high in fruits, vegetables, and low-fat dairy foods. The DASH eating plan includes whole grains, poultry, fish, and nuts, and has low amounts of fats, red meats, sweets, and sugared beverages. It is also high in potassium, calcium, and magnesium, as well as protein and fiber. Eating foods lower in salt and sodium also can reduce blood pressure.

Table 19.5 gives the servings and food groups for the DASH eating plan. The number of servings that is right for you may vary, depending on your caloric need.

The DASH eating plan has more daily servings of fruits, vegetables, and grains than you may be used to eating. Those foods are high in fiber, and eating more of them may temporarily cause bloating and

Table 19.5. The DASH Eating Plan

Food Group	Daily Servings (except as noted)	Serving Sizes
Grains and grain products	7–8	1 slice bread 1 cup ready-to-eat cereal[a] ½ cup cooked, rice, pasta, or cereal
Vegetables	4–5	1 cup raw leafy vegetable ½ cup cooked vegetable 6 ounces vegetable juice
Fruits	4–5	1 medium fruit ¼ cup dried fruit ½ cup fresh, frozen, or canned fruit 6 ounces fruit juice
Low-fat or fat-free dairy foods	2–3	8 ounces milk 1 cup yogurt 1½ ounces cheese
Lean meats,	2 or fewer	3 ounces cooked lean meat, skinless poultry, and fish
Nuts, seeds, and dry beans	4–5 per week	1/3 cup or 1½ ounces nuts 1 tablespoon or ½ ounce seeds ½ cup cooked dry beans
Fats and oils[b]	2–3	1 teaspoon soft margarine 1 tablespoon low-fat mayonnaise 2 tablespoons light salad dressing 1 teaspoon vegetable oil
Sweets	5 per week	1 tablespoon sugar 1 tablespoon jelly or jam ½ ounce jelly beans 8 ounces lemonade

Note: The DASH eating plan is based on 2,000 calories a day. The number of daily servings in a food group may vary from those listed, depending upon your caloric needs.

[a] Serving sizes vary between ½ cup and 1¼ cups. Check the product's nutrition label.

[b] Fat content changes serving counts for fats and oils: For example, 1 tablespoon of regular salad dressing equals 1 serving, 1 tablespoon of low-fat salad dressing equals ½ serving, and 1 tablespoon of fat-free salad dressing equals 0 servings.

diarrhea. To get used to the DASH eating plan, gradually increase your servings of fruits, vegetables, and grains. Later in this chapter we will offer some tips on how to adopt the DASH eating plan.

A good way to change to the DASH eating plan is to keep a diary of your current eating habits. Write down what you eat, how much, when, and why. Note whether you snack on high-fat foods while watching television or if you skip breakfast and eat a big lunch. Do this for several days. You'll be able to see where you can start making changes.

If you're trying to lose weight, you should choose an eating plan that is lower in calories. You can still use the DASH eating plan, but follow it at a lower calorie level. (See the section "How to Lose Weight on the DASH Eating Plan.") Again, a food diary can be helpful. It can tell you if there are certain times that you eat but aren't really hungry or when you can substitute low-calorie foods for high-calorie foods.

Tips on Switching to the DASH Eating Plan

- Change gradually. Add a vegetable or fruit serving at lunch and dinner.

- Use only half the butter or margarine you do now.

- If you have trouble digesting dairy products, try lactase enzyme pills or drops—they're available at drugstores and groceries. Or buy lactose-free milk or milk with lactase enzyme added to it.

- Get added nutrients such as the B vitamins by choosing whole grain foods, including whole wheat bread or whole grain cereals.

- Spread out the servings. Have two servings of fruits or vegetables at each meal, or add fruits as snacks.

- Treat meat as one part of the meal, instead of the focus. Try casseroles, pasta, and stir-fry dishes. Have two or more meatless meals a week.

- Use fruits or low-fat foods as desserts and snacks.

How to Lose Weight on the DASH Eating Plan

The DASH eating plan was not designed to promote weight loss. However, it is rich in low-calorie foods such as fruits and vegetables. You can make it lower in calories by replacing high-calorie foods with more fruits and vegetables—and that also will make it easier for you to reach your DASH eating plan goals. Here are some examples.

To increase fruits:

- Eat a medium apple instead of four shortbread cookies. You'll save 80 calories.

- Eat ¼ cup of dried apricots instead of a 2-ounce bag of pork rinds. You'll save 230 calories.

To increase vegetables:

- Have a hamburger that's 3 ounces instead of 6 ounces. Add a ½ cup serving of carrots and a ½ cup serving of spinach. You'll save more than 200 calories.

- Instead of 5 ounces of chicken, have a stir fry with 2 ounces of chicken and 1½ cups of raw vegetables. Use a small amount of vegetable oil. You'll save 50 calories.

To increase low-fat or fat-free dairy products:

- Have a ½ cup serving of low-fat frozen yogurt instead of a 1½-ounce milk chocolate bar. You'll save about 110 calories.

And don't forget these calorie-saving tips:

- Use low-fat or fat-free condiments, such as fat-free salad dressings.
- Eat smaller portions—cut back gradually.
- Choose low-fat or fat-free dairy products to reduce total fat intake.
- Use food labels to compare fat content in packaged foods. Items marked low-fat or fat-free are not always lower in calories than their regular versions. See Figure 19.1 on how to read and compare food labels.
- Limit foods with lots of added sugar, such as pies, flavored yogurts, candy bars, ice cream, sherbet, regular soft drinks, and fruit drinks.
- Eat fruits canned in their own juice.
- Snack on fruit, vegetable sticks, unbuttered and unsalted popcorn, or bread sticks.
- Drink water or club soda.

Spice It Up and Use Less Sodium

Use More Spices and Less Salt

An important part of healthy eating is choosing foods that are low in salt (sodium chloride) and other forms of sodium. Using less sodium is key to keeping blood pressure at a healthy level.

Most Americans use more salt and sodium than they need. Some people, such as African Americans and the elderly, are especially sensitive to salt and sodium and should be particularly careful about how much they consume.

Most Americans should consume no more than 2.4 grams (2,400 milligrams) of sodium a day. That equals 6 grams (about 1 teaspoon) of table salt a day. For someone with high blood pressure, the doctor may advise less. The 6 grams includes all salt and sodium consumed, including that used in cooking and at the table.

Before trying salt substitutes, you should check with your doctor, especially if you have high blood pressure. These contain potassium chloride and may be harmful for those with certain medical conditions.

Tips to Reduce Salt and Sodium

- Buy fresh, plain frozen, or canned "with no salt added" vegetables.

- Use fresh poultry, fish, and lean meat, rather than canned or processed types.

- Use herbs, spices, and salt-free seasoning blends in cooking and at the table.

- Cook rice, pasta, and hot cereal without salt. Cut back on instant or flavored rice, pasta, and cereal mixes, which usually have added salt.

- Choose "convenience" foods that are low in sodium. Cut back on frozen dinners, pizza, packaged mixes, canned soups or broths, and salad dressings—these often have a lot of sodium.

- Rinse canned foods, such as tuna, to remove some sodium.

- When available, buy low- or reduced-sodium or no-salt-added versions of foods—see Figure 19.1 for guidance on how to use food labels.

- Choose ready-to-eat breakfast cereals that are low in sodium.

With herbs, spices, garlic, and onions, you can make your food spicy without salt and sodium. There's no reason why eating less sodium should make your food any less delicious! See Table 19.6 for some great ideas on using spices.

Table 19.6. Tips for Using Herbs and Spices

Herb or Spice	Use in
Basil	Soups and salads, vegetables, fish, and meats
Cinnamon	Salads, vegetables, breads, and snacks
Chili Powder	Soups, salads, vegetables, and fish
Cloves	Soups, salads, and vegetables
Dill Weed and Dill Seed	Fish, soups, salads, and vegetables
Ginger	Soups, salads, vegetables, and meats
Marjoram	Soups, salads, vegetables, beef, fish, and chicken
Nutmeg	Vegetables, meats, and snacks
Oregano	Soups, salads, vegetables, meats, and snacks
Parsley	Salads, vegetables, fish, and meats
Rosemary	Salads, vegetables, fish, and meats
Sage	Soups, salads, vegetables, meats, and chicken
Thyme	Salads, vegetables, fish, and chicken

Experiment with these and other herbs and spices. To start, use small amounts to find out if you like them.

Shopping for Foods That Will Help You Lower Your Blood Pressure

By paying close attention to food labels when you shop, you can consume less sodium. Sodium is found naturally in many foods. But processed foods account for most of the salt and sodium that Americans consume. Processed foods that are high in salt include regular canned vegetables and soups, frozen dinners, lunchmeats, instant and ready-to-eat cereals, and salty chips and other snacks.

Use food labels to help you choose products that are low in sodium. Figure 19.1 shows you how to read and compare food labels.

As you read food labels, you may be surprised that many foods contain sodium, including baking soda, soy sauce, monosodium glutamate (MSG), seasoned salts, and some antacids.

Easy on the Alcohol

Drinking too much alcohol can raise blood pressure. It also can harm the liver, brain, and heart. Alcoholic drinks also contain calories, which matters if you are trying to lose weight.

If you drink alcoholic beverages, drink only a moderate amount— one drink a day for women, two drinks a day for men.

What counts as a drink?

- 12 ounces of beer (regular or light, 150 calories),
- 5 ounces of wine (100 calories), or
- 1½ ounces of 80-proof whiskey (100 calories).

Compare Labels

Food labels can help you choose items lower in sodium, as well as calories, saturated fat, total fat, and cholesterol. Figure 19.1 illustrates some of the information found on food labels.

Manage Your Blood Pressure Drugs

If you have high blood pressure, the lifestyle habits noted here may not lower your blood pressure enough. If they don't, you'll need to take drugs.

Even if you need drugs, you still must make the lifestyle changes. Doing so will help your drugs work better and may reduce how much of them you need.

There are many drugs available to lower blood pressure. They work in various ways. Many people need to take two or more drugs to bring their blood pressure down to a healthy level.

See Table 19.7 for a rundown on the main types of drugs and how they work.

When you start on a drug, work with your doctor to get the right drug and dose level for you. If you have side effects, tell your doctor so the drugs can be adjusted. If you're worried about cost, tell your doctor or pharmacist—there may be a less expensive drug or a generic form that you can use instead.

FROZEN PEAS	
Nutrition Facts	
Serving Size: ½ cup	
Servings Per Container: about 3	

Amount Per Serving	
Calories: 60	Calories from Fat: 0

	% Daily Value*
Total Fat 0g	0%
Saturated Fat 0g	0%
Cholesterol 0mg	0%
Sodium 125mg	5%
Total Carbohydrate 11g	4%
Dietary Fiber 6g	22%
Sugars 5g	
Protein 5g	

Vitamin A 15%	•	Vitamin C	30%
Calcium 0%	•	Iron	6%

* Percent Daily Values are based on a 2,000 calorie diet.

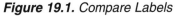

Amount per serving
Nutrient amounts are provided for one serving. If you eat more or less than a serving, add or subtract amounts. For example, if you eat 1 cup of peas, you need to double the nutrient amounts on the label.

Number of servings
There may be more than one serving in the package, so be sure to check serving size.

Nutrients
You'll find the milligrams of sodium in one serving.

Percent daily value
Percent daily value helps you compare products and tells you if the food is high or low in sodium. Choose products with the lowest percent daily value for sodium.

CANNED PEAS	
Nutrition Facts	
Serving Size: ½ cup	
Servings Per Container: about 3	

Amount Per Serving	
Calories: 60	Calories from Fat: 0

	% Daily Value*
Total Fat 0g	0%
Saturated Fat 0g	0%
Cholesterol 0mg	0%
Sodium 380mg	16%
Total Carbohydrate 12g	4%
Dietary Fiber 3g	14%
Sugars 4g	
Protein 4g	

Vitamin A 6%	•	Vitamin C	10%
Calcium 2%	•	Iron	8%

* Percent Daily Values are based on a 2,000 calorie diet

? **Which product is lower in sodium?**
Answer: The frozen peas. The canned peas have three times more sodium than the frozen peas.

***Figure 19.1.** Compare Labels*

It's important that you take your drugs as prescribed. That can prevent a heart attack, stroke, and congestive heart failure, which is a serious condition in which the heart cannot pump as much blood as the body needs.

It's easy to forget to take medicines, but just like putting your socks on in the morning and brushing your teeth, taking your medicine can become part of your daily routine.

Tips to Help You Remember to Take Your Blood Pressure Drugs

- Put a favorite picture of yourself or a loved one on the refrigerator with a note that says, "Remember to take your high blood pressure drugs."

- Keep your high blood pressure drugs on the nightstand next to your side of the bed.

- Take your high blood pressure drugs right after you brush your teeth, and keep them with your toothbrush as a reminder.

- Put "sticky" notes in visible places to remind yourself to take your high blood pressure drugs. You can put notes on the refrigerator, on the bathroom mirror, or on the front door.

- Set up a buddy system with a friend who also is on daily medication and arrange to call each other every day with a reminder to "take your blood pressure drugs."

- Ask your child or grandchild to call you every day with a quick reminder. It's a great way to stay in touch, and little ones love to help the grown-ups.

- Place your drugs in a weekly pillbox, available at most pharmacies.

- If you have a personal computer, program a start-up reminder to take your high blood pressure drugs, or sign up with a free service that will send you a reminder e-mail every day.

Table 19.7 Blood Pressure Drugs

Drug Category	How They Work
Diuretics	These are sometimes called "water pills" because they work in the kidney and flush excess water and sodium from the body through urine.
Beta-blockers	These reduce nerve impulses to the heart and blood vessels. This makes the heart beat less often and with less force. Blood pressure drops, and the heart works less hard.
Angiotensin converting enzyme inhibitors	These prevent the formation of a hormone called angiotensin II, which normally causes blood vessels to narrow. The blood vessels relax, and pressure goes down.
Angiotensin antagonists	These shield blood vessels from angiotensin II. As a result, the blood vessels open wider, and pressure goes down.
Calcium channel blockers	These keep calcium from entering the muscle cells of the heart and blood vessels. Blood vessels relax, and pressure goes down.
Alpha-blockers	These reduce nerve impulses to blood vessels, allowing blood to pass more easily.
Alpha-beta-blockers	These work the same way as alpha-blockers but also slow the heartbeat, as beta-blockers do.
Nervous system inhibitors	These relax blood vessels by controlling nerve impulses.
Vasodilators	These directly open blood vessels by relaxing the muscle in the vessel walls.

- Remember to refill your prescription. Each time you pick up a refill, make a note on your calendar to order and pick up the next refill one week before the medication is due to run out.

You can be taking drugs and still not have your blood pressure under control. Everyone—and older Americans in particular—must be careful to keep his or her blood pressure below 140/90 mmHg. If your blood pressure is higher than that, talk with your doctor about adjusting your drugs or making lifestyle changes to bring your blood pressure down.

Some over-the-counter drugs, such as arthritis and pain drugs, and dietary supplements, such as ephedra, ma haung, and bitter orange, can raise your blood pressure. Be sure to tell your doctor about any nonprescription drugs that you're taking and ask whether they may make it harder for you to bring your blood pressure under control.

Action Items to Help Lower Your Blood Pressure

1. Maintain a healthy weight

   - Check with your health care provider to see if you need to lose weight.
   - If you do, lose weight slowly using a healthy eating plan and engaging in physical activity.

2. Be physically active

   - Engage in physical activity for a total of thirty minutes on most days of the week.
   - Combine everyday chores with moderate-level sporting activities, such as walking, to achieve your physical activity goals.

3. Follow a healthy eating plan

   - Set up a healthy eating plan with foods low in saturated fat, total fat, and cholesterol, and high in fruits, vegetables, and low-fat dairy foods such as the DASH eating plan.
   - Write down everything that you eat and drink in a food diary. Note areas that are successful or need improvement.
   - If you are trying to lose weight, choose an eating plan that is lower in calories.

4. Reduce sodium in your diet
   - Choose foods that are low in salt and other forms of sodium.
   - Use spices, garlic, and onions to add flavor to your meals without adding more sodium.

5. Drink alcohol only in moderation
   - In addition to raising blood pressure, too much alcohol can add unneeded calories to your diet.
   - If you drink alcoholic beverages, have only a moderate amount—one drink a day for women, two drinks a day for men.

6. Take prescribed drugs as directed
   - If you need drugs to help lower your blood pressure, you still must follow the lifestyle changes mentioned above.
   - Use notes and other reminders to help you remember to take your drugs. Ask your family to help you with reminder phone calls and messages.

Questions to Ask Your Doctor If You Have High Blood Pressure

- What is my blood pressure reading in numbers?
- What is my goal blood pressure?
- Is my blood pressure under adequate control?
- Is my systolic pressure too high (over 140)?
- What would be a healthy weight for me?
- Is there a diet to help me lose weight (if I need to) and lower my blood pressure?
- Is there a recommended healthy eating plan I should follow to help lower my blood pressure (if I don't need to lose weight)?
- Is it safe for me to start doing regular physical activity?
- What is the name of my blood pressure medication? Is that the brand name or the generic name?
- What are the possible side effects of my medication? (Be sure the doctor knows about any allergies you have and any other

medications you are taking, including over-the-counter drugs, vitamins, and dietary supplements.)

- What time of day should I take my blood pressure medicine?

- Should I take it with food?

- Are there any foods, beverages, or dietary supplements I should avoid when taking this medicine?

- What should I do if I forget to take my blood pressure medicine at the recommended time? Should I take it as soon as I remember or should I wait until the next dosage is due?

Chapter 20

Heart Health for People with Diabetes

Diabetes Overview

What is diabetes?

Diabetes is a disorder of metabolism—the way our bodies use digested food for growth and energy. Most of the food we eat is broken down into glucose, the form of sugar in the blood. Glucose is the main source of fuel for the body.

After digestion, glucose passes into the bloodstream, where it is used by cells for growth and energy. For glucose to get into cells, insulin must be present. Insulin is a hormone produced by the pancreas, a large gland behind the stomach.

When we eat, the pancreas is supposed to automatically produce the right amount of insulin to move glucose from blood into our cells. In people with diabetes, however, the pancreas either produces little or no insulin, or the cells do not respond appropriately to the insulin that is produced. Glucose builds up in the blood, overflows into the urine, and passes out of the body. Thus, the body loses its main source of fuel even though the blood contains large amounts of glucose.

Excerpted from "Diabetes Overview," National Diabetes Information Clearinghouse, a service of the National Institute of Diabetes and Digestive and Kidney Diseases, National Institutes of Health, NIH Publication No. 04-3873, April 2004, and "Prevent Diabetes Problems: Keep Your Heart and Blood Vessels Healthy," National Diabetes Information Clearinghouse, NIH Publication No. 03-4283, September 2003.

What are the types of diabetes?

The three main types of diabetes are

- type 1 diabetes
- type 2 diabetes
- gestational diabetes

Type 1 Diabetes: Type 1 diabetes is an autoimmune disease. An autoimmune disease results when the body's system for fighting infection (the immune system) turns against a part of the body. In diabetes, the immune system attacks the insulin-producing beta cells in the pancreas and destroys them. The pancreas then produces little or no insulin. Someone with type 1 diabetes needs to take insulin daily to live.

At present, scientists do not know exactly what causes the body's immune system to attack the beta cells, but they believe that autoimmune, genetic, and environmental factors, possibly viruses, are involved. Type 1 diabetes accounts for about 5 to 10 percent of diagnosed diabetes in the United States.

Type 1 diabetes develops most often in children and young adults, but the disorder can appear at any age. Symptoms of type 1 diabetes usually develop over a short period, although beta cell destruction can begin years earlier.

Symptoms include increased thirst and urination, constant hunger, weight loss, blurred vision, and extreme fatigue. If not diagnosed and treated with insulin, a person can lapse into a life-threatening diabetic coma, also known as diabetic ketoacidosis.

Type 2 Diabetes: The most common form of diabetes is type 2 diabetes. About 90 to 95 percent of people with diabetes have type 2. This form of diabetes is associated with older age, obesity, family history of diabetes, previous history of gestational diabetes, physical inactivity, and ethnicity. About 80 percent of people with type 2 diabetes are overweight. Type 2 diabetes is increasingly being diagnosed in children and adolescents. However, nationally representative data on prevalence of type 2 diabetes in youth are not available.

When type 2 diabetes is diagnosed, the pancreas is usually producing enough insulin, but, for unknown reasons, the body cannot use the insulin effectively, a condition called insulin resistance. After several years, insulin production decreases. The result is the same as for type 1 diabetes—glucose builds up in the blood and the body cannot make efficient use of its main source of fuel.

The symptoms of type 2 diabetes develop gradually. They are not as sudden in onset as in type 1 diabetes. Some people have no symptoms. Symptoms may include fatigue or nausea, frequent urination, unusual thirst, weight loss, blurred vision, frequent infections, and slow healing of wounds or sores.

Gestational Diabetes: Gestational diabetes develops only during pregnancy. Like type 2 diabetes, it occurs more often in African Americans, American Indians, Hispanic Americans, and among women with a family history of diabetes. Women who have had gestational diabetes have a 20 to 50 percent chance of developing type 2 diabetes within 5 to 10 years.

Prevent Diabetes Problems: Keep Your Heart and Blood Vessels Healthy

What are diabetes problems?

Too much glucose (sugar) in the blood for a long time can cause diabetes problems. This high blood glucose (also called blood sugar) can damage many parts of the body, such as the heart, blood vessels, eyes, and kidneys. Heart and blood vessel disease can lead to heart attacks and strokes, the leading causes of death for people with diabetes. You can do a lot to prevent or slow down diabetes problems.

This part of the chapter is about heart and blood vessel problems caused by diabetes. You will learn the things you can do each day and during each year to stay healthy and prevent diabetes problems.

What should I do each day to stay healthy with diabetes?

1. Follow the healthy eating plan that you and your doctor or dietitian have worked out.

2. Be active a total of thirty minutes most days. Ask your doctor what activities are best for you.

3. Take your diabetes medicines at the same times each day.

4. Check your blood glucose every day. Each time you check your blood glucose, write the number in your record book.

5. Check your feet every day for cuts, blisters, sores, swelling, redness, or sore toenails.

6. Brush and floss your teeth and gums every day.

7. Don't smoke.

What do my heart and blood vessels do?

Your heart and blood vessels make up your circulatory system. Your heart is a big muscle that pumps blood through your body. Your heart pumps blood carrying oxygen to large blood vessels, called arteries, and small blood vessels, called capillaries. Other blood vessels, called veins, carry blood back to the heart.

What can I do to prevent heart disease and stroke?

You can do a lot to prevent heart disease and stroke.

- **Keep your blood glucose under control.** You can see if it is under control by having an A1C test at least twice a year. The A1C test tells you your average blood glucose for the past two to three months. The target for most people is below 7.

- **Keep your blood pressure under control.** Have it checked at every doctor visit. The target for most people is below 130/80.

- **Keep your cholesterol under control.** Have it checked at least once a year. The targets for most people are
  - LDL (bad) cholesterol: below 100
  - HDL (good) cholesterol: above 40 in men and above 50 in women
  - Triglycerides (another type of fat in the blood): below 150

- **Make physical activity a part of your daily routine.** Aim for at least thirty minutes of exercise most days of the week. Check with your doctor to learn what activities are best for you. Take a half-hour walk every day, or walk for ten minutes after each meal. Use the stairs instead of the elevator. Park at the far end of the lot.

- **Make sure that the foods you eat are "heart-healthy."** Include foods high in fiber, such as oat bran, oatmeal, whole-grain breads and cereals, fruits, and vegetables. Cut back on foods high in saturated fat or cholesterol, such as meats, butter, dairy products with fat, eggs, shortening, lard, and foods with palm oil or coconut oil.

- **Lose weight if you need to.** If you are overweight, try to exercise most days of the week. See a registered dietitian for help in planning meals and lowering the fat and calorie content of your diet to reach and maintain a healthy weight.

- **If you smoke, quit.** Your doctor can tell you about ways to help you quit smoking.

- **Ask your doctor whether you should take an aspirin every day.** Studies have shown that taking a low dose of aspirin every day can help reduce your risk of heart disease and stroke.

- **Take your medicines as directed.**

How do my blood vessels get clogged?

Several things, including having diabetes, can make your blood cholesterol level too high. Cholesterol is a substance that is made by the body and used for many important functions. It is also found in some food derived from animals. When cholesterol is too high, the insides of large blood vessels become narrowed, even clogged. This problem is called atherosclerosis.

Narrowed and clogged blood vessels make it harder for enough blood to get to all parts of your body. This can cause problems.

What can happen when blood vessels are clogged?

When arteries become narrowed and clogged, you may have heart problems:

- **Chest pain,** also called angina. When you have angina, you feel pain in your chest, arms, shoulders, or back. You may feel the pain more when your heart beats faster, such as when you exercise. The pain may go away when you rest. You also may feel very weak and sweaty. If you do not get treatment, chest pain may happen more often. If diabetes has damaged the heart nerves, you may not feel the chest pain.

- **Heart attack.** A heart attack happens when a blood vessel in or near the heart becomes blocked. Not enough blood can get to that part of the heart muscle. That area of the heart muscle stops working, so the heart is weaker. During a heart attack, you may have chest pain along with nausea, indigestion, extreme weakness, and sweating.

What are the warning signs of a heart attack?

You may have one or more of the following warning signs:

143

- chest pain or discomfort
- pain or discomfort in your arms, back, jaw, or neck
- indigestion or stomach pain
- shortness of breath
- sweating
- nausea or vomiting
- light-headedness

Or, you may have no warning signs at all. Or they may come and go.

How does heart disease cause high blood pressure?

Narrowed blood vessels leave a smaller opening for blood to flow through. It is like turning on a garden hose and holding your thumb over the opening. The smaller opening makes the water shoot out with more pressure. In the same way, narrowed blood vessels lead to high blood pressure. Other factors, such as kidney problems and being overweight, also can lead to high blood pressure.

Many people with diabetes also have high blood pressure. If you have heart, eye, or kidney problems from diabetes, high blood pressure can make them worse.

You will see your blood pressure written with two numbers separated by a slash. For example: 120/70. Keep your first number below 130 and your second number below 80.

If you have high blood pressure, ask your doctor how to lower it. Your doctor may ask you to take blood pressure medicine every day. Some types of blood pressure medicine can also help keep your kidneys healthy.

To lower your blood pressure, your doctor may also ask you to lose weight; eat more fruits and vegetables; eat less salt and high-sodium foods such as canned soups, luncheon meats, salty snack foods, and fast foods; and drink less alcohol.

What are the warning signs of a stroke?

A stroke happens when part of your brain is not getting enough blood and stops working. Depending on the part of the brain that is damaged, a stroke can cause:

- sudden weakness or numbness of your face, arm, or leg on one side of your body

- sudden confusion, trouble talking, or trouble understanding
- sudden dizziness, loss of balance, or trouble walking
- sudden trouble seeing in one or both eyes or sudden double vision
- sudden severe headache

Sometimes, one or more of these warning signs may happen and then disappear. You might be having a "mini-stroke," also called a TIA (transient ischemic attack). If you have any of these warning signs, tell your doctor right away.

How can clogged blood vessels hurt my legs and feet?

Peripheral vascular disease can happen when the openings in your blood vessels become narrow and not enough blood gets to your legs and feet. You may feel pain in your buttocks, the back of your legs, or your thighs when you stand, walk, or exercise.

What can I do to prevent or control peripheral vascular disease?

- Don't smoke.
- Keep blood pressure under control.
- Keep blood fats close to normal.
- Exercise.

You also may need surgery to treat this problem.

Chapter 21

Physical Activity Fundamental in Preventing Obesity and Cardiovascular Disease

Regular physical activity, fitness, and exercise are critically important for the health and well-being of people of all ages. Research has demonstrated that virtually all individuals can benefit from regular physical activity, whether they participate in vigorous exercise or some type of moderate health-enhancing physical activity. Even among frail and very old adults, mobility and functioning can be improved through physical activity.[1] Therefore, physical fitness should be a priority for Americans of all ages.

Regular physical activity has been shown to reduce the morbidity and mortality from many chronic diseases. Millions of Americans suffer from chronic illnesses that can be prevented or improved through regular physical activity:

- 12.6 million people have coronary heart disease[2];

- 1.1 million people suffer from a heart attack in a given year[2];

- 17 million people have diabetes; about 90% to 95% of cases are type 2 diabetes, which is associated with obesity and physical inactivity[3]; approximately 16 million people have "pre-diabetes";

- 107,000 people are newly diagnosed with colon cancer each year[4,5];

- 300,000 people suffer from hip fractures each year[6];

Excerpted from "Physical Activity Fundamental to Preventing Disease," Office of the Assistant Secretary for Planning and Evaluation, U.S. Department of Health and Human Services, June 2002.

- 50 million people have high blood pressure[2]; and

- Nearly 50 million adults (between the ages of 20 and 74), or 27 percent of the adult population, are obese; overall more than 108 million adults, or 61 percent of the adult population are either obese or overweight.[7,8]

In a 1993 study, 14 percent of all deaths in the United States were attributed to activity patterns and diet.[9] Another study linked sedentary lifestyles to 23 percent of deaths from major chronic diseases.[10] For example, physical activity has been shown to reduce the risk of developing or dying from heart disease, diabetes, colon cancer, and high blood pressure. On average, people who are physically active outlive those who are inactive.[11–16]

Despite the well-known benefits of physical activity, most adults and many children lead a relatively sedentary lifestyle and are not active enough to achieve these health benefits. A sedentary lifestyle is defined as engaging in no leisure-time physical activity (exercises, sports, physically active hobbies) in a two-week period. Data from the National Health Interview Survey shows that in 1997–98 nearly four in ten (38.3 percent) adults reported no participation in leisure-time physical activity.[17]

Approximately one-third of persons age sixty-five or older lead a sedentary lifestyle. Older women are generally less physically active than older men. Fifty-four percent of men and 66 percent of women age seventy-five and older engage in no leisure-time physical activity.[17]

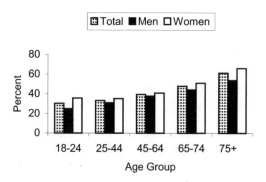

Figure 21.1. Physically Inactive Adults, by Age Group. Source: 1997–98 National Health Interview Survey.

In general, African American older adults are less active than white older adults. In the mid-1990s, 37 percent of white men age seventy-five and older reported no leisure-time physical activity, compared to 59 percent of African American men age seventy-five and older; 47 percent of white women age seventy-five and older reported no leisure-time physical activity, compared to 60 percent of African American women age seventy-five and older.[18]

More than one-third of young people in grades nine through twelve do not regularly engage in vigorous physical activity. Furthermore, 43 percent of students in grades nine through twelve watch television more than two hours per day.[19] Physical activity declines dramatically over the course of adolescence, and girls are significantly less likely than boys to participate regularly in vigorous physical activity.

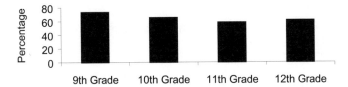

Figure 21.2. *Vigorous Physical Activity of Adolescents by Grade Level, 1999. Vigorous physical activity is defined as exercise that made the respondent sweat and breathe hard for at least twenty minutes on three or more of the seven days preceding the survey. Source: Youth Risk Behavior Surveillance System (YRBSS), CDC, NCCDPHP.*

Physical Activity and Good Physical Health

Participation in regular physical activity—at least thirty minutes of moderate activity on at least five days per week, or twenty minutes of vigorous physical activity at least three times per week—is critical to sustaining good health. Youth should strive for at least one hour of exercise a day. Regular physical activity has beneficial effects on most (if not all) organ systems, and consequently it helps to prevent a broad range of health problems and diseases. People of all ages, both male and female, derive substantial health benefits from physical activity.

Regular physical activity reduces the risk of developing or dying from some of the leading causes of illness in the United States. Regular physical activity improves health in the following ways[22]:

- Reduces the risk of dying prematurely from heart disease and other conditions;

- Reduces the risk of developing diabetes;

- Reduces the risk of developing high blood pressure;

- Reduces blood pressure in people who already have high blood pressure;

- Reduces the risk of developing colon and breast cancer[5];

- Helps to maintain a healthy weight;

- Helps build and maintain healthy bones, muscles, and joints;

- Helps older adults to become stronger and better able to move about without falling;

- Reduces feelings of depression and anxiety; and

- Promotes psychological well-being.

Regular physical activity is associated with lower mortality rates for both older and younger adults.[22] Even those who are moderately active on a regular basis have lower mortality rates than those who are least active. Regular physical activity leads to cardiovascular fitness, which decreases the risk of cardiovascular disease mortality in general and coronary artery disease mortality in particular. High blood pressure is a major underlying cause of cardiovascular complications and mortality. Regular physical activity can prevent or delay the development of high blood pressure, and reduces blood pressure in persons with hypertension.

Regular physical activity is also important for maintaining muscle strength, joint structure, joint functioning, and bone health.[22] Weight-bearing physical activity is essential for normal skeletal development during childhood and adolescence and for achieving and maintaining peak bone mass in young adults. Among postmenopausal women, exercise, especially muscle strengthening (resistance) activity, may protect against the rapid decline in bone mass. However, data on the effects of exercise on postmenopausal bone loss are not clear-cut and the timing of the intervention (e.g., stage of menopausal transition) can influence the response. Regardless, physical activity including muscle-strengthening exercise appears to protect against falling and fractures among the elderly, probably by increasing muscle strength and balance.[22] In addition, physical activity may be beneficial for many people with arthritis.

Regular physical activity can help improve the lives of young people beyond its effects on physical health. Although research has not been conducted to conclusively demonstrate a direct link between physical activity and improved academic performance, such a link might be expected. Studies have found participation in physical activity increases adolescents' self-esteem and reduces anxiety and stress.[22] Through its effects on mental health, physical activity may help increase students' capacity for learning. One study found that spending more time in physical education did not have harmful effects on the standardized academic achievement test scores of elementary school students; in fact, there was some evidence that participation in a two-year health-related physical education program had several significant favorable effects on academic achievement.[24]

Participation in physical activity and sports can promote social well-being, as well as good physical and mental health, among young people. Research has shown that students who participate in interscholastic sports are less likely to be regular and heavy smokers or use drugs,[25] and are more likely to stay in school and have good conduct and high academic achievement.[26] Sports and physical activity programs can introduce young people to skills such as teamwork, self-discipline, sportsmanship, leadership, and socialization. Lack of recreational activity, on the other hand, may contribute to making young people more vulnerable to gangs, drugs, or violence.

Physical Activity (Along with a Nutritious Diet) Is Key to Maintaining Energy Balance and a Healthy Weight

Regular physical activity along with a nutritious diet is key to maintaining a healthy weight. In order to maintain a healthy weight, there must be a balance between calories consumed and calories expended through metabolic and physical activity. Although overweight and obesity are caused by many factors, in most individuals, weight gain results from a combination of excess calorie consumption and inadequate physical activity.

Even though a large portion of a person's total caloric requirement is used for basal metabolism and processing food, an individual's various physical activities may account for as much as 15 to 40 percent of the calories he or she burns each day. While vigorous exercise uses calories at a higher rate, any physical activity will burn calories. For example, a 140-pound person can burn 175 calories in thirty minutes of moderate bicycling, and 322 calories in thirty minutes of moderate jogging. The same person can also burn 105 calories by vacuuming or raking leaves for the same amount of time.

The Epidemic of Overweight and Obesity

As a result of lifestyle and dietary changes, overweight and obesity have reached epidemic proportions in the United States. The Body

$$BMI = \left\{ \frac{WEIGHT\ (pounds)}{HEIGHT\ (inches)^2} \right\} \times 703$$

Weight in Pounds

Height	120	130	140	150	160	170	180	190	200	210	220	230	240	250
4'6	29	31	34	36	39	41	43	46	48	51	53	56	58	60
4'8	27	29	31	34	36	38	40	43	45	47	49	52	54	56
4'10	25	27	29	31	34	36	38	40	42	44	46	48	50	52
5'0	23	25	27	29	31	33	35	37	39	41	43	45	47	49
5'2	22	24	26	27	29	31	33	35	37	38	40	42	44	46
5'4	21	22	24	26	28	29	31	33	34	36	38	40	41	43
5'6	19	21	23	24	26	27	29	31	32	34	36	37	39	40
5'8	18	20	21	23	24	26	27	29	30	32	34	35	37	38
5'10	17	19	20	22	23	24	26	27	29	30	32	33	35	36
6'0	16	18	19	20	22	23	24	26	27	28	30	31	33	34
6'2	15	17	18	19	21	22	23	24	26	27	28	30	31	32
6'4	15	16	17	18	20	21	22	23	24	26	27	28	29	30
6'6	14	15	16	17	19	20	21	22	23	24	25	27	28	29
6'8	13	14	15	17	18	19	20	21	22	23	24	25	26	28

Height in Feet and Inches

■ Healthy Weight   ■ Overweight   ■ Obese

Figure 21.3. BMI Weight Chart. Source: Surgeon General's Call to Action to Prevent and Decrease Overweight and Obesity, 2001.

Mass Index (BMI) is the most commonly used measure to define overweight and obesity. BMI is a measure of weight in relation to height. BMI is calculated as weight in pounds divided by the square of the height in inches, multiplied by 703.

According to the National Institutes of Health Clinical Guidelines, overweight in adults is defined as a BMI between 25 lbs/in^2 and 29.9 lbs/in^2; and obesity in adults is identified by a BMI of 30 lbs/in^2 or greater.[28] These definitions are based on evidence that suggests that health risks are greater at or above a BMI of 25 lbs/in^2 compared to those at a BMI below that level. The risk of premature death increases with an increasing BMI. This increase in mortality tends to be modest until a BMI of 30 lbs/in^2 is reached.

Overweight and obesity are increasing in both genders and among all population groups. In 1999, an estimated 61 percent of adults in the United States were overweight or obese; this contrasts with the late 1970s, when an estimated 47 percent of adults were overweight or obese.[7] Figure 21.4 demonstrates the increasing prevalence of obesity among adults throughout the United States.

Among women, the prevalence of overweight and obesity generally is higher in women who are members of racial and ethnic minority populations than in non-Hispanic white women.[7] Among men, Mexican Americans have a higher prevalence of overweight and obesity than non-Hispanic whites or non-Hispanic blacks. For non-Hispanic men, the prevalence of overweight and obesity among whites is slightly greater than among blacks (see Figure 21.5).

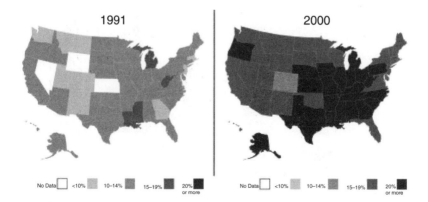

Figure 21.4. Obesity among U.S. Adults

Disparities in prevalence of overweight and obesity also exist based on socioeconomic status.[7] For all racial and ethnic groups combined, women of lower socioeconomic status (income less than 130 percent of the poverty threshold) are approximately 50 percent more likely to be obese than those with higher socioeconomic status (income greater than 130 percent of the poverty threshold). Men are about

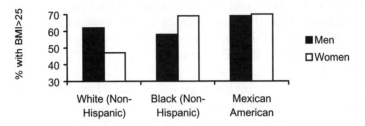

Figure 21.5. *Age-Adjusted Prevalence of Overweight or Obesity in Selected Groups, 1988–94 (Source: Surgeon General's Call to Action to Prevent and Decrease Overweight and Obesity, 2001).*

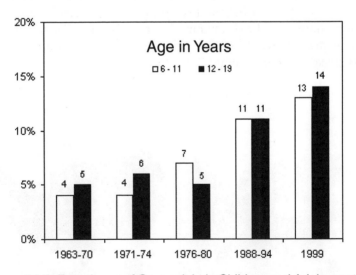

Figure 21.6. *Prevalence of Overweight in Children and Adolescents Ages 6–19 (Source: CDC/NCHS, NHES, and NHANES. Excludes pregnant women starting with 1971–74. Pregnancy status not available for 1963–70. Data for 1963–65 are for children 6–11 years of age; data for 166–70 are for adolescents 12–17 years of age, not 12–19 years.)*

equally likely to be obese whether they are in a low or a high socio-economic group.

The overweight and obesity epidemic is not limited to adults. What is particularly alarming is that the percentage of young people who are overweight has almost doubled in the last twenty years for children aged six to eleven, and almost tripled for adolescents aged twelve to nineteen. In children and adolescents, overweight has been defined as a sex- and age-specific BMI at or above the ninety-fifth percentile for a reference population, based on Centers for Disease Control and Prevention (CDC) growth charts (see Figure 21.6).

Associated Health Risks of Not Maintaining a Healthy Weight

Epidemiological studies show an increase in mortality associated with overweight and obesity. Approximately three hundred thousand deaths a year in this country are currently associated with overweight and obesity.[29] Morbidity from obesity may be as great as from poverty, smoking, or problem drinking.[20] Overweight and obesity are associated with an increased risk for developing various medical conditions including cardiovascular disease, certain cancers (endometrial, colon, postmenopausal breast, kidney, and esophageal),[5] high blood pressure, arthritis-related disabilities and type 2 diabetes.[7]

According to the Surgeon General's Call to Action to Prevent and Decrease Overweight and Obesity (2001), the health risks associated with obesity are:

- premature death
- type 2 diabetes
- heart disease
- stroke
- hypertension
- gallbladder disease
- osteoarthritis (degeneration of cartilage and bone in joints)
- sleep apnea
- asthma
- breathing problems
- cancer (endometrial, colon, kidney, esophageal, and postmenopausal breast cancer)

- high blood cholesterol
- complications of pregnancy
- menstrual irregularities
- hirsutism (presence of excess body and facial hair)
- stress incontinence (urine leakage caused by weak pelvic-floor muscles)
- increased surgical risk
- psychological disorders such as depression
- psychological difficulties due to social stigmatization

It is also important for individuals who are currently at a healthy weight to strive to maintain it since both modest and large weight gains are associated with significantly increased risk of disease. For example, a weight gain of eleven to eighteen pounds increases a person's risk for developing type 2 diabetes to twice that of individuals who have not gained weight, while those who gain forty-four pounds or more have four times the risk of type 2 diabetes.[30]

Recent research studies have shown that a gain of ten to twenty pounds resulted in an increased risk of coronary heart disease (which can result in nonfatal heart attacks and death) of 1.25 times in women[31] and 1.6 times in men.[32] In these studies, weight increases of twenty-two pounds in men and forty-four pounds in women resulted in a increased coronary heart disease risk of 1.75 and 2.65, respectively. In one study among women with a BMI of 34 or greater, the risk of developing endometrial cancer was increased by more than six times.[33] Overweight and obesity are also known to exacerbate many chronic conditions such as hypertension and elevated cholesterol. Overweight and obese individuals also may suffer from social stigmatization, discrimination, and poor body image.

Although obesity-associated morbidities occur most frequently in adults, important consequences of excess weight as well as antecedents of adult disease occur in overweight children and adolescents. Overweight children and adolescents are more likely to become overweight or obese adults. As the prevalence of overweight and obesity increases in children and adolescents, type 2 diabetes, high blood lipids, and hypertension as well as early maturation and orthopedic problems are occurring with increased frequency. A common consequence of childhood overweight is psychosocial—specifically discrimination.[34]

Call to Action

Because physical inactivity is a risk factor for many diseases and conditions, making physical activity an integral part of daily life is crucial. Physical activity need not be strenuous to be beneficial. People of all ages benefit from moderate physical activity, such as thirty minutes of walking five or more times a week. In addition, physical activity does not need to be sustained for long periods of time in order to provide health benefits. Repeated shorter bursts of moderate-intensity activity also yield health benefits. In other words, walking in two fifteen-minute segments or three ten-minute segments is beneficial.

There is a pressing need to encourage a more active lifestyle among the American people. Clearly, the goal of a more active population will be a challenge, requiring a commitment to change on the part of individuals, families, workplaces, and communities. Both the public and private sectors will need to band together to promote more healthy habits for those of all ages.[7] Encouraging more activity can be as simple as establishing walking programs at schools, at worksites, and in the community. Some communities have an existing infrastructure that supports physical activity, such as sidewalks and bicycle trails, and worksites, schools, and shopping areas in close proximity to residential areas. In many other areas, such community amenities need to be developed to foster walking, cycling, and other types of exercise as a regular part of daily activity. Schools provide many opportunities to engage children in physical activity as well as healthy eating. For adults, worksites provide opportunities to reinforce the adoption and maintenance of healthy lifestyle behaviors. Perhaps the most important change, however, is at the individual and family level. Each person must understand the value of physical activity for his or her health and well-being and commit to a lifestyle that is truly active.

References

1. Butler RN, Davis R, Lewis CB, et al. Physical fitness: benefits of exercising for the older patient. *Geriatrics* 53(10):46–62. 1998.

2. American Heart Association. *2002 heart and stroke statistical update*. Dallas, TX: American Heart Association, 2001.

3. Centers for Disease Control and Prevention. *National diabetes fact sheet: general information and national estimates on diabetes in the United States, 2000*. Atlanta, GA: U.S. Department

of Health and Human Services, Centers for Disease Control and Prevention, 2002.

4. American Cancer Society. *Cancer facts & figures 2002*. Atlanta, GA: American Cancer Society, Inc., 2002.

5. Vainio H, Bianchini F, eds. Weight control and physical activity. *IARC Handbooks of Cancer Prevention*. IARC Press Vol. 6, 2002.

6. Popovic JR. 1999 National Hospital Discharge Survey: Annual summary with detailed diagnosis and procedure data. National Center for Health Statistics. *Vital Health Statistics* 13(151). 2001.

7. U.S. Department of Health and Human Services. *The Surgeon General's call to action to prevent and decrease overweight and obesity*. Rockville, MD: U.S. Department of Health and Human Services, Public Health Service, Office of the Surgeon General; 2001. (Available from U.S. GPO, Washington.)

8. U.S. Census Bureau. Resident population estimates of the United States by age and sex, July 1, 1999. Accessed on June 17, 2002, on the Internet at: http://eire.census.gov/popest/archives/national/nation2/intfile2-1.txt

9. McGinnis JM, Foege WH. Actual causes of death in the United States. *JAMA* 270(18):207–12.1993.

10. Hahn RA, Teuesch SM, Rothenberg RB, et. al. Excess deaths from nine chronic diseases in the United States, 1986. *JAMA* 264(20):2554–59. 1998.

11. Paffenbarger RS, Hyde RT, Wing AL, et al. The association of changes in physical-activity level and other lifestyle characteristics with mortality among men. *N Engl J Med* 328(8): 538–45. 1993.

12. Sherman SE, D'Agostino RB, Cobb JL, et al. Physical activity and mortality in women in the Framingham Heart Study. *Am Heart J* 128(5):879–84. 1994.

13. Kaplan GA, Strawbridge WJ, Cohen RD, et al. Natural history of leisure-time physical activity and its correlates: Associations with mortality from all causes and cardiovascular diseases over 28 years. *Am J Epid* 144(8):793–97. 1996.

14. Kushi LH, Fee RM, Folsom AR, et al. Physical activity and mortality in postmenopausal women. *JAMA* 277:1287–92. 1997.

15. Lee CD, Blair SN, Jackson AS. Cardiorespiratory fitness, body composition, and all-cause and cardiovascular disease mortality in men. *Am J Clin Nutr* 69 (3):373–80. 1999.

16. Wei M, Kampert JB, Barlow CE, et al. Relationship between low cardiorespiratory fitness and mortality in normal-weight, overweight, and obese men. *JAMA* 282(16):1547–53. 1999.

17. U. S. Department of Health and Human Services. Leisuretime physical activity among adults: United States, 1997–98. U.S. Department of Health and Human Services, Centers for Disease Control and Prevention, National Center for Health Statistics, 2002.

18. Centers for Disease Control and Prevention. CDC Surveillance Summaries, December 17, 1999. *MMWR* 48(No. SS-8). 1999.

19. Kann L, et al. Youth risk behavior surveillance–United States, 1999. In: CDC Surveillance Summaries, June 9, 2000. *MMWR* 49(No. SS-5):1-96. 2000.

20. Strum R. The effects of obesity, smoking and problem drinking on chronic medical problems and health care costs. *Health Affairs* 21(2):245–53. 2002.

21. Pratt M, Macera CA, Wang G. Higher direct medical costs associated with physical inactivity. *The Physician and Sportsmedicine* 28:63–70. 2000.

22. U.S. Department of Health and Human Services. *Physical activity and health: a report of the Surgeon General*. Atlanta, GA: U.S. Department of Health and Human Services, Centers for Disease Control and Prevention, National Center for Chronic Disease Prevention and Health Promotion, 1996.

23. Freudenheim M.. Employers focus on weight as workplace health issue. *New York Times*. September 6, 1999.

24. Sallis JF, McKenzie TL, Kolody B, Lewis M, Marshall S, Rosengard P. Effects of health-related physical education on academic achievement: project SPARK. *Research Quarterly for Exercise and Sport* 70(2):127–34. 1999.

25. Escobedo LG, Marcus SE, Holtzman D, Giovino GA. Sports participation, age at smoking initiation and the risk of smoking among U.S. high school students. *Journal of the American Medical Association* 269:1391–95. 1993.

26. Zill N, Nord CW, Loomis LS. *Adolescent time use, risky behavior and outcomes: an analysis of national data*. Rockville, MD: Westat, 1995.

27. U.S. Preventive Services Task Force. *Guide to Clinical Preventive Services*, 2nd ed. Baltimore: Williams and Wilkins, 611–24. 1996.

28. U.S. Department of Health and Human Services, National Institutes of Health, National Heart, Lung, and Blood Institute. Clinical guidelines on the identification, evaluation, and treatment of overweight and obesity in adults; evidence report. HHS, PHS; Pub No. 98-4083. 1998.

29. Allison DB, Fontaine KR, Manson JE, Stevens J, VanItallie TB. Annual deaths attributable to obesity in the United States. *JAMA* Oct 27;282(16):1530–38. 1999.

30. Ford ES, Williamson DF, Liu S. Weight change and diabetes incidence: Findings from a national cohort of U.S. adults. *Am J Epidemiol* 146(3):214–22. August 1, 1997.

31. Willett WC, Manson JE, Stampfer MJ, et al. Weight, weight change and coronary heart disease in women. Risk within the 'normal' weight range. *JAMA* 273(6):461–65. February 8, 1995.

32. Galanis DJ, Harris T, Sharp DS, et al. Relative weight, weight change, and risk of coronary heart disease in the Honolulu Heart Program. *Am J Epidimiol* 147(4):379–86. February 15, 1998.

33. Weiderpass E, Persson I, Adami HO, et al. Body size in different periods of life, diabetes, hypertension, and risk of postmenopausal endometrial cancer. *Cancer Causes Control* 11(2):185–92. February 2000.

34. Dietz WH. Health consequences of obesity in youth: Childhood predictors of adult disease. *Pediatrics* 101(3)Supp:518–25. March 1998.

Chapter 22

Young Adult Fitness Protects Heart Health in Middle Age

Cardiorespiratory fitness in early adulthood significantly decreases the chance of developing high blood pressure and diabetes—both major risk factors for heart disease and stroke—in middle age, according to a new study supported by the National Heart, Lung, and Blood Institute (NHLBI), part of the National Institutes of Health. Fitness also reduces the risk for the metabolic syndrome, a constellation of factors that includes excess abdominal fat, elevated blood pressure and triglycerides, and low levels of the high-density lipoprotein, the "good" cholesterol.

Further, improving fitness in healthy young adults can cut by as much as 50 percent the risk for diabetes and the metabolic syndrome.

The research is the first large observational study to look at the role of fitness on healthy young adults' development of risk factors for heart disease. Prior studies had examined the relationship between fitness and death from heart disease and stroke.

Its findings appear in the December 17, 2003, issue of *The Journal of the American Medical Association*. The study was done by researchers at Northwestern University in Chicago; Nemours Cardiac Center in Wilmington, Delaware; the Kaiser Permanente Division of Research in Oakland, California; the University of Minnesota School of Public Health in Minneapolis, Minnesota; and the University of Alabama at Birmingham.

Reprinted from "Young Adult Fitness Protects Heart Health in Middle Age," National Heart, Lung, and Blood Institute (NHLBI), National Institutes of Health, press release dated December 16, 2003.

"This study underscores the importance of both fitness and maintaining a healthy weight in the fight against heart disease and stroke and their risk factors," said NHLBI acting director Dr. Barbara Alving. "Americans need to become physically active early in life and continue to be active as they age in order to remain as healthy as possible."

"Given the epidemic of obesity in the United States and the decline in people's physical activity, it's important that Americans take steps to improve their physical fitness," cautioned Dr. Mercedes Carnethon, of the Department of Preventive Medicine at Northwestern University in Chicago. "If all the young adults in our study had been fit, there would have been nearly a third fewer cases of high blood pressure, diabetes, and metabolic syndrome."

Heart disease and stroke are the first and third leading causes of death for Americans. Nearly thirteen million Americans have heart disease and nearly five million have had a stroke.

Data came from the Coronary Artery Risk Development in Young Adults (CARDIA) study, which began in January 1984 and ended in December 2001. The fitness study involved 4,487 black and white men and women, who were ages eighteen to thirty at the time of their enrollment. They participated through four clinical centers—in Birmingham, Alabama; Chicago, Illinois; Minneapolis, Minnesota; and Oakland, California. Birmingham also served as the study's Coordinating Center.

All participants were followed for fifteen years, but 2,478 of them had their cardiopulmonary fitness tested again after seven years in order to measure changes in fitness.

Cardiopulmonary fitness was measured with an exercise treadmill test, which included up to nine, two-minute stages of progressive difficulty. Women were classified as "low" in fitness if they completed less than six minutes of exercise and men if they completed less than ten minutes. Women who completed six to nine minutes of exercise were classified as "moderately" fit and men if they completed ten to twelve minutes. Those who completed more exercise were classified as "highly" fit.

Other findings include:

- Results were the same for black and white adults, as well as men and women.

- Those who were low in fitness or moderately fit had twice the risk of high blood pressure, diabetes, and metabolic syndrome as those who were highly fit. Moreover, the risk increased directly as fitness level dropped.

- Weight gain was inversely related to fitness over the course of the study.

- Of those who retook the treadmill test after seven years, the average weight gain was about fifteen pounds. The average weight gain after fifteen years was about twenty-eight pounds.

- Those who were obese tended to be less fit: Of those who were obese, 68 percent were low in fitness, 29 percent were moderately fit, and 4 percent were highly fit. Of those who were not obese, 13 percent were low in fitness, 36 percent were moderately fit, and 51 percent were highly fit.

- Fitness did not protect those who were highly fit and obese at the start of the study from developing diabetes or the metabolic syndrome later in life.

"The key point from this study is that the development of risk factors for heart disease and stroke isn't just the natural result of aging," said Carnethon. "All Americans—including women and minorities—can protect themselves against those risks by maintaining their physical fitness.

"Americans don't have to run marathons to improve their physical fitness," said Cheryl Nelson, NHLBI project officer for the study. "They should try to engage in at least thirty minutes of a moderate-intensity physical activity such as brisk walking on most and, preferably, all days of the week. Being physically active will not only improve their fitness but also help them maintain a healthy weight, which in turn will protect their heart health."

Chapter 23

What You Should Know before Using Aspirin to Lower Cardiovascular Risks

Only a health professional can safely decide if the regular use of aspirin to prevent a heart attack or stroke is right for you.

Aspirin

It's often thought of as one of those harmless over-the-counter drugs that you've relied on for years to fight pain, swelling, headache, and fever. Now you're hearing that it can also lower your risk of a heart attack, some kinds of strokes, and other very specific heart and blood vessel diseases. Then why not use an aspirin a day? No need to bother your health professional with questions about something so simple, right? Wrong. Although aspirin may seem like a quick and easy solution to any fears you might have, it's not as simple as you think.

If you're using aspirin to lower your chance of a heart attack or clot-related stroke and you haven't talked with a health professional about it, read on. The information here could help you avoid risks and stay healthy.

Aspirin: What the Studies Show

It's been about one hundred years since aspirin was created, and in that time, it has played a major role in treating headaches, fevers,

Reprinted from "Before Using Aspirin to Lower Your Risk of Heart Attack or Stroke, Here is What You Should Know," U.S. Food and Drug Administration, Center for Drug Evaluation and Research, March 13, 2003.

and minor aches and pains for millions of people. Now there are studies that show it is also helpful in lowering the chance of a heart attack or clot-related stroke, and for increasing blood flow to the brain in people with evidence of poor circulation.

Most health professionals agree that long-term aspirin use to prevent a heart attack or stroke in healthy people is unnecessary. If you are using aspirin to lower the risk of a heart attack or stroke and you have not yet talked with a health professional about it, you may be putting your health at risk. You should use aspirin daily *only* under the guidance of a health professional.

Aspirin: Not Without Risks

Aspirin has been known to help people that are living with some kinds of heart and blood vessel diseases. It can help prevent a heart attack or clot-related stroke by lowering the clotting action of the blood's platelets. The same properties that make aspirin work in stopping blood from clotting may also cause unwanted side effects, such as stomach bleeding, bleeding in the brain, kidney failure, and other kinds of strokes. If your health professional agrees to your use of daily aspirin treatment, you'll need his or her medical knowledge and guidance to help you prevent unwanted side effects.

Aspirin is a drug that can mix badly with other medicines (prescription and over-the-counter), vitamins, and herbal or dietary supplements. People who are already using a prescribed medication to thin the blood should talk to a health professional before using aspirin, even occasionally. Additionally, there are a number of vitamins and dietary supplements that are known to thin blood. Discuss the use of all medicines, vitamins, and dietary supplements with your health professional before using aspirin daily.

Aspirin: Dose Matters

Whether you are using aspirin daily to lower the risk of a heart attack or clot-related stroke, or you're using it for any other purpose that is not listed on the aspirin's label, the dose you use does matter. It's important to your health that the dose you use and the frequency with which you use it are right for you. You can rely on your health professional to provide you with the dosing and directions that will give you the most benefit with the fewest side effects. Also, discuss with your health professional the different forms of aspirin products that might be best suited for you.

Remember, not all over-the-counter pain relievers are the same. Aspirin products have been found to lower the risk of heart attack and clot-related stroke for people who already have evidence of poor blood flow to the heart or brain. However, not all over-the-counter pain relievers contain aspirin. Read the label carefully. Some drug products combine aspirin with other pain relievers or with certain other ingredients and should not be used for long-term aspirin treatment. If you have questions, talk to your health professional.

Before you use aspirin to lower your risk of heart attack and stroke, talk to a health professional. It could save your life.

Chapter 24

Cardiac Rehabilitation

Cardiac rehabilitation (rehab) services are designed to help patients with heart disease recover faster and return to full and productive lives. Cardiac rehab includes exercise, education, counseling, and learning ways to live a healthier life. Together with medical and surgical treatments, cardiac rehab can help you feel better and live a healthier life.

You can benefit from cardiac rehab if you:

- Have heart disease, such as angina or heart failure, or have had a heart attack.

- Have had coronary bypass surgery or a balloon catheter (PTCA) procedure on your heart.

- Have had a heart transplant.

Cardiac rehab can make a difference. It is a safe and effective way to help you:

- Feel better faster.
- Get stronger.
- Reduce stress.

Excerpted from "Recovering from Heart Problems through Cardiac Rehabilitation: Patient Guide," Agency for Healthcare Research and Quality (formerly Agency for Health Care Policy and Research), Publication No. 96-0674, October 1995. Reviewed by David A. Cooke, M.D., August 2004.

- Reduce the risks of future heart problems.
- Live longer.

Almost everyone with heart disease can benefit from some type of cardiac rehab. No one is too old or too young. Women benefit from cardiac rehab as much as men.

This chapter can help you learn how to lower your risk for future heart problems. You will also learn tips for finding a cardiac rehab plan that is right for you. Most important, you will learn what you can do to be healthier.

When you have heart disease, breaking old habits and learning new ones can be stressful. Wondering about your future health can be stressful, too. Yet the support of family and friends, as well as health care providers, can make a big difference in how well you adjust to these changes.

The Cardiac Rehab Team

Cardiac rehab services can involve many health care providers. Your team may include:

- Doctors (your family doctor, a heart specialist, perhaps a surgeon);
- Nurses;
- Exercise specialists;
- Physical and occupational therapists;
- Dietitians;
- Psychologists or other behavior therapists.

Sometimes a primary care provider, such as your family doctor or nurse practitioner, works alone, playing many roles, or refers patients to other health care specialists as needed.

Yet the most important member of your cardiac rehab team is you. No one else can make you exercise. Or quit smoking. Or eat a more healthful diet.

To be an active member of the cardiac rehab team:

- Learn about your heart condition.
- Learn what you can do to help your heart.
- Follow the treatment plan.

- Feel free to ask questions.
- Report symptoms or problems.

A support network can help you. Your support network may be family, friends, or a group of other people with heart problems. Family members and friends can make a difference. They may want to learn more about heart problems so their help can be even more valuable. For example, family members may have to learn to let you do things for yourself. Or they may want to learn about preparing heart-healthy meals. Your family and friends can give you emotional support as you adjust to a new, healthier lifestyle. You may also want the support of other people who have heart disease. Ask your cardiac rehab team if they know of a support group you can join.

How Do I Get Started?

Cardiac rehab often begins in the hospital after a heart attack, heart surgery, or other heart treatment. It continues in an outpatient setting after you leave the hospital. Once you learn the habits of heart-healthy living, stick with them for life.

In an Outpatient Setting

Outpatient rehab may be located at the hospital, in a medical or professional center, in a community facility such as the YMCA, or at your place of work. You may even have cardiac rehab at home. You will be advised to increase the amount of exercise you do. You will also receive education and encouragement to control your risk factors.

For Life

After you have learned the skills of heart-healthy living, you should continue to use them for life. You need your doctor's approval to get started in cardiac rehab. Tell your doctor or nurse that you're interested in cardiac rehab and ask which rehab services or plans are best for you.

How Does Cardiac Rehab Work?

Cardiac rehab has two major parts:

- **Exercise training:** To help you learn how to exercise safely, strengthen your muscles, and improve your stamina. Your exercise plan will be based on your individual ability, needs, and interests.

- **Education, counseling, and training:** To help you understand your heart condition and find ways to reduce your risk of future heart problems. The cardiac rehab team will help you learn how to cope with the stress of adjusting to a new lifestyle and to deal with your fears about the future.

Cardiac rehab often takes place in groups. However, each patient's plan is based on his or her specific risk factors and special needs.

Cardiac rehab helps you recognize and change unhealthy habits you may have and establish new, more healthy ones. Your rehab may last six weeks, six months, or even longer. It is important that you complete the recommended rehab plan.

No matter how difficult it seems, your hard work in cardiac rehab will have lifetime benefits.

Is It Safe for Me?

Cardiac rehab is safe. Studies show that serious health problems caused by cardiac rehab exercise are rare. The cardiac rehab team is trained to handle emergencies. Your health care provider can help you choose a plan that is safe for you. Many patients can safely exercise without supervision, once they learn their own exercise plan.

Checking how your heart reacts and adapts to exercise is an important part of cardiac rehab. You may be connected to an EKG transmitter while you exercise. If your cardiac rehab is done at home, you may be connected to an EKG machine by telephone, or you may phone the cardiac rehab team to let them know how you are doing. In some settings, you check your own pulse rate or estimate how hard you are exercising.

What's in It for Me?

The goals of cardiac rehab are different for each patient. In helping set your personal goals, your health care team will look at your general health, your personal heart problem, your risks for future heart problems, your doctor's recommendations, and, of course, your own preferences.

Cardiac rehab can reduce your symptoms and your chances of having more heart problems. It also has many other benefits:

- Exercise tones your muscles and improves your energy level and spirits. It helps both your heart and your body get stronger and work better. Exercise also can get you back to work and other activities faster.

- Aerobic exercise raises your pulse rate and makes you perspire. It helps improve the flow of oxygen-rich blood throughout your body. Strength training, such as using weights, improves your muscle strength and your stamina. Both types of exercise in the right amount are safe and important for your heart health.

- A healthy diet can lower blood cholesterol, control weight, and help prevent or control high blood pressure and other problems such as diabetes. Plus, you will feel better and have more energy.

- Cardiac rehab can help you quit smoking. Kicking the habit means less risk of lung cancer, emphysema, and bronchitis, as well as less risk of heart attack, stroke, and other heart and blood vessel problems. It means more energy, and it means better health for your loved ones.

- You can learn to manage stress instead of letting it manage you. You will feel better and improve your heart health.

Make a habit of the heart-healthy lifestyle you learn in cardiac rehab. Your life depends on it!

How Do I Find a Plan That's Right for Me?

Your doctor or nurse may recommend a cardiac rehab plan or help you to arrange for exercise training, education, counseling, and other services. Many hospitals and outpatient health care centers offer cardiac rehab—so do some local schools and community centers. You can also check the Yellow Pages of your telephone book.

When choosing a cardiac rehab plan, ask about:

- **Time:** Is it offered when you can get there without causing added stress? Cardiac rehab services offered at the workplace are sometimes an option.

- **Place:** Is it easy to get to? Keep in mind that traffic problems can add to your stress. Is there parking? Public transportation?

- **Setting:** Is it an individual or group plan? Is it home-based or in a facility? Think about whether you want to be in a group with professional supervision.

- **Services:** Does it offer a wide range of services? More importantly, does it include the areas you need help with, such as quitting smoking?

- **Cost:** Is it affordable? Is it covered by insurance? Your insurance may cover all or part of the cost of some cardiac rehab services but not others. Find out what will be covered and for how long. Consider what you can afford and for how long.

Cardiac rehab has lifelong favorable effects, so choose a plan that will serve your needs. For example, if you smoke, look for a plan that will help you quit. Choose a plan that includes activities you enjoy, such as regular walking in a shopping mall or park. Before you sign up, visit and resolve any questions you might have.

How Can I Get the Most Out of Cardiac Rehabilitation?

Studies show that controlling your risk factors for heart disease can help you lead a healthier life. So make sure your cardiac rehab plan works for you. Here's how:

- **Plan:** Work with your health care team to design or change your services to meet your needs.

- **Communicate:** Ask questions. If you don't understand the answers, keep asking until you do. Report changes in your feelings or symptoms.

- **Take charge of your recovery:** No one else can do it for you. Your new lifestyle is healthy for your heart, so stick with it—for life.

To gain more control over your cardiac rehab, remember your goals and keep important information where you can find it. You may want to have a special calendar just for your rehab activities or keep a notebook for this.

Sometimes people who have big changes in their lives feel depressed. Some people with heart problems feel depressed when they find out about their disease or after surgery. Cardiac rehab may help you feel better, but if you are seriously depressed you will need additional help. When you are depressed, it is hard to do things to help yourself get better, such as going to cardiac rehab or getting back to your usual activities. If you are depressed, tell your doctor. Depression can be treated.

Chapter 25

Information about Sexual Activity for Heart Patients

Many heart patients and their partners may feel anxious about resuming their sex life after heart surgery or a heart attack. Those feelings are normal and, in fact, if you're recovering from a heart problem, feelings of anxiety, depression, or lack of desire may occur. The good news is many concerns about physical activity are unfounded. You can still enjoy sex while you're a heart patient and after.

Sex and Your Heart

To most people, sexual activity means sexual intercourse. But sex is more than that. You can express your interest in sex in a lot of ways. You may just want your mate near you. Or you may like to touch and hold. While many heart patients are physically able to resume sexual intercourse, emotionally they may not be ready. Knowing the facts about how intercourse affects your body may help your understanding.

Several physical changes occur in your body during sex, and you may be more aware of them now. Rest assured that these, too, are normal and can include:

- As you get aroused, your breathing slowly increases. Your skin also gets flushed. Your heart rate and blood pressure also become slightly elevated.

"So You'll Know: Sex and Heart Disease," reprinted with permission from the St. Luke's Heart Institute, http://www.stlukesonline.org/services/heart © 2000. St. Luke's Regional Medical Center. All rights reserved.

- As you get more excited, sexual tension builds. Both heart rate and blood pressure rise even more. (Your heart rate can increase anywhere from 90 to 145 beats per minute.) During orgasm, you release this pent-up tension and your heart rate, blood pressure, and breathing return to resting levels.

Sex after Heart Attack or Heart Surgery

Usually, you can resume sex within a few weeks after a heart attack or heart surgery. More people resume sex after heart surgery than after a heart attack. But some are less active. This may be due to anxiety, depression, or lack of desire. Medical care and counseling may help.

When you recover from a heart attack, you may be more aware of your heartbeat, breathing, and muscle tightening or tension. This is normal, so don't worry. Intercourse takes slightly more energy than other sexual activities, so your doctor may tell you to wait until you feel stronger before you have intercourse again.

You can touch, hold, and caress without the goal of orgasm. You and your spouse can feel loved and secure without demands to perform. As you get more confident, you will feel more at ease with yourself and your partner.

How do Psychological Factors Affect Sex?

Many heart patients find emotional barriers to sex stronger than any physical limitations. These feelings can include:

- Being depressed.
- Having trouble sleeping or sleeping too much, especially during the day.
- Eating more or less than usual.
- Being less interested in life.
- Feeling tired all the time (especially after activity).

These feelings are common. But in most cases, they go away within three months after a heart attack or surgery. Problems with sex may increase if you remain depressed. This loss of desire is often added to a false fear that sex will cause a heart problem. If you find that you stop having sex or have prolonged periods between when you normally would have intercourse, you may want to seek counseling. A counselor can help address your fears and concerns as well as those of your partner.

Will Medicines Affect Sex?

Many medicines for heart problems can affect sexual desire and how you perform. These include:

- Blood pressure medicines
- Fluid pills
- Tranquilizers
- Antidepressants and some medications used for chest pain or irregular heartbeat

Such medications may affect your sex drive and function. Male sex problems may include the inability to achieve or maintain an erection (impotence). Some men also may have premature ejaculations or none at all. A woman may not have enough vaginal fluid, which can make intercourse painful. Some women may not get sexually aroused or be able to have an orgasm.

Preparing for Sex

Developing a healthy lifestyle and emotional understanding is important for daily living. But you may find that the following suggestions can put you on the road to a healthy sex life as well:

- **Have a healthy daily balance** of diet, exercise, rest, and medicine.
- **Exercise** boosts health and confidence. Aerobic exercises include walking, jogging, swimming, bicycling, and dancing. These activities can decrease your chance of rapid heart rate, lack of breath, or chest pain during sex.
- **If you smoke, stop.** Many hospitals have a smoking cessation program that can help.
- **Be patient.** Try to understand your emotions. You or your partner may feel vulnerable after a heart attack or surgery. Your emotions may change quickly from tears to laughter or from joy to anger. These sudden mood swings are generally temporary. So try to be patient with each other. A good sense of humor helps.

- **Adjust what you expect from each other** sexually. You may have had a good sex life before your heart problem. You may be afraid to resume sex, but don't let it stop you from enjoying each other again.

- **Avoid rushing into sex** to prove things are "back to normal." If you and your spouse have sex before you're ready, it may only reinforce your fears.

Finally, resuming sex often makes you closer to your partner. It lets you rekindle tenderness and romance. Sex after a heart attack or surgery may ease stress, and it can boost your self-esteem.

Coping as a Couple

Heart patients aren't the only victims of heart disease. Often their partners can become anxious or depressed. The mixed emotions of two people can add tension to your marriage. Both of you should recognize, respect, and try to understand what the other is feeling.

Often a patient's partner fights to balance being overprotective and not helping enough. In most cases, spouses are overprotective. If you and your family are depressed and anxious, serious conflicts can develop. Often a partner is concerned about the risk of sex and cardiac symptoms during sex. A couple may have already had problems with sex. These may get worse after a heart attack or surgery.

As a rule, the more often a couple complained about sex before the illness, the less often they have sex afterward. Talk about the problems. Couples who discuss their sexual needs and concerns seem to cope better.

Suggestions for Resuming Sex

- Choose a time when you're both rested and free from stress.

- It's best to wait one to three hours after eating a full meal before having sex. This allows your food to digest. Like any other physical activity, digesting food requires more blood.

- Find a familiar, peaceful place.

- For some, it's more comfortable for the heart patient to be on the bottom. However, this has nothing to do with physical ability. Most couples don't feel the need to change the way they engage in foreplay or sexual positions.

What If I Experience Symptoms During Sex?

You'll likely experience normal changes during sex—flushed skin, increased heart rate—but be aware of the following symptoms which may indicate your heart can't handle the stress:

- Pressure, pain, or discomfort in your jaw, neck, chest, arm, or stomach.
- Marked shortness of breath.
- Very rapid or irregular heart beats.

If you have any of these symptoms during sex, tell your partner, reduce your activity, and rest. Nitroglycerin tablets may help. Check with your doctor. If the symptoms aren't relieved by medicine, or if they recur after resuming sex, get medical help.

Myths

There are more misconceptions about sex than any actual physical problems that result from intercourse. Common myths include:

Myth: *Sex after a heart attack often causes sudden death.*

Fact: This rarely happens. When it does, it usually occurs when one has sex outside of marriage. Extramarital sex is probably more stressful than sex with a spouse. Often there's an unexpressed need to perform with a new partner. This can be complicated by heavy quantities of food and alcohol, which place additional stress on the heart. Sex outside of marriage usually occurs in a new place, adding to the stress.

Myth: *Alcohol is a sexual stimulant.*

Fact: In fact, alcohol is a strong depressant. While small amounts may help reduce tension in the long run, it may hurt performance.

Myth: *It's best for the heart patient to be on the bottom during sex.*

Fact: Studies show that there is no advantage to this position. For some, it may be more comfortable. It also may be more comfortable to lie on your side. These positions put less pressure on the chest wall and can make it easier to breathe.

Myth: *Decline in sex drive and function after a heart attack or surgery is because of the physical demands sex places on the heart.*

Fact: The biggest impact is psychological. Physically, having sex is similar to walking up two flights of stairs at a brisk pace.

Myth: *If chest pain occurs during sex, you should quit having sex forever.*

Fact: While chest pain can occur during sex, it's rarely severe. Check with your doctor, who may prescribe nitroglycerin or other medication or suggest an exercise regimen to help you build up strength.

Final Thoughts

When both you and your partner have a greater understanding of both the fears and desires involved in your sex life, you may begin to feel better about sex as well as other areas of your life.

The reality is, heart disease may alter your life in ways you hadn't considered. But it also can allow you to reflect on what's important. In the process, you may learn more about yourself and those around you.

Part Three

Facts about Heart Diseases and Disorders

Chapter 26

Facts about Coronary Heart Disease

Coronary heart disease (CHD) is the most common form of heart disease, the leading cause of death for Americans. About 12.6 million Americans suffer from CHD, which often results in a heart attack. About 1.1 million Americans suffer a heart attack each year—about 515,000 of these heart attacks are fatal.

Fortunately, CHD can be prevented or controlled. This chapter gives an overview of CHD and its prevention, diagnosis, and treatment. It describes the steps that Americans can take to protect their heart health.

What Is Coronary Heart Disease?

The heart is a muscle that works twenty-four hours a day. To perform well, it needs a constant supply of oxygen and nutrients, which is delivered by the blood through the coronary arteries.

That blood flow can be reduced by a process called atherosclerosis, in which plaques or fatty substances build up inside the walls of blood vessels. The plaques attract blood components, which stick to the inside surface of the vessel walls. Atherosclerosis can affect any blood vessel, and causes them to narrow and harden. It develops over many years and can begin early, even in childhood.

Reprinted from "Facts about Coronary Heart Disease," National Heart, Lung, and Blood Institute, National Institutes of Health, NIH Publication No. 02-2265, revised October 2003.

In CHD, atherosclerosis affects the coronary arteries. The fatty buildup, or plaque, can break open and lead to the formation of a blood clot. The clot covers the site of the rupture, also reducing blood flow. Eventually, the clot becomes firm. The process of fatty buildup, plaque rupture, and clot formation recurs, progressively narrowing the arteries. Ever less blood reaches the heart muscle.

When too little blood reaches a part of the body, the condition is called ischemia. When this occurs with the heart, it's called cardiac ischemia. If the blood supply is nearly or completely, and abruptly, cut off, a heart attack results and cells in the heart muscle that do not receive enough oxygen begin to die. The more time that passes without treatment to restore blood flow, the greater the damage to the heart. Because heart cells cannot be replaced, the cell loss is permanent.

Who Gets Coronary Heart Disease?

Certain behaviors and conditions increase the risk that someone will develop CHD. They also can increase the chance that CHD, if already present, will worsen. They are called "risk factors," and, while some cannot be modified, most can.

Risk factors that cannot be modified are: age (45 or older for men; 55 or older for women) and a family history of early CHD (a father or brother diagnosed before age 55, or a mother or sister diagnosed with heart disease before age 65).

Factors that can be modified are: cigarette smoking, high blood cholesterol, high blood pressure, overweight/obesity, physical inactivity, and diabetes.

Risk factors do not add their effects in a simple way. Rather, they multiply each other's effects. Generally, each risk factor alone doubles a person's chance of developing CHD. Someone who has high blood cholesterol and high blood pressure and smokes cigarettes is eight times more likely to develop CHD than someone who has no risk factors. So, it is important to prevent or control risk factors that can be modified—see the "Lifestyle" section for how to do this.

What Are the Symptoms of CHD?

Symptoms of CHD vary. Some persons feel no discomfort, while others have chest pain or shortness of breath. Sometimes, the first symptom of CHD is a heart attack or cardiac arrest (a sudden, abrupt loss of heart function).

184

Chest pain also can vary in its occurrence. It happens when the blood flow to the heart is critically reduced and does not match the demands placed on the heart. Called angina, the pain can be mild and intermittent, or more pronounced and steady. It can be severe enough to make normal everyday activities difficult. The same inadequate blood supply also may cause no symptoms, a condition called silent ischemia.

Often, particularly in men, angina is felt behind the breastbone and may radiate up the left arm or neck. It may also be felt in the shoulder, elbows, jaw, or back. Angina is usually brought on by exercise, lasts two to five minutes, does not change with breathing, and is eased by rest.

Women may get a less typical form of angina that feels like shortness of breath or indigestion, and can linger or occur in a different location than behind the breastbone. This less typical form may not be brought on by exertion or be eased by rest. In fact, it may occur only at rest.

A person who has any symptoms should talk with his or her doctor. Without treatment, the symptoms may return, worsen, become unstable, or progress to a heart attack.

What to Do in a Heart Attack

Those with CHD should talk with their doctor about the symptoms of a heart attack and the appropriate steps to take to get emergency care. The key to surviving a heart attack is fast action. Learn the heart attack warning signs and, if you or someone else experiences any of them, call 9-1-1 fast. Do not wait for more than a few minutes—five minutes at most.

Heart Attack Warning Signs

When a heart attack happens, every minute counts. Know the warning signs:

- Chest discomfort. Most heart attacks involve discomfort in the center of the chest that lasts for more than a few minutes, or goes away and comes back. The discomfort can feel like uncomfortable pressure, squeezing, fullness, or pain.

- Discomfort in arm(s), back, neck, jaw, or stomach.

- Shortness of breath. Often comes along with chest discomfort. But it also can occur before chest discomfort.

- Cold sweat, nausea, or lightheadedness.

Most heart attacks are not sudden and intense, but start slowly, with only mild pain or discomfort. It may not be clear what's wrong—even for those who have had a heart attack before. Signs can change for each attack. So, when in doubt, check it out. Don't wait more than a few minutes—five at most—to call 9-1-1. Fast action can save lives.

Fast treatment is critical: Treatments to restore blood flow to the heart are most effective if given within one hour of the start of symptoms. The sooner treatment is begun, the greater the chance for survival and a full recovery.

The most common warning sign—chest discomfort—is the same for men and women. However, women are somewhat more likely than men to have some of the other common symptoms, particularly shortness of breath, nausea and vomiting, and back or jaw pain. Also, women tend to be about ten years older than men when they have a heart attack and to have other conditions as well, such as diabetes, high blood pressure, and congestive heart failure. So it is vital that women receive treatment fast.

Calling 9-1-1 is the best way to get fast treatment. It is like bringing the hospital to you. Emergency medical personnel can begin treatment immediately—even before arrival at the hospital. They also have equipment to start the heart beating if it stops during the heart attack. Furthermore, patients who use the ambulance tend to receive faster treatment on their arrival at the hospital.

If, for some reason, you are having heart attack symptoms and cannot call 9-1-1, have someone else drive you at once to the hospital. Never drive yourself to the hospital, unless you absolutely have no other choice.

You also can increase your chance of surviving a heart attack by preparing ahead of time, especially if you have CHD. Talk with your doctor about what to do if you experience any warning signs and how to reduce your heart attack risk. Fill out a heart attack survival plan (see Figure 26.1) and keep it in a handy place, such as your wallet or purse. Make sure your family and friends know about the warning signs and to call 9-1-1 within five minutes.

What Are the Tests for CHD?

There is no single, simple test for CHD. Which diagnostic tests are done depends on a number of factors, especially the severity of the symptoms and the likelihood that their cause is CHD. After taking a

Figure 26.1. Heart Attack Survival Plan

Write down the following information and keep it in a handy place. You may want to photocopy it and keep a copy at home, at work, and in your wallet or purse. Share the information with emergency medical personnel and hospital staff.

Medicines you are taking:

1. _____

2. _____

3. _____

Medicines you are allergic to:

1. _____

2. _____

3. _____

If symptoms stop completely in less than 5 minutes, you should still call your health care provider:

Phone number during office hours: _____

Phone number after office hours: _____

Person to contact if you go to the hospital:

Name: _____   Work phone: _____

Home phone: _____

careful medical history and doing a physical examination, the doctor may use some of the following tests to rule out other causes for the symptoms, and to confirm the presence and check the severity of CHD:

- **Electrocardiogram (ECG or EKG):** This is a graphic record of the electrical activity of the heart as it contracts and relaxes. The ECG can detect abnormal heartbeats, some areas of damage, inadequate blood flow, and heart enlargement.

- **Stress test:** The stress test is used to check for problems that show up only when the heart is working hard. There are different types of stress test. One is called the exercise test (also called a treadmill test or bicycle exercise ECG); another uses a drug instead of exercise to increase blood flow. The latter is used for persons, such as those with arthritis, who cannot exercise. In both cases, the blood pressure and heartbeat response are continuously monitored and periodically recorded. An ECG rate and blood pressure are taken before, during, and after the test. For an exercise stress test, breathing and oxygen consumption also may be measured. Still another type of stress test uses a nuclear scan (see next bullet) to assess heart muscle contraction or blood flow in the heart. Stress tests are useful but not 100 percent reliable. False positives (showing a problem where none exists) and false negatives (showing no problem when something is wrong) can occur. For instance, gender and race can affect the measurements of exercise stress tests.

- **Nuclear scan:** This also is called a thallium stress test. It is sometimes used to show areas of the heart that lack blood flow and are damaged, as well as problems with the heart's pumping action. A small amount of a radioactive material called thallium is injected into a vein, usually in the arm. A scanning camera positioned over the heart records whether the nuclear material is taken up by the heart muscle (healthy areas) or not (damaged areas). The camera also can evaluate how well the heart muscle pumps blood. This test can be done during both rest and exercise, enhancing the usefulness of its results.

- **Coronary angiography (or arteriography):** This test is used to detect blockages and narrowed areas inside coronary arteries. A fine tube (catheter) is threaded through an artery of an arm or leg into position in the heart vessel. A dye that shows up on x-ray is then injected into the blood vessel, and the vessels and heart are filmed as the heart pumps. The picture is called an angiogram or arteriogram.

- **Ventriculogram:** This is a picture of the heart's main pumping chamber, the left ventricle. It is taken by following a procedure similar to the one described for an angiogram. For a ventriculogram, the catheter is positioned in the left ventricle.

- **Intracoronary ultrasound:** This uses a catheter that can measure blood flow. It gives a picture of the coronary arteries that shows the thickness and character of the artery wall. This lets the doctor assess blood flow and blockages.

How Is CHD Treated?

There are three main types of treatment for CHD: lifestyle, medication, and, for advanced atherosclerosis, special procedures. The first two types of treatment also can help prevent the development of CHD. A discussion of each type of treatment follows.

Lifestyle

Six key steps can help prevent or control CHD: stop smoking cigarettes, lower high blood pressure, reduce high blood cholesterol, lose extra weight, become physically active, and manage diabetes.

Cigarette Smoking

There is no safe way to smoke. Although low-tar and low-nicotine cigarettes may somewhat reduce the risk for lung cancer, they do not lessen the risk for CHD. In fact, smoking accelerates atherosclerosis. It also increases the risk for stroke.

The risk for CHD increases along with the number of cigarettes smoked daily. Quitting sharply lowers the risk, even in the first year and no matter what a person's age. Quitting also reduces the risk for a second heart attack in those who have already had one.

The U.S. Food and Drug Administration has approved five medications that can help persons stop smoking and lessen the urge to smoke. These are: Bupropion SR (available only by prescription), which has no nicotine and reduces the craving for cigarettes; nicotine supplements, which include gum (available over the counter); a nicotine patch (available both over the counter and by prescription); a nicotine inhaler (available only by prescription); and a nicotine nasal spray (available only by prescription).

For more about how to stop smoking, check the Virtual Office of the U.S. Surgeon General at www.surgeongeneral.gov/tobacco.

High Blood Pressure

Also known as hypertension, high blood pressure usually has no symptoms. Once developed, it typically lasts a lifetime. If uncontrolled, it can lead to heart and kidney diseases, and stroke.

Blood pressure is given as two numbers—the systolic pressure over the diastolic pressure—and both are important. A measurement of 140/90 mmHg (millimeters of mercury) or above is called high blood pressure—but if either number is high, that, too, is hypertension. A healthy blood pressure is around 120/80.

Lifestyle steps often can prevent or control high blood pressure: lose excess weight; become physically active; follow a healthy eating plan, including foods lower in salt and sodium; and limit alcohol intake. Some of these steps are the same as those needed to reduce the risk for CHD and are discussed later.

A key ingredient of healthy eating is choosing foods lower in salt (sodium chloride) and other forms of sodium. Most Americans should consume no more than 2,400 milligrams of sodium (which equals about 6 grams of salt, or about 1 teaspoon) in a day. This is the amount listed as a Daily Value on the Nutrition Facts label on food items. Recent research shows that it's even better to consume no more than 1,500 milligrams of sodium (which equals about 4 grams of salt, or about 2/3 teaspoon) in a day. This includes *all* salt—that in processed foods or added in cooking or at the table.

An overall eating plan also should be low in saturated fat and cholesterol, and moderate in total fat. It also should include plenty of fruits and vegetables—most are naturally low in salt and calories.

One such healthy eating plan has been shown to reduce elevated blood pressure. It's called the DASH diet. DASH stands for Dietary Approaches to Stop Hypertension. The eating plan emphasizes fruits, vegetables, and low-fat dairy products. It is reduced in red meat, sweets, and sugar-containing drinks. It is rich in potassium, calcium, magnesium, fiber, and protein. See chapter 19 for more information on the DASH diet.

Those who consume alcoholic beverages should do so in moderation. Alcoholic beverages supply calories but few nutrients. They are harmful when consumed in excess, and some persons should not drink at all. Furthermore, drinking alcoholic beverages increases the risk of some serious health problems. For example, even one drink a day can slightly raise the risk of breast cancer. While drinking alcoholic beverages in moderation may lower the risk of CHD— mainly among men over age forty-five and women over age fifty-five—there are other factors that reduce the risk of heart disease. These include a healthy diet, physical activity, avoidance of smoking, and maintenance of a healthy weight.

Moderate drinking is defined as no more than two drinks a day for men and no more than one drink a day for women. One drink equals 1.5 ounces of 80-proof whiskey, or 5 ounces of wine, or 12 ounces of beer (regular or light).

Those who drink alcoholic beverages should be aware that they may affect medications taken. They should talk about this with their doctor or pharmacist.

High Blood Cholesterol

Cholesterol is a soft, waxy substance involved in normal cell function. Normally, the body makes all the cholesterol it needs. Excess saturated fat and cholesterol in the diet cause the fatty buildup in blood vessels, which contributes to atherosclerosis.

Cholesterol travels through the blood in packages called lipoproteins. There are two main types of lipoprotein that affect the risk for CHD: low-density lipoprotein (LDL), also called the "bad" cholesterol, which causes deposits in blood vessels; and high-density lipoprotein (HDL), also called the "good" cholesterol, which helps remove cholesterol from the blood. It's important to have a low level of LDL and a high level of HDL.

Healthy adults age twenty and older should have a lipoprotein analysis once every five years to measure their levels of total cholesterol, LDL, HDL, and triglycerides, another fatty substance in the blood.

To help prevent or control high blood cholesterol, follow a healthy eating plan such as that mentioned previously, become physically active, and lose excess weight. Those who already have CHD should be especially careful to control their cholesterol and may need to follow an eating plan more restricted in saturated fat and cholesterol.

Overweight and Obesity

About 65 percent of American adults are overweight or obese. Being overweight or obese increases the risk not only for heart disease, but also for other conditions, including stroke, gallbladder disease, arthritis, and breast, colon, and other cancers.

191

Overweight and obesity are determined by two key measures—body mass index, or BMI, and waist circumference. BMI relates height to weight.

Here is a shortcut way to calculate your BMI:

1. Multiply Your Weight in pounds by 703

2. Divide the answer in step 1 by your height in inches

3. Divide the answer in step 2 by your height in inches again to get your BMI

Example: For a person who is 5 feet 5 inches tall (65 inches) and weighs 180 pounds, the BMI is 29.9, calculated as follows: 180 x 703 = 126,540; 126,540/65 = 1,946; 1,946/65 = 29.9.

A normal BMI is 18.5–24.9; an overweight BMI is 25–29.9; and an obese BMI is 30 and over. Heart disease risk increases if waist circumference is greater than thirty-five inches for women or greater than forty inches for men.

Those who are overweight or obese should aim for a healthy weight in order to reduce CHD risk. Even a small weight loss—just 10 percent of current weight—will help to lower CHD risk and that of the other conditions too. Those who cannot lose should at least try not to gain more weight.

There are no quick fixes to lose weight. To be successful, weight loss must be viewed as a change of lifestyle and not as a temporary effort to drop pounds quickly. Otherwise, the weight will probably be regained. Do not try to lose more than 1/2 to 2 pounds a week.

To lose weight, follow a heart-healthy eating plan. Eat a variety of nutritious foods in moderate amounts. Choose foods that are lower in calories and fat. It's also important to become physically active. This helps use calories and, so, aids weight loss. It also helps keep the weight off for life.

Physical Activity

Physical activity is one of the best ways to help prevent and control CHD. It can lower LDL and raise HDL. It also lowers blood pressure for those who are overweight.

To become physically active, do thirty minutes of a moderate activity on most and, preferably, all days. Examples of moderate activities are brisk walking and dancing. If thirty minutes is too much time, break it up into periods of at least ten minutes each. Those who have been inactive should start slowly. Begin at a lower level of physical activity and slowly increase the time and intensity of the effort.

Those with CHD or who have a high risk for it should check with their doctor before starting a physical activity program. Others who should consult a doctor first include those with chronic health problems, men over age forty, and women over age fifty. The doctor can give advice on how rigorous the exercise should be.

Those who have had a heart attack benefit greatly from physical activity. Many hospitals have a cardiac rehabilitation program. The doctor can offer advice about a suitable program.

Diabetes

Diabetes mellitus affects more than seventeen million Americans. It damages blood vessels, including the coronary arteries of the heart. Up to 75 percent of those with diabetes develop heart and blood vessel diseases. Diabetes also can lead to stroke, kidney failure, and other problems.

Diabetes occurs when the body is not able to use sugar as it should for growth and energy. The body gets sugar when it changes food into glucose (a form of sugar). A hormone made in the pancreas and called insulin is needed for the glucose to be taken up and used by the body. In diabetes, the body cannot make use of the glucose in the blood because either the pancreas cannot make enough insulin or the insulin that is available is not effective.

Symptoms of diabetes include: increased thirst and urination (including at night), weight loss, blurred vision, hunger, fatigue, frequent infections, and slow healing of wounds or sores.

There are two main types of diabetes—type 1 and type 2. Type 1 usually appears suddenly and most commonly in those under age thirty. Type 2 diabetes occurs gradually and most often in those over age forty. Up to 95 percent of those with diabetes have type 2.

You're more likely to develop type 2 if you are overweight or obese, especially with extra weight around the middle, over age forty, or have high blood pressure or a family history of diabetes. Diabetes is particularly prevalent among African Americans, Asians, and American Indians.

Because of the link with heart disease, it's important for those with diabetes to prevent or control heart disease and its risk factors. Fortunately, new research shows that the same steps that reduce the risk of CHD also lower the chance of developing type 2 diabetes. And, for those who already have diabetes, those steps, along with taking any prescribed medication, also can delay or prevent the development of complications of diabetes, such as eye or kidney disease and nerve damage.

According to the research, a 7 percent loss of body weight and 150 minutes of moderate physical activity a week can reduce the chance of developing diabetes by 58 percent in those who are at high risk. The lifestyle changes cut the risk of developing type 2 diabetes regardless of age, ethnicity, gender, or weight.

Steps that reduce the risk of developing diabetes—as well as CHD—are to:

• Follow a healthy eating plan, which is low in saturated fat and cholesterol, and moderate in total fat.

• Aim for a healthy weight.

• Be physically active each day—thirty minutes of moderate physical activity on most and, preferably, all days of the week.

• Not smoke.

• Prevent or control high blood pressure.

• Prevent or control high blood cholesterol.

Those who already have diabetes can delay its progression, or prevent or slow the development of heart, blood vessel, and other complications by following the steps given previously as well as to:

• Eat meals and snacks at around the same times each day.

• Check with the doctor about the best physical activities.

• Take prescribed medicine for diabetes at the same times each day.

• Check blood sugar every day. Each time blood sugar is checked, the number should be written in a record book. The doctor should be called if the numbers are too high or too low for two to three days.

• Check the feet every day for cuts, sores, bumps, or red spots.

• Brush and floss teeth and gums every day.

• Take any prescribed medication for other conditions, such as CHD.

• For those who have CHD, check with the doctor about whether or not to take aspirin each day.

Medications

Sometimes, in addition to making lifestyle changes, medications may be needed to prevent or control CHD. For instance, medications may be used to control a risk factor such as high blood pressure or high blood cholesterol and so help prevent the development of CHD. Or, medication may be used to relieve the chest pain of CHD.

If prescribed, medications must be taken as directed. Drugs can have side effects. If side effects occur, they should be reported to the doctor. Often, a change in the dose or type of a medication, or the use of a combination of drugs, can stop the side effect.

Drugs used to treat CHD and its risk factors include:

- **Aspirin:** helps to lower the risk of a heart attack for those who have already had one. It also helps to keep arteries open in those who have had a previous heart bypass or other artery-opening procedure such as coronary angioplasty. Because of its risks, aspirin is not approved by the Food and Drug Administration for the prevention of heart attacks in healthy persons. It may be harmful for some persons, especially those with no risk of heart disease. Patients must be assessed carefully to make sure the benefits of taking aspirin outweigh the risks. Each person should talk to his or her doctor about whether or not to take aspirin. Aspirin also is given to patients who arrive at a hospital emergency department with a suspected heart attack.

- **Digitalis:** helps the heart contract better and is used when the heart's pumping function has been weakened; it also slows some fast heart rhythms.

- **ACE (angiotensin converting enzyme) inhibitor:** stops production of a chemical produced by the body that makes blood vessels narrow. It is used for high blood pressure and damaged heart muscle. It also can prevent kidney damage in some patients with diabetes.

- **Beta blocker:** slows the heart and makes it beat with less force, lowering blood pressure and making the heart work less hard. It is used for high blood pressure, chest pain, and to prevent a repeat heart attack.

- **Nitrate (including nitroglycerin):** relaxes blood vessels and stops chest pain/angina.

- **Calcium-channel blocker:** relaxes blood vessels, and is used for high blood pressure and chest pain/angina.

- **Diuretic:** decreases fluid in the body and is used for high blood pressure. Diuretics are sometimes referred to as "water pills."

- **Blood cholesterol-lowering agents:** decrease LDL levels in the blood. Some can increase HDL.

- **Thrombolytic agents:** also called "clot-busting drugs," they are given during a heart attack to dissolve a blood clot in a coronary artery in order to restore blood flow. They must be given immediately after heart attack symptoms begin. To be most effective, they need to be given within one hour of the start of heart attack symptoms.

Special Procedures

Advanced atherosclerosis may require a special procedure to open an artery and improve blood flow. This is usually done to ease severe chest pain, or to clear major or multiple blockages in blood vessels.

Two commonly used procedures are coronary angioplasty and coronary artery bypass graft operation.

Coronary Angioplasty, or Balloon Angioplasty

In this procedure, a fine tube, or catheter, is threaded through an artery into the narrowed heart vessel. The catheter has a tiny balloon at its tip. The balloon is repeatedly inflated and deflated to open and stretch the artery, improving blood flow. The balloon is then deflated, and the catheter is removed.

Doctors often insert a stent during the angioplasty. A wire mesh tube, the stent is used to keep an artery open after an angioplasty. The stent stays in the artery permanently.

Angioplasty is not surgery. It is done while the patient is awake and may last one to two hours.

In about a third of those who have an angioplasty, the blood vessel becomes narrowed or blocked again within six months. Vessels that reclose may be opened again with another angioplasty or a coronary artery bypass graft. An artery with a stent also can reclose.

Coronary Artery Bypass Graft Operation

Also known as "bypass surgery," the procedure uses a piece of vein taken from the leg, or of an artery taken from the chest or wrist. This piece is attached to the heart artery above and below the narrowed area, thus making a bypass around the blockage. Sometimes, more than one bypass is needed.

Bypass surgery may be needed due to various reasons, such as an angioplasty that did not sufficiently widen the blood vessel, or blockages that cannot be reached by, or are too long or hard for, angioplasty. In certain cases, bypass surgery may be preferred to angioplasty. For instance, it may be used for persons who have both CHD and diabetes.

A bypass also can close again. This happens in about 10 percent of bypass surgeries, usually after ten or more years.

Other Procedures

Other procedures also may be used to open coronary arteries:

- *Atherectomy:* A specially equipped catheter is threaded through an artery to a blockage, where thin strips of plaque are shaved off and removed. Balloon angioplasty or insertion of a stent may be done as well.

- *Laser angioplasty:* A catheter with a laser tip is inserted into an artery to burn, vaporize, or break down plaque. The procedure may be used alone or along with balloon angioplasty.

It is important to understand that these procedures relieve the symptoms of CHD but do not cure the disease. Lifestyle changes must still be followed and any necessary medications must continue to be taken.

Chapter 27

Angina

What is angina and how will I know if I have it?

Angina, or angina pectoris, refers to symptoms such as chest pain or discomfort caused by reduced blood flow to the heart. Angina is often the first sign of heart disease.

The heart is a muscle that gets blood from blood vessels called the coronary arteries. If one or more of your coronary arteries has a blockage that reduces blood flow to your heart from time to time, you may have angina.

Narrowed and blocked arteries are usually due to a gradual buildup of fatty deposits called plaque inside the arteries. This process is called atherosclerosis.

People with angina usually feel discomfort (often a pressure-like pain) in or around the chest, shoulders, jaw, neck, back, or arms. It may feel like a squeezing, pressing sensation in the chest. Angina pain is usually caused and made worse by exercise and eased by rest. The pain usually lasts two to five minutes. If you have this kind of chest pain, you should contact your health care provider. You can take medicine that will help your angina. If you suspect you might be having a heart attack (see following warning signs), call or have someone else call 9-1-1.

Not all chest discomfort is angina. For example, acid reflux (heartburn) and lung infection or inflammation can cause chest pain.

Reprinted from "Angina," National Women's Health Information Center (www.4woman.gov), published in March 2002.

Here are some signs that your angina is very serious and you may be having a heart attack. If you have any of these signs, call 9-1-1 immediately:

- Pain or discomfort that is very bad, gets worse, and lasts longer than twenty minutes.

- Pain or discomfort along with weakness, feeling sick to your stomach, sweating, or fainting.

- Pain or discomfort that does not go away when you take angina medicine.

- Pain or discomfort that is worse than you have ever had before.

Does angina mean I'm having a heart attack?

Not necessarily. An episode of angina is not a heart attack, but it does mean that you have a greater chance of having a heart attack. Angina pain means that some of the heart muscle is not getting enough blood temporarily. A heart attack, on the other hand, occurs when the blood flow to a part of the heart is suddenly and permanently cut off, usually by a blood clot. This can lead to serious heart damage.

Is all angina the same?

No. There are two main kinds of angina—common or stable angina and unstable angina. Both kinds of angina mean an increased risk of heart attack, but unstable angina is often a major warning sign that a heart attack can happen soon.

People with common or stable angina have episodes of chest discomfort that usually occur in an expected pattern. Common angina occurs when you are exerting more than usual activity (such as running to catch a bus) or are under mental and emotional stress. The level of activity or stress that causes the angina is somewhat predictable, and the pattern changes only slowly. Resting or relaxing usually eases the discomfort.

Unstable angina, instead of appearing gradually, may first appear as a very severe episode or as frequently recurring bouts of angina. The chest pain of unstable angina is unexpected and usually occurs at rest, or may wake a person in the night. Sometimes an established stable pattern of angina may change sharply. For example, it may be provoked by far less exercise than in the past. Unstable angina should be treated as an emergency because it can lead quickly to a heart attack, dangerous heart rhythms, or even sudden death.

Are there other types of angina besides stable (common) and unstable angina?

There are two other forms of angina. One, Prinzmetal's or variant angina, is quite rare, but causes discomfort almost always when a person is at rest. It is caused by a spasm that narrows the coronary artery and lessens the flow of blood to the heart. The other is called microvascular angina. This type of angina occurs in people who have chest pain but have no apparent coronary artery blockage. The pain from microvascular angina results from poorly functioning blood vessels. Microvascular angina can be treated with the same medicines as common angina.

How is angina diagnosed?

Health care providers can usually find out if you have angina by listening to you talk about your symptoms and their patterns. They may also order some tests to further evaluate your angina. Tests may include x-rays; an electrocardiogram (ECG or EKG) at rest, and during and after exercise; a nuclear stress test; and coronary angiography. Variant angina can be diagnosed using a Holter monitor. Holter monitoring gets a nonstop reading of your heart rate and rhythm over a twenty-four-hour period (or longer). You wear a recording device (the Holter monitor), which is connected to small metal disks called electrodes that are placed on your chest. With certain types of monitors, you can push a "record" button to capture a rhythm when you feel the symptoms of angina.

What should I do if I start to have unexpected chest pains while resting?

If you have unexpected chest pain at rest, seek immediate medical help. Call or have someone else call 9-1-1. This kind of pain may mean that clots are forming in an artery and are about to cause a heart attack. Medicine is available at the hospital that can stop clots from forming and dissolve existing clots.

How is angina treated?

Lifestyle changes and medicine are the most common ways to control stable angina. Although angina may be brought on by exercise, this does not mean that you should stop exercising. In fact, you should keep doing an exercise program that has been approved by your health care provider.

Risk factors for coronary artery disease should be controlled, including high blood pressure, cigarette smoking, high blood cholesterol, and excess weight. By eating healthfully, not smoking, limiting how much alcohol you drink, and avoiding stress, you may live more comfortably and with fewer angina attacks. You may need medicine to help lower your blood pressure or your cholesterol.

Drugs are often used to control angina. The most commonly used drug for angina is nitroglycerin, which relieves pain by relaxing blood vessels. This allows more blood to flow to the heart muscle and also decreases the workload of the heart. Nitroglycerin is taken when discomfort occurs or is expected. Your health care provider may prescribe other drugs to be taken every day to help reduce the heart's workload. Two types of drugs often used are called beta-blockers and calcium channel blockers.

What lifestyle changes can help with angina?

Talk to your health care provider about changes you can make to improve your heart health and your angina. You may benefit from:

- weight loss
- increasing your physical activity
- eating healthy foods and not overeating
- controlling stress in your life
- quitting smoking
- drinking less alcohol

What if lifestyle changes and medicine fail to control angina?

If lifestyle changes and drugs fail to ease angina, or if your risk of heart attack is high, you may need additional tests and treatment. One common test is cardiac catheterization. This test involves inserting a catheter (a thin tube) into a forearm or groin artery and threading the catheter into the heart. A dye can be injected and tracked by computerized x-ray (coronary angiography or arteriography) to show where the arteries are blocked. Balloon angioplasty may be used to open up narrowed arteries. This procedure uses a tiny balloon that is inflated briefly inside the artery. Sometimes a stent (a tiny metal mesh tube) is put in to help keep the artery open.

Chapter 28

Heart Attack

What is a heart attack?

A heart attack occurs when the supply of blood and oxygen to an area of heart muscle is blocked, usually by a clot in a coronary artery. Often, this blockage leads to arrhythmias (irregular heartbeat or rhythm) that cause a severe decrease in the pumping function of the heart and may bring about sudden death. If the blockage is not treated within a few hours, the affected heart muscle will die and be replaced by scar tissue.

A heart attack is a life-threatening event. Everyone should know the warning signs of a heart attack and how to get emergency help. Many people suffer permanent damage to their hearts or die because they do not get help immediately.

Each year, more than a million persons in the U.S. have a heart attack and about half (515,000) of them die. About one-half of those who die do so within one hour of the start of symptoms and before reaching the hospital.

Emergency personnel can often stop arrhythmias with emergency CPR (cardiopulmonary resuscitation), defibrillation (electrical shock), and prompt advanced cardiac life support procedures. If care is sought soon enough, blood flow in the blocked artery can be restored in time to prevent permanent damage to the heart. Yet, most people do not

Reprinted from "Heart Attack," Diseases and Conditions Index, National Heart, Lung, and Blood Institute, National Institutes of Health, 2004.

seek medical care for two hours or more after symptoms begin. Many people wait twelve hours or longer.

A heart attack is an emergency. Call 9-1-1 if you think you (or someone else) may be having a heart attack. Prompt treatment of a heart attack can help prevent or limit lasting damage to the heart and can prevent sudden death.

Are there other names for a heart attack?

- Myocardial infarction or MI
- Acute myocardial infarction or AMI
- Acute coronary syndrome
- Coronary thrombosis
- Coronary occlusion

What causes a heart attack?

Most heart attacks are caused by a blood clot that blocks one of the coronary arteries (the blood vessels that bring blood and oxygen to the heart muscle). When blood cannot reach part of your heart, that area starves for oxygen. If the blockage continues long enough, cells in the affected area die.

Coronary Artery Disease (CAD) is the most common underlying cause of a heart attack. CAD is the hardening and narrowing of the coronary arteries by the buildup of plaque in the inside walls (atherosclerosis). Over time, plaque buildup in the coronary arteries can:

- Narrow the arteries so that less blood flows to the heart muscle
- Completely block the arteries and the flow of blood
- Cause blood clots to form and block the arteries.

A less common cause of heart attacks is a severe spasm (tightening) of the coronary artery that cuts off blood flow to the heart. These spasms can occur in persons with or without CAD. Artery spasm can sometimes be caused by:

- Taking certain drugs, such as cocaine
- Emotional stress
- Exposure to cold
- Cigarette smoking.

What makes a heart attack more likely?

Certain factors make it more likely that you will develop CAD and have a heart attack. These are called risk factors. Risk factors you cannot change include:

- Your age
  - Men: over age forty-five
  - Women: over age fifty-five
- Having a family history of early heart disease
  - Heart disease diagnosed in father or brother before age fifty-five
  - Heart disease diagnosed in mother or sister before age sixty-five
- Having a personal history of CAD
  - Angina
  - A previous heart attack
  - A surgical procedure (angioplasty, heart bypass) to increase blood flow to your heart.

Risk factors that you can change include:

- Smoking
- High blood pressure
- High blood cholesterol
- Obesity
- Being physically inactive
- Diabetes (high blood sugar)

How can I prevent a heart attack?

Most heart attacks are caused by coronary artery disease (CAD). You can help prevent a heart attack by knowing about your risk factors for CAD and heart attack and taking action to lower your risks.

You can lower your risk of having a heart attack, even if you have already had a heart attack or are told that your chances of having a heart attack are high.

To prevent a heart attack, you will most likely need to make lifestyle changes. You may also need to get treatment for conditions that raise your risk.

Make Lifestyle Changes

You can lower your risk for CAD and a heart attack by making healthy lifestyle choices:

- Eat a healthy diet to prevent or reduce high blood pressure and high blood cholesterol, and maintain a healthy weight
- If you smoke, quit
- Exercise as directed by your doctor
- Lose weight if you are overweight or obese

Treat Related Conditions

In addition to making lifestyle changes, you can help prevent heart attacks by treating conditions you have that make a heart attack more likely:

- *High blood cholesterol.* If you have high cholesterol, follow your doctor's advice about lowering your cholesterol. Take medications to lower your cholesterol as directed.
- *High blood pressure.* If you have high blood pressure, follow your doctor's advice about keeping your blood pressure under control. Take blood pressure medications as directed.
- *High blood sugar (diabetes).* If you have diabetes, follow your doctor's advice about keeping your blood sugar levels under control. Take medications as directed.

Prevent a Second Heart Attack

If you have already had a heart attack, it is very important to follow your doctor's advice to prevent a second heart attack:

- Make lifestyle changes as directed
- Take your medications as directed
- Follow any other treatment recommended by your doctor, such as cardiac rehabilitation.

By taking these steps, you can prevent or reduce the chance of another heart attack and related complications, such as heart failure.

Make sure that you have an emergency action plan in case you have signs of a second heart attack. Talk to your doctor about making your plan, and talk with your family about it. The plan should include:

- The signs and symptoms of a heart attack
- Instructions for the prompt use of aspirin and nitroglycerin
- How to access emergency medical services in your community (most people dial 9-1-1)
- The location of the nearest hospital that offers twenty-four-hour emergency heart care.

Remember, the symptoms of a second heart attack may not be the same as those of a first heart attack. If in doubt, call 9-1-1.

What are the signs and symptoms of a heart attack?

The warning signs and symptoms of a heart attack can include:

- **Chest discomfort.** Most heart attacks involve discomfort in the center of the chest that lasts for more than a few minutes, or goes away and comes back. The discomfort can feel like uncomfortable pressure, squeezing, fullness, or pain. Heart attack pain can sometimes feel like indigestion or heartburn.
- **Discomfort in other areas of the upper body.** Can include pain, discomfort, or numbness in one or both arms, the back, neck, jaw, or stomach.
- **Shortness of breath.** Often comes along with chest discomfort, but it also can occur before chest discomfort.
- **Other symptoms** may include breaking out in a cold sweat, having nausea and vomiting, or feeling light-headed or dizzy.

Signs and symptoms vary from person to person. In fact, if you have a second heart attack, your symptoms may not be the same as for the first heart attack. Some people have no symptoms. This is called a "silent" heart attack.

The symptoms of angina can be similar to those of a heart attack. If you have angina and notice a change or a worsening of your symptoms, talk with your doctor right away.

Know the warning signs of a heart attack so you can act fast to get treatment. Many heart attack victims wait two hours or more after their symptoms begin before they seek medical help. This delay can result in death or lasting heart damage.

If you think you may be having a heart attack, or if your angina pain does not go away as usual when you take your angina medicine as directed, call 9-1-1 for help. You can begin to receive life-saving treatment in the ambulance on the way to an emergency room.

How is a heart attack diagnosed?

Diagnosis (and treatment) of a heart attack can begin when emergency medical personnel arrive after you call 9-1-1. Don't put off calling 9-1-1 because you are not sure that you are having a heart attack.

At the hospital emergency room, doctors will work fast to find out if you are having or have had a heart attack. They will consider your symptoms, medical and family history, and test results. Initial tests will be quickly followed by treatment if you are having a heart attack.

Tests used include:

- **Electrocardiogram (ECG or EKG).** This test is used to measure the rate and regularity of your heartbeat. A twelve-lead EKG is used in diagnosing a heart attack.

- **Blood tests.** When cells in the heart die, they release enzymes into the blood. They are called markers or biomarkers. Measuring the amount of these markers in the blood can show how much damage was done to your heart. These tests are often repeated at intervals to check for changes. The specific blood tests are:

  - **Troponin test.** This test checks the troponin levels in the blood. It is considered the most accurate blood test to see if a heart attack has occurred and how much damage was done to the heart.

  - **CK or CK-MB test.** These tests check for the amount of the different forms of creatine kinase in the blood.

  - **Myoglobin test.** This test checks for the presence of myoglobin in the blood. Myoglobin is released when the heart or other muscle is injured.

- **Nuclear heart scan.** This test uses radioactive tracers (technetium or thallium) to outline heart chambers and major blood vessels leading to and from the heart. A nuclear heart scan shows any damage to your heart muscle.

- **Cardiac catheterization.** A thin flexible tube (catheter) is passed through an artery in the groin or arm to reach the coronary arteries. Your doctor can determine pressure and blood flow in the heart's chambers, collect blood samples from the heart, and examine the arteries of the heart by x-ray.

- **Coronary angiography.** This test is usually performed along with cardiac catheterization. A dye that can be seen using x-ray is injected through the catheter into the coronary arteries. Your doctor can see the flow of blood through the heart and see where there are blockages.

How is a heart attack treated?

A heart attack is a medical emergency. Delaying treatment can mean lasting damage to your heart or even death. The sooner treatment begins, the better your chances of recovering. Your treatment may begin in the ambulance or in the emergency room and continue in a special area called a coronary care unit or CCU.

In the Hospital

If you are having a heart attack, doctors will:

- Work quickly to restore blood flow to the heart
- Continuously monitor your vital signs to detect and treat complications

Restoring blood flow to the heart is vital to prevent or limit damage to the heart muscle and to prevent another heart attack. The main treatments are the use of thrombolytic ("clot-busting") drugs and procedures such as angioplasty.

- Thrombolytic drugs ("clot-busters") are used to dissolve blood clots that are blocking blood flow to the heart. When given soon after a heart attack begins, these drugs can limit or prevent permanent damage to the heart. To be most effective, they need to be given within one hour after of the start of heart attack symptoms.
- Angioplasty procedures are used to open blocked or narrowed coronary arteries. A stent, which is a tiny metal mesh tube, may be placed in the artery to help keep it open.
- Coronary artery bypass surgery uses arteries or veins from other areas in your body to bypass your blocked coronary arteries.

The CCU is specially equipped with monitors that continuously measure your vital signs. Those that can show signs of complications include:

- EKG, which detects any heart rhythm (arrhythmia) or functional problems
- Blood pressure
- Pulse oximetry, which measures the amount of oxygen in the blood and provides an early warning sign of a low level of oxygen in the blood.

Medications used in treating heart attacks include:

- *Beta blockers* to decrease the workload on your heart by slowing your heart rate. This makes your heart beat with less force and lowers your blood pressure. Some beta blockers are also used to relieve angina (chest pain) and in heart attack patients to help prevent additional heart attacks. They are also used to correct irregular heartbeat.
- *Angiotensin-converting enzyme (ACE) inhibitors* to lower blood pressure and reduce the strain on your heart. They are used in some patients after a heart attack to increase survival rate and help slow down further weakening of the heart.
- *Nitrates*, such as nitroglycerin, to relax blood vessels and stop chest pain.
- *Anticoagulants* to thin the blood and prevent clots from forming in your arteries.
- *Antiplatelet medications* (such as aspirin and clopidogrel) to stop platelets from clumping together to form clots. These medications are given to people who have had a heart attack, have angina, or who experience angina after angioplasty.
- *Glycoprotein IIb-IIIa inhibitors*, which are potent antiplatelet medicines given intravenously to prevent clots from forming in your arteries.
- *Medicines to relieve pain and anxiety.*
- *Medicines to treat arrhythmias* (irregular heart rhythms), which often occur during a heart attack.
- *Oxygen therapy.*

The length of your hospital stay after a heart attack depends on your condition and response to treatment. Most people spend several days in the hospital after a heart attack. While in the hospital, your heart will be monitored, and you will receive needed medications. You will probably have further testing, and you will be treated for any complications that arise.

While you are still in the hospital or after you go home after your heart attack, your doctor may order other tests, such as:

- *Echocardiogram.* In this test, ultrasound is used to make an image of your heart that can be seen on a video monitor. It shows how well the heart is filling with blood and pumping it to the rest of the body.

- *Exercise stress test.* This test shows how well your heart pumps at higher workloads when it needs more oxygen. EKG and blood pressure readings are taken before, during, and after exercise to see how your heart responds to exercise. The first EKG and blood pressure reading are done to get a baseline. Readings are then taken while you walk on an exercise treadmill or pedal a stationary bicycle. The test continues until you reach a heart rate set by your doctor. The exercise part is stopped if chest pain or a very sharp rise in blood pressure occurs. Monitoring continues for ten to fifteen minutes after exercise or until your heart rate returns to baseline.

Cardiac Rehabilitation (Rehab)

Your doctor may prescribe cardiac rehabilitation (rehab) to help you recover from a heart attack and help prevent another heart attack. Almost everyone who has survived a heart attack can benefit from rehab.

The cardiac rehab team may include:

- Doctors
    - Your family doctor
    - A heart specialist
    - A surgeon
- Nurses
- Exercise specialists
- Physical therapists and occupational therapists
- Dietitians
- Psychologists or other behavior therapists.

Rehab has two parts:

- *Exercise training* to help you learn how to exercise safely, strengthen your muscles, and improve your stamina. Your exercise plan will be based on your individual ability, needs, and interests.

- *Education, counseling, and training* to help you understand your heart condition and find ways to reduce your risk of future heart problems. The cardiac rehab team will help you learn how to cope with the stress of adjusting to a new lifestyle and to deal with your fears about the future.

After You Leave the Hospital

After a heart attack, your treatment may include cardiac rehab in the first weeks or months, checkups and tests, lifestyle changes, and medications. You will need to see your doctor for checkups and tests to see how your heart is doing. Your doctor will most likely recommend lifestyle changes, such as quitting smoking, losing weight, changing your diet, or increasing your physical activity.

After a heart attack, most people take daily medications. These may include:

- Aspirin
- Medicines that lower your cholesterol or your blood pressure
- Other medicines to help reduce your heart's workload

Always take medications as your doctor directs.

How does life change after a heart attack?

There are millions of people who have survived a heart attack. Many recover fully and are able to lead normal lives.

If you have already had a heart attack, your goals are to:

- Recover and resume normal activities as much as possible
- Prevent another heart attack
- Prevent complications, such as heart failure or cardiac arrest.

After a heart attack, you will need to see your doctor regularly for checkups and tests to see how your heart is doing. Your doctor will also most likely recommend:

- Lifestyle changes, such as quitting smoking, changing your diet, or increasing your physical activity

- Medications such as aspirin, nitroglycerin tablets for angina, medicines to lower your cholesterol or blood pressure, and medicines to help reduce your heart's workload
- That you participate in a cardiac rehabilitation program.

Exercise is good for your heart muscle and overall health. It can help you lose weight, keep your cholesterol and blood pressure under control, reduce stress, and lift your mood. If you have angina after your heart attack, you will need to learn when to rest and when and how to take medicine for angina.

Returning to Usual Activities

After a heart attack, most people are able to return to their normal activities. Ask your doctor when you should go back to:

- Driving
- Physical activity
- Work
- Sexual activity
- Strenuous activities (running, heavy lifting, etc.)
- Air travel.

Most people without chest pain following an uncomplicated heart attack can safely return to most of their usual activities within a few weeks. Most can begin walking immediately. Sexual activity with the usual partner can also begin within a few weeks for most patients without chest pain or other complications. Driving can usually begin within a week for most patients without chest pain or other complications if allowed by state law. Each state has rules for driving a motor vehicle following a serious illness. Patients with complications or chest pain should not drive until their symptoms have been stable for a few weeks. Your doctor will tell you when you should return to each of these activities.

Anxiety and Depression after a Heart Attack

After a heart attack, many people worry about having another heart attack. They often feel depressed and may have trouble adjusting to a new lifestyle. You should discuss your feelings of anxiety or depression with your doctor. Your doctor can give you medicine for anxiety or depression, if needed. Spend time with family, friends, and even pets. Affection can make you feel better and less lonely. Most people do not continue to feel depressed after they have fully recovered.

Know How and When to Seek Medical Attention

Having a heart attack increases your chances of having another one. Therefore, it is very important that you and your family know how and when to seek medical attention. Talk to your doctor about making an emergency action plan, and talk with your family about it. The plan should include:

- The signs and symptoms of a heart attack
- Instructions for the prompt use of aspirin and nitroglycerin
- How to access emergency medical services in your community
- The location of the nearest hospital that offers twenty-four-hour emergency heart care.

Many heart attack survivors also have chest pain or angina. The pain usually occurs after exertion and goes away in a few minutes when you rest or take your angina medicine (nitroglycerin) as directed. In a heart attack, the pain is usually more severe than angina, and it does not go away when you rest or take your angina medicine. If in doubt whether your chest pain is angina or a heart attack, call 9-1-1.

Unfortunately, most heart attack victims wait two hours or more after their symptoms begin before they seek medical help. This delay can result in death or lasting heart damage.

Chapter 29

Sudden Cardiac Death

What Is Sudden Cardiac Death (SCD)?

- Sudden cardiac death is a sudden, unexpected death caused by loss of heart function.

- It is the largest cause of natural death in the United States, causing about 250,000 adult deaths each year.

What Causes Sudden Cardiac Death?

Most sudden cardiac deaths are caused by arrhythmias (abnormal heart rhythms). The most common life-threatening arrhythmia is ventricular fibrillation, an erratic, disorganized firing of impulses from the ventricles. When this occurs, the heart is unable to pump blood, and death will occur within minutes, if left untreated.

Certain traits put one at increased risk for SCD:

- Coronary artery disease (80 percent of SCD is linked to coronary artery disease)

- Ventricular tachycardia (abnormally rapid heart rhythm) or ventricular fibrillation (fluttering or quivering of the lower chambers of the heart) after a heart attack

- Those with certain risk factors for coronary artery disease:
  - cigarette smoking
  - family history
  - high cholesterol
  - high blood pressure with heart enlargement
- History of heart defects
- History of syncope (fainting)
- Heart failure with ejection fraction less than 30 percent
- Hypertrophic cardiomyopathy (an increased growth in thickness of the wall of the left ventricle)
- Dilated cardiomyopathy (an abnormally enlarged heart) may be the cause of SCD in about 10 percent of cases
- History of certain abnormal heart rhythms:
  - Long QT syndrome
  - Ventricular tachycardia
  - Ventricular fibrillation
  - Wolff Parkinson White syndrome
  - Extremely slow heart rates or heart block
- First six to eighteen months after a coronary event (heart attack)
- Obesity
- Diabetes

Statistics

- 80 percent of SCD is associated with coronary artery disease.
- About half of deaths from coronary heart disease are sudden.
- About 250,000 sudden cardiac deaths occur each year among adults in the United States.
- SCD occurs mostly in adults (mid-thirties to forties).
- SCD affects men twice as much as women.
- SCD occurs in only 1 to 2 per 100,000 children per year.

Is Sudden Cardiac Death a Heart Attack?

Sudden cardiac death is not a heart attack. A heart attack occurs due to blockage in one or more of the coronary arteries that feed the heart muscle, resulting in lack of blood flow to the heart muscle. The heart becomes damaged.

In contrast, during sudden cardiac death, the electrical system to the heart suddenly becomes irregular. The ventricles may flutter or quiver (ventricular fibrillation), and blood is not delivered to the body. Of greatest concern in the first few minutes is that blood flow to the brain will be reduced so drastically, a person will lose consciousness. Death follows unless emergency treatment is begun immediately.

Emergency Treatment for Sudden Cardiac Death

Sudden cardiac death can be treated and reversed, but emergency action must take place almost immediately. Survival can be as high as 90 percent if treatment is initiated within the first minutes after SCD. The rate decreases by about 10 percent each minute longer. Those who survive have a good long-term outlook.

The American Heart Association promotes using the four steps, called "the chain of survival."

1. *Early Access to Care.* Quick contact with emergency care is essential. If someone experiences SCD, call 911 (in most communities) or your local emergency number immediately.

2. *Early Cardiopulmonary Resuscitation (CPR).* If performed properly, CPR can help save a life, as the procedure keeps blood and oxygen circulating through the body until emergency medical help arrives.

3. *Early Defibrillation.* In most adults, sudden cardiac death is related to ventricular fibrillation. Quick defibrillation (delivery of an electrical shock) is necessary to return the heart rhythm to a normal heartbeat. The shorter the time until defibrillation, the greater the chance the person will survive. Emergency squads use portable defibrillators and frequently there are public access defibrillators (AEDs) in public locations that are intended to be available for use by citizens who observed the cardiac arrest (see following for more information).

4. *Early Advanced Care.* After successful defibrillation, most patients require hospital care to treat and prevent future events.

These four steps can increase survival as high as 90 percent if initiated within the first minutes after SCD. Survival decreases by about

10 percent each minute longer. Those who survive have a good long-term outlook.

To Learn CPR

Learning CPR is the largest gift you can give your family and friends. CPR is easy for most adults and teens to learn. It is a technique designed to temporarily circulate oxygenated blood through the body of a person whose heart has stopped. It involves:

- Assessing the airway
- Breathing for the person
- Determining if the person is pulseless and applying pressure to the chest to circulate blood

To learn more about CPR:

- Contact your local American Heart Association
- Call the national American Heart Association at 1-800-AHA-USA1, or
- Go to the American Heart Association website at www.americanheart.org.
- Home training programs are available through a program called CPR prompt. See www.complient.com for more information.

More about Automatic External Defibrillators

Automatic external defibrillators (AEDs) are defibrillators with computers that are able to recognize ventricular fibrillation (VF), advise the operator that a shock is needed, and deliver the shock. AEDs are designed to be used by a wide range of personnel such as fire department personnel, police officers, lifeguards, flight attendants, security guards, teachers, and even family members of high-risk persons. The goal is to provide access to defibrillation when needed as quickly as possible. CPR along with AEDs can dramatically increase survival rates for sudden cardiac death.

Can SCD Be Prevented?

If you have any of the risk factors for SCD, it is important that you speak with your doctor about possible steps to reduce the risk of SCD. Sudden cardiac death (SCD) events are prevented by:

- Evaluation
- Prevention Strategies

Evaluation

Your doctor will want to evaluate you if you have risk factors for SCD or have had a SCD event. Evaluation includes:

- History—Information by the patient and those who have witnessed the patient's SCD event (if the patient has had one) is very helpful to prevent future risk. The doctor will ask about:
  - Prior history of SCD
  - Family history of SCD, Long QT syndrome, or cardiomyopathies
  - Use of medications that may prolong the QT interval
  - Symptoms: syncope (fainting, dizziness), dyspnea (shortness of breath), chest pain, palpitations (fluttering in chest)
  - History of any of the risk factors for SCD mentioned previously
- Diagnostic tests—these tests help determine what caused the SCD event: ECG, ejection fraction, ambulatory monitoring, echocardiography, cardiac catheterization, electrophysiology study

Prevention

Primary Prevention

The goal of primary prevention is to decrease the risk of sudden cardiac death in those who have never had an event. Treatment is aimed at identifying those at high risk and treating the risk factors. If you have any of the risk factors listed previously, it is important to speak to your doctor about possible steps to reduce your risk.

- *Medications*: To help reduce the risk of SCD occurring, doctors may prescribe medications to patients who have had heart attacks, heart failure, or those with specific arrhythmias (irregular heart rhythms). If your doctor prescribes a medication, he or she will tell you more about why you are taking it. It is important to know:
  - the names of your medications
  - what they are for
  - how often and at what times to take them

- *Risk factor modification*: If you have coronary artery disease, and even if you do not, there are certain lifestyle changes that can be made to reduce the risk of SCD. These include reducing high blood pressure and cholesterol, quitting smoking, losing weight, exercising regularly, and eating a healthy diet. Patients and families should know the signs and symptoms for coronary artery disease and the steps to take if symptoms occur. If you have any questions about risk factors for heart disease or how to make these changes, ask your doctor for advice.

- *Implantable cardioverter-defibrillator (ICD)*: For patients whose risk factors put them at great risk for SCD (history of ventricular tachycardia, post heart attack with poor left ventricular function [ejection fraction], or those with specific genetic heart defects), an ICD may be inserted as a primary prevention treatment. The ICD is a small machine, similar to a pacemaker, that is designed to constantly monitor the heart rhythm. When it detects a very fast or slow abnormal heart rhythm, it delivers energy to the heart muscle to cause the heart to beat in a normal rhythm again. The ICD also records the data of each abnormal heartbeat, which can be viewed by the doctor through a third part of the system kept at the hospital.

- *Interventional procedures or coronary artery bypass surgery*: For patients with known coronary artery disease, a procedure such as angioplasty or bypass surgery may be needed to improve blood flow to the heart muscle and prevent future coronary events.

Secondary Prevention

Once someone has survived sudden cardiac death, the goal is to decrease the risk of future events:

- *Medications*: Antiarrhythmic medications are given to prevent future ventricular tachycardia or fibrillation. Because everyone is different, it may take trials of several medications and doses to find the one that works best for you.

- *Risk factor modification*: Those at risk for cardiac events should target risk factors and treat them through lifestyle changes and medications. Patients and families should know the signs and symptoms for coronary artery disease and the steps to take if symptoms occur.

- *Implantable cardioverter-defibrillator (ICD)*

- *Interventional procedures or coronary artery bypass surgery*: For those who have significant coronary artery disease, decreased blood flow to the heart can cause areas of ischemia (lack of oxygen-rich blood flow to the heart muscle). These areas of heart muscle can be more irritable, causing life-threatening heart rhythms. Bypass surgery or angioplasty returns blood flow to the heart muscle. These procedures, combined with an ICD, can be a life-saving treatment.

- *LV reconstruction surgery combined with ablation*: When a heart attack occurs in the left ventricle (left lower pumping chamber of the heart), a scar forms. The scarred tissue may make the heart more prone to ventricular tachycardia. The electrophysiologist (doctor specializing in electrical disorders of the heart) can determine the exact area causing the arrhythmia. The electrophysiologist, working with your surgeon, may combine ablation (the use of high-energy electrical energy to "disconnect" abnormal electrical pathways within the heart) with surgical removal of the infarcted (dead) area of heart tissue.

A Note about SCD and Athletes

One cannot discuss SCD without touching upon SCD and athletes. Although SCD occurs rarely in athletes, when it does happen, it often affects us with shock and disbelief. How can this happen to someone who is so "healthy?"

- **Cause:** Most cases of SCD are related to undetected heart disease. In the younger population, it is often due to congenital heart defects, while in older athletes (thirty-five years and older), the cause is more often related to coronary artery disease.

- **Prevalence:** SCD in athletes occurs rarely; however the media often makes it seem like it happens more often. It is estimated that in the younger population, most SCD occurs while playing team sports, in about 1 in 100,000 to 1 in 300,000 athletes, and more often in males. In older athletes, it occurs more often during running or jogging and in approximately 1 in 15,000 joggers and 1 in 50,000 marathon runners.

- **Screening:** The American Heart Association recommends cardiovascular screening for high school and collegiate athletes and should include:

- Complete and careful personal and family history
- Physical exam

Screening should be repeated every two years with a history obtained every year.

Men older than forty years and women older than fifty years should also have an:

- Exercise stress test
- Education about cardiac risk factors and symptoms

If heart problems are identified or suspected, the athlete should be referred to a cardiologist for further evaluation and treatment guidelines prior to participating in sports.

What to Do If You Witness Sudden Cardiac Death

Dial your local emergency personnel immediately (9-1-1 in most areas) and initiate CPR. If done properly, CPR can save a person's life.

If there is a public access defibrillator (AED) available, the best chance of survival includes defibrillation with that device.

CPR plus defibrillation = rescue.

After successful defibrillation, most people require hospital care.

Sources

Sra, J., Dhala, A., Blanck, Z., Deshpande, S., Cooley, R., Akhtar, M. (1999) Sudden Cardiac Death, *Cardiology,* 24, 461–540.

Kern, K. B., Paraskos, J. A. (2000) Task Force 1: Cardiac Arrest, *JACC,* 35, 832–53.

AHA (1998) CPR (on-line). Available: www.americanheart.org/Heart/CPR/PAD/brochure.html

AHA (1996) Cardiovascular Preparticipation Screening of Competitive Athletes: A Statement for Health Professionals From the Sudden Death Committee and Congenital Cardiac Defects Committee, *Circulation,* 94, 850–56, (on-line). Available: http://www.americanheart.org/Scientific/statements/1996/089601.html

Wilkoff, B. Sudden Cardiac Death, *Cleveland Clinic Health Talk,* 2002.

Chapter 30

Silent Ischemia

Cardiac ischemia happens when an artery becomes narrowed or blocked for a short time, preventing oxygen-rich blood from reaching the heart. If ischemia is severe or lasts too long, it can cause a heart attack (myocardial infarction) and can lead to the death of heart tissue. In most cases, a temporary blood shortage to the heart causes angina pectoris. But in certain other cases, there is no pain. These cases are called silent ischemia.

Silent ischemia may also disturb the heart's rhythm. Abnormal rhythms such as ventricular tachycardia or ventricular fibrillation can interfere with the heart's pumping ability and can cause fainting or even sudden cardiac death.

How common is silent ischemia, and who is at risk?

An estimated four million Americans—mostly men over age sixty-five—have episodes of silent ischemia. People who have had previous heart attacks or those who have diabetes are especially at risk for silent ischemia. Heart muscle disease (cardiomyopathy) that is caused by silent ischemia is among the four most common causes of heart failure in the United States.

Major risk factors include

- Previous heart attacks

Reprinted from "Silent Ischemia," © 2000 Norfolk County Cardiology Associates, www.nocard.com. Reprinted with permission.

223

- Coronary artery disease
- Diabetes
- High blood pressure (Hypertension)
- Smoking
- Obesity
- Cardiomyopathy
- Alcohol and drug abuse

What are the symptoms of silent ischemia?

Silent ischemia has no symptoms, but researchers have found that if you have noticeable chest pain, you may also have episodes of silent ischemia.

How is silent ischemia diagnosed?

The following tests can be used to diagnose silent ischemia:

- An exercise stress test can show blood flow through your coronary arteries in response to exercise, usually walking on a treadmill.

- Holter monitoring records your heart rate and rhythm over a twenty-four-hour period (or more). You wear a recording device (the Holter monitor), which is connected to disks on your chest. Doctors can then look at the printout of the recording to find out if you have had episodes of silent ischemia.

How is ischemia treated?

Lifestyle Changes

Treatment for ischemia is similar to that for any form of cardiovascular disease and usually begins with the following lifestyle changes:

- If you smoke, quit.
- Control high blood pressure, cholesterol, and diabetes.
- Limit how much alcohol you drink.
- Adopt healthy eating habits.
- Start an exercise program that has been approved by your doctor.

Medicines and Surgery

Treatment focuses on improving blood flow to your heart and on reducing your heart's oxygen demands. You may receive aspirin, blood-thinning medicines (anticoagulants), or other blood-thinning agents to prevent blood clots from forming. Oxygen may be given to increase the oxygen content of the blood still flowing through your heart. Pain-killers may be used for pain.

Some patients receive drugs aimed at slowing their heart rate, opening and relaxing their blood vessels, and otherwise reducing the burden on the heart. Most patients respond well to these medicines. Those who do not respond well may need a transcatheter intervention (such as balloon angioplasty), coronary artery bypass surgery, or a related procedure.

Chapter 31

Arrhythmias

The Normal Cardiac Cycle

During each heartbeat, the two upper chambers (right and left atria) contract, followed by contraction of the two lower pumping chambers (right and left ventricles). This action is coordinated by the heart's electrical system.

Normal electrical activation of the heart occurs in an orderly fashion. With each beat, the electrical impulse starts in the sinus (or sinoatrial) node (in the right atrium). The impulse spreads through the atria, stimulating the atria to contract. The impulse then reaches the atrioventricular node (AV node), an electrical bridge that allows impulses to go from the atria to the ventricles. There is a short delay in conduction before the impulse goes on to the ventricles. From the AV node, the impulse travels through a pathway of fibers called the His-Purkinje system. This network sends the impulse into the muscular walls of the ventricles and causes them to contract. The contraction pumps blood out of the heart to the lungs and throughout the body.

The rate at which the normal heart beats depends on the body's need for oxygen-rich blood. When at rest, the body needs less oxygen-rich blood, so the heart rate may be slower. However, during activity or exercise, the body needs more oxygen-rich blood, and the sinus node causes the heart rate to increase. Taking a pulse tells how fast the heart is beating.

Taking Your Pulse

You can feel your pulse on your wrist. Place your index and middle finger on the inner wrist of your other arm, just below the base of your thumb. Your heart rate, or pulse, is the number of beats felt in one minute. You can count the number of beats in 10 seconds and multiply by 6 to determine your heart rate in beats per minute. By feeling your pulse, you can also tell if your heart rhythm is regular or not.

Your Heart Rate = Pulse in 10 seconds x 6 = _____ beats per minute

What Is an Arrhythmia?

An arrhythmia (also called dysrhythmia or irregular heart rhythm) is an irregular or abnormal heartbeat.

Arrhythmias may have many causes, including coronary artery disease, changes in the heart muscle (cardiomyopathy), valve disorders, electrolyte imbalances in your blood (such as sodium or potassium), injury from a heart attack, or the healing process after heart surgery. A fast or slow heart rate does not always mean your heart rhythm is abnormal. Fast or slow heart rates are also related to normal causes, including anxiety, activity, medications, or other normal causes.

Common Types of Arrhythmias

A normal heart rate is fifty to one hundred beats per minute. Here are some common arrhythmias:

- **Tachycardia:** a fast heart rhythm with a rate of more than 100 beats per minute.

- **Bradycardia:** a slow heart rhythm with a rate below 60 beats per minute.

- **Supraventricular arrhythmias:** arrhythmias that begin above the ventricles, such as in the upper chambers, or atria. "Supra" means above; "ventricular" refers to the lower chambers of the heart (ventricles).

- **Premature atrial contractions (PACs):** early, extra beats that originate in the upper chambers of the heart (atria).

- **Paroxysmal supraventricular tachycardia (PSVT):** a rapid, usually regular rhythm originating from above the ventricles. PSVT begins and ends suddenly.

- **Accessory pathway tachycardias** (e.g., Wolff-Parkinson-White syndrome): a fast heart rhythm due to an extra abnormal electrical pathway or connection between the atria and ventricles. The impulses travel through the extra pathways as well as the usual route. This allows the impulses to travel around the heart very quickly, causing the heart to beat unusually fast.

- **AV nodal reentrant tachycardia (AVNRT):** a fast heart rate due to having more than one pathway through the atrioventricular (AV) node.

- **Atrial tachycardia:** a rapid heart rhythm originating in the atria.

- **Atrial fibrillation:** a very common irregular heart rhythm. Many impulses begin and spread through the atria, competing for a chance to travel through the AV node. The resulting rhythm is disorganized, rapid, and irregular. Because the impulses are traveling through the atria in a disorderly fashion, there is a loss of coordinated atrial contraction.

- **Atrial flutter:** an atrial arrhythmia due to one or more rapid circuits in the atrium. Atrial flutter is usually more organized and regular than atrial fibrillation.

- **Ventricular arrhythmias:** arrhythmias that begin in the lower chambers of the heart.

- **Premature ventricular contractions (PVCs):** early, extra beats beginning in the lower chambers of the heart. PVCs are common. Most of the time they cause no symptoms and require no treatment. In some people, they can be related to stress, too much caffeine or nicotine, or exercise. But sometimes, PVCs can be caused by heart disease or electrolyte imbalance. People who have a lot of PVCs, or symptoms associated with them, should be evaluated by a cardiologist (heart doctor).

- **Ventricular tachycardia (V-tach):** a rapid rhythm originating from the lower chambers of the heart. The rapid rate prevents the heart from filling adequately with blood, and less blood is able to pump through the body. This can be a more serious arrhythmia, especially in people with heart disease, and may be associated with more symptoms. This condition should be evaluated by a cardiologist.

- **Ventricular fibrillation:** an erratic, disorganized firing of impulses from the ventricles. The ventricles quiver and cannot generate an effective contraction, causing an inability to deliver blood to the body. This is a medical emergency that must be treated with cardiopulmonary resuscitation (CPR) and defibrillation as soon as possible.

- **Long QT:** the QT interval is the area on the electrocardiogram (ECG or EKG) that represents the time it takes the for the heart muscle to contract and then recover, or for the electrical impulse to fire and then recharge. When the QT interval is longer than normal, it increases the risk for "torsade de pointes," a life-threatening form of ventricular tachycardia.

- **Bradyarrhythmias:** slow heart rhythms which may arise from disease in the heart's conduction system, such as the sinus (or sinoatrial, SA) node, AV node or, HIS-Purkinje system.

- **Sinus node dysfunction:** slow heart rhythms due to an abnormal SA node.

- **Heart block:** a delay or complete block of the electrical impulse as it travels from the sinus node to the ventricles. The level of the block or delay may occur in the AV node or HIS-Purkinje system. The heart may beat irregularly and often, more slowly.

What Are the Symptoms of an Arrhythmia?

An arrhythmia may be "silent" and not cause any symptoms. A doctor can detect an irregular heartbeat during an examination by taking the person's pulse or through a test called an electrocardiogram (ECG).

If symptoms occur, they may include:

- Palpitations: a feeling of skipped heart beats, fluttering, "flip-flops," or feeling that the heart is "running away"
- Pounding in the chest
- Dizziness or feeling lightheaded
- Fainting
- Shortness of breath

- Chest discomfort
- Weakness or fatigue (feeling very tired)

How Are Arrhythmias Diagnosed?

After evaluating a patient's symptoms and performing a physical examination, the cardiologist may perform a variety of diagnostic tests to help confirm the presence of an arrhythmia and indicate its causes.

Some tests that may be done to confirm the presence of an arrhythmia include:

- **Electrocardiogram (ECG):** a picture, on graph paper, of the electrical impulses traveling through the heart muscle, recorded by electrodes attached to the chest, arms, and legs.

- **Ambulatory monitors:** there are several types:
  - A **Holter monitor** is a small portable recorder that is attached to electrodes on the chest and that can record the heart rhythm continuously for twenty-four hours at a time.
  - A **transtelephonic monitor** records events when the patient is hooked to electrode leads connected to a device that can transmit the rhythm over a telephone.
  - A **transtelephonic monitor with a memory loop** can be worn continuously for prolonged periods and records and saves the rhythm around the time that an event button is activated. After recording, the rhythm recorded and saved can be transmitted over the telephone.

- **Stress test:** an exercise test which may be particularly useful in recording arrhythmias that can be brought on with stress or exercise. This test may also be helpful in determining if there is underlying heart disease or coronary artery disease associated with an arrhythmia.

- **Echocardiogram:** an ultrasound of the heart may be useful in determining if there is any associated heart muscle or valve disease that may be causing an arrhythmia.

Cardiac catheterization: during this test, using local anesthetics, a catheter is inserted into a blood vessel and guided to the heart with the aid of an x-ray machine. A contrast dye is injected through the catheter so that x-ray movies of the coronary arteries, heart chambers, and valves may be taken. This test may be ordered by a physician to determine if the cause of an arrhythmia is coronary artery disease and to give information about how well the heart muscle and valves are working.

- **Electrophysiology study (EPS):** a special heart catheterization that studies the heart's electrical system. The catheters inserted can record the electrical activity within the heart and are used to help find the cause of the rhythm disturbance and the best treatment. During the test, the arrhythmia may be safely reproduced and terminated.

- **Head upright tilt test (HUT):** a test used to safely reproduce fainting spells in people that may be prone to these episodes. During the test, the patient is tilted on a special table to 60 or more degrees upright. Blood pressure and heart rhythm are recorded. In susceptible individuals, a fainting spell may be provoked. A medication that may bring on these spells may also be used during the tilt procedure.

How Are Arrhythmias Treated?

Treatment depends on the type and seriousness of the arrhythmia. In some cases, no treatment is necessary. Treatment options may include medications, lifestyle changes, cardioversion, pacemakers, implantable cardioverter-defibrillators, catheter ablation, or surgery.

Medications

Antiarrhythmic drugs are medications used to convert the arrhythmia to sinus rhythm. Other medications include heart-rate control drugs; anticoagulant or antiplatelet therapy (drugs, such as warfarin—a "blood thinner"—or aspirin, that reduce the risk of clots forming or strokes.)

It is important to know the names of your medications, what they are for, and how often and at what times to take them.

Lifestyle Changes

If you notice that your irregular heart rhythm occurs more often with certain activities, you should avoid them.

- If you smoke, stop.
- Limit your intake of alcohol.

- Limit or stop using caffeine. Some people are sensitive to caffeine and may notice more symptoms when using caffeinated products (such as tea, coffee, colas, and some over-the-counter medications).

- Beware of stimulants used in cough and cold medications. Some of these medications contain ingredients that promote irregular heart rhythms. Read the label and ask your doctor or pharmacist what medication would be best for you.

Electrical Cardioversion

In patients with persistent arrhythmias (such as atrial fibrillation), a normal rhythm may not be achieved with drug therapy alone. After administration of a short-acting anesthesia, an electrical shock is delivered to your chest wall that synchronizes the heart and allows the normal rhythm to restart.

Permanent Pacemaker

A device that sends small electrical impulses to the heart muscle to maintain a normal heart rate. Pacemakers primarily prevent the heart from beating too slowly. The pacemaker has a pulse generator (which houses the battery and a tiny computer) and leads (wires) that send impulses from the pulse generator to the heart muscle, as well as sense the heart's electrical activity. Newer pacemakers have many sophisticated features that are designed to help with the management of arrhythmias and to optimize heart-rate-related function as much as possible.

Implantable Cardioverter-Defibrillator (ICD)

A sophisticated device used primarily to treat ventricular tachycardia and ventricular fibrillation, two life-threatening heart rhythms. The ICD constantly monitors the heart rhythm. When it detects a very fast, abnormal heart rhythm, it delivers energy to the heart muscle to cause the heart to beat in a normal rhythm again.

There are several ways an ICD can restore a normal heart rhythm:

- **Anti-tachycardia pacing, or ATP:** When the heart beats too fast, a series of small electrical impulses may be delivered to the heart muscle to restore a normal heart rate and rhythm.

- **Cardioversion:** a low-energy shock may be delivered at the same time as the heartbeat to restore a normal heart rhythm.

- **Defibrillation:** when the heart is beating dangerously fast or irregularly, a higher energy shock may be delivered to the heart muscle to restore a normal rhythm.

- **Anti-bradycardia pacing:** many ICDs provide backup pacing to prevent too slow a heart rhythm

Catheter Ablation

During an ablation, energy is delivered through a catheter to a small area of tissue inside the heart that causes the abnormal heart rhythm. This energy "disconnects" the pathway of the abnormal rhythm. Ablation is used to treat PSVTs, atrial flutter, and some atrial and ventricular tachycardias. It can also be used to disconnect the electrical pathway between the atria and the ventricles, which may be useful in people with atrial fibrillation. Ablation may be combined with other procedures to achieve optimal treatment.

Heart Surgery

This may be needed to correct a heart problem that may be causing the arrhythmia. The Maze procedure is a type of surgery used to correct atrial fibrillation. During this procedure, a series of incisions are made in the right and left atria to confine the electrical impulses to defined pathways.

Chapter 32

Heart Failure

Heart failure (sometimes known as congestive heart failure [CHF]) is a serious condition in which the heart is not pumping well enough. In late stages, the heart is unable to meet the body's demand for oxygen. Heart failure is so named because the heart is failing to pump efficiently, which often results in congestion in the lungs. As a result, the heart tries to work harder, which only makes the problem worse.

Conditions that could lead to heart failure include the following:

- Coronary artery disease
- High blood pressure (hypertension)
- Heart attack
- Diabetes mellitus
- Cardiomyopathy
- Heart valve disease (e.g., valvular stenosis or valvular regurgitation)
- Infection in the heart valves (valvular endocarditis) or of the heart muscle (myocarditis)
- Congenital heart disease (cardiac conditions present since birth)

- Severe lung disease (e.g., pulmonary hypertension) or obstructive sleep apnea
- Pericardial disease (pericarditis)

According to current statistics from the American Heart Association, there are about five million heart failure patients in the United States, and 550,000 new cases of heart failure diagnosed in the United States every year. This includes ten out every one thousand people over the age of sixty-five. Of newly diagnosed patients under the age of sixty-five, 80 percent of the men and 70 percent of the women will die within eight years. In people diagnosed with heart failure, sudden cardiac death occurs at six to nine times the rate of the general population.

What is heart failure?

Heart failure is a serious condition in which the heart is not pumping well enough. In late stages, the heart is unable to meet the body's demand for oxygen. Like a traffic jam, this can lead to congestion within the lungs as blood flows backward from the heart. Once this congestion begins, the patient may experience shortness of breath (dyspnea) that initially occurs only during exercise, and later even while at rest.

Affecting about five million Americans, heart failure has been called an "American Epidemic." The prevalence of heart failure in the United States is due in part to the increasing age of the population— the risk of heart failure increases as one ages. Additionally, while fewer people are dying from heart disease because of the range of treatments available (e.g., medication, angioplasty and stenting, surgery), more people are living with disability from heart disease (e.g., heart muscle damage from a heart attack that leads to heart failure).

In spite of its name, heart failure does not necessarily indicate that the heart has completely stopped, which is the case when someone has gone into cardiac arrest. Heart failure means the heart is operating at a decreased efficiency level and, therefore, is working harder to try and make up for the shortcoming in function. For example, the heart may pump more frequently to compensate for its weakened pumping ability. The longer the heart overworks itself to compensate for its shortcomings, the more its pumping ability is damaged and the more likely that serious pumping failure will result. The increased workload of the heart may lead to changes in various parts of the body, as they try to compensate for the heart's weakened ability to function. These changes can include the following:

- **Remodeling**. A significant physical change known as remodeling occurs with heart failure. Remodeling is most notably characterized by enlargement of the heart's left ventricle. In addition, the left ventricle becomes thinner. There is an increased use of oxygen, greater degree of mitral valve regurgitation, and decreased ejection fraction. The process is a complex one. Contributing factors include the release of hormones in response to inflammation brought on by heart failure, or the extent to which a person's genes determine how the heart adapts after it is injured or diseased. Whatever the causes, left ventricular remodeling sets in motion an unhealthy domino effect, as progressive damage to heart cells leads to reduced cardiac output and more severe heart disease. This weakening may be "global," as in cardiomyopathy, or regional, affecting only part of the left ventricle (e.g., heart attack).

- **Hypertrophy** of the heart walls. The heart walls may thicken in an attempt to strengthen their pumping ability.

- **Tachycardia**. An abnormally fast heartbeat that could result from the heart's attempt to function more efficiently.

- **Kidney malfunction**. Initially, the kidneys respond to the heart's low volume output by retaining water and salt. The kidneys perceive a low-volume state, as if the person is dehydrated, and respond in kind. Unfortunately, the kidneys' response actually worsens the fluid buildup, and can contribute to high blood pressure. This places added stress on the filters in the kidneys (nephrons), and is a major cause of kidney failure.

Although the term "heart failure" usually refers to the chronic condition described in this chapter, there is also a condition known as acute heart failure. It is sudden in onset and usually results from a sudden catastrophic change in the heart (e.g., massive heart attack, endocarditis, ruptured or torn heart valve leaflets, aortic dissection). In acute heart failure, the heart muscle does not have time to hypertrophy and enlarge. This condition is often fatal, even if emergency medical treatment is received immediately.

Which conditions could lead to heart failure?

There are a variety of conditions that could lead, or are associated with, heart failure. These conditions include the following:

- **Coronary artery disease (CAD)**. One of the most common causes of heart failure in the United States. CAD is a chronic disease in which there is a "hardening" of the arteries (atherosclerosis) on the surface of the heart. The term "hardening" refers to a condition that causes the arteries to become so narrowed and stiff that they block the free flow of blood. Severely reduced blood flow to the heart may weaken the heart muscle.

- **Arrhythmia**. A serious arrhythmia (abnormal heart rhythm) can diminish the effectiveness of the heart's pumping ability.

- **Heart attack** (myocardial infarction). Following a heart attack, part of the heart muscle is replaced with scar tissue that prevents the heart from working efficiently. As the weakened heart muscle struggles to pump blood, the muscle fibers of the heart stretch, resulting in enlarged and weakened chambers in the heart (remodeling). The AHA estimates that about 22 percent of patients who suffer a heart attack will become disabled with heart failure within six years.

- **High blood pressure** (hypertension). High blood pressure has been called the single most common risk factor for the development of heart failure. Nearly 75 percent of all heart failure cases involve patients with previously diagnosed hypertension. Uncontrolled high blood pressure causes the heart muscle to overwork itself in order to pump blood under high pressure throughout the body. Increases in blood pressure are also associated with a greater incidence of heart attack.

- **Cardiomyopathy**. A type of chronic heart disease in which the heart muscle becomes abnormally enlarged, thickened, or stiffened. As a result, the heart muscle's ability to pump blood can become increasingly weakened, leading to heart failure. This condition is seen with viral infections or alcohol abuse, but in many patients, the cause is never found.

- **Valvular heart disease**. Narrowing (stenosis) or leaking (regurgitation) of one or more of the heart's four valves. The resulting blood flow restriction (in stenosis) or overload of blood (in regurgitation) can lead to heart failure. These patients are initially treated with medication, but will often require valve surgery. There may also be an infection in the heart valves (valvular endocarditis). Valvular disease is most often a result of the aging process, but may also be a type of congenital heart disease (present from birth). Less commonly, it results from rheumatic heart disease.

- **Congenital heart disease**. A heart-related problem that is present from birth. It involves one or more defects in the heart (e.g., ventricular septal defect, atrial septal defect), the veins leading to the heart, the arteries leaving the heart, or connections among these various parts of the body. Heart failure may develop if the congenital defect creates a blood flow problem (e.g., because of a hole in the heart) or a heart muscle strength problem (e.g., because of a narrowed valve).

- Severe **lung disease** (e.g., pulmonary hypertension). When the right side of the heart cannot generate enough force to pump blood through a diseased pair of lungs, heart failure can result.

Other conditions that are associated with heart failure include:

- **Obstructive sleep apnea (OSA)**. A condition commonly found among individuals with heart failure. Muscles in the back of the throat normally work to keep the throat open, but the airway can become blocked if the muscles relax during sleep. When the brain detects a drop in oxygen from not breathing, it quickly sends a signal to the chest muscles and diaphragm to gulp in air. As a result, the sleeper makes a gasping or snorting sound and is awakened. This struggle to breathe and arousal from sleep causes tension in the left ventricle and increases in heart rate, blood pressure, and the body's demand for oxygen. This increases the risk for developing ischemia, arrhythmia, chronic high blood pressure, pulmonary hypertension, and carotid artery disease. Treatment includes continuous positive airflow pressure (CPAP), in which a bedside machine delivers air continuously through a plastic mask over the nose. The predetermined air pressure acts as a splint to keep the airway open, while still allowing the person to exhale. CPAP has been shown to be effective in lowering blood pressure and increasing ejection fraction, suggesting that the relief of obstructive sleep apnea can also impact on symptoms of heart failure.

- **Anemia**. Anemia is a deficiency in red blood cells or hemoglobin, the iron-rich, oxygen-carrying molecules in red blood cells. Chronic, severe anemia can be a cause of heart failure, and can worsen as heart failure progresses. Even mild to moderate anemia is a common finding in patients with heart failure. This is because the heart must work harder in order to circulate a decreased number of red blood cells throughout the body. Studies have shown that correcting anemia can improve heart failure. Patients treated with a combination of intravenous (IV) iron and injections of erythropoietin (a protein that increases red blood cell production) have exhibited an increased ejection fraction, decreased need for diuretics, and improved New York Heart Association (NYHA) class.

- **Clinical depression.** There appears to be a link between clinical depression and overall cardiovascular health, with recent studies showing that heart failure patients who suffer from depression are more likely to experience an increase in their heart failure symptoms and a decrease in their overall quality of life over time. It is believed that clinical depression may trigger higher levels of stress hormones (e.g., adrenaline), which may help to explain why the hearts of clinically depressed people beat faster, even during sleep. Studies have also shown that people with both heart disease and clinical depression have reduced heart rate variability (the heart's ability to handle stress).

- **Diabetes mellitus.** Diabetes is a strong risk factor for developing coronary artery disease or heart attack, which may lead to heart failure and also cardiomyopathy. In addition, people with diabetes who also have heart failure should use caution when taking thiazolidinediones (TZDs), a class of drugs for patients with type 2 diabetes. TZDs may increase fluid retention in some people with heart failure. Joint recommendations from the American Heart Association and the American Diabetes Association state that people with moderate to severe (New York Heart Association [NYHA] class III or IV) heart failure should not take TZDs. Patients who are taking medications for diabetes are encouraged to discuss their condition with their physician.

Other conditions that are associated with heart failure include lupus, rheumatoid arthritis, hyperthyroidism, certain chemotherapy drugs, alcohol abuse, and abuse of some types of drugs (primarily amphetamines and cocaine).

The risk of developing heart failure is also increased by the presence of certain risk factors, which include the following:

- Smoking
- Obesity (a body mass index [BMI] of 30 or greater)
- Lack of exercise

- Dietary habits, such as high salt intake or the failure to take medication properly
- Uncontrolled high blood pressure
- Arrhythmias
- Worsening lung disease (emphysema) or pulmonary embolism
- Infection
- Emotional distress
- Certain medications
- Fluid overload
- Hyper- or hypothyroidism (thyroid diseases)

What are the different types of heart failure?

There are a number of different types of heart failure, which are classified according to which side of the heart is more affected, which phase of the heartbeat is more affected, and how severe the condition is.

Two types of heart failure are identified according to which side of the heart is most affected:

- Left-sided heart failure occurs when the left ventricle cannot adequately pump oxygen-rich blood from the heart to the rest of the body. The main symptoms for this condition include shortness of breath, fatigue, and coughing, especially at night or while lying down. There may also be lung congestion (with both blood and fluid).

- Right-sided heart failure (cor pulmonale) takes place when the right ventricle is not pumping adequately, which tends to cause fluid buildup in the veins and swelling (edema) in the legs and ankles. Right-sided heart failure usually occurs as a direct result of left-sided heart failure. It can also be caused by severe lung disease (e.g., chronic obstructive pulmonary disease, pulmonary hypertension) in which the right side of the heart cannot generate enough force to pump blood through a diseased pair of lungs.

Two other types of heart failure are identified according to which phase of the heart's pumping cycle is more affected:

- Systolic heart failure means that the heart is unable to pump out adequate amounts of blood during its contraction (systole).

Lung congestion and swelling (edema) of the lower extremities are typical symptoms of systolic heart failure.

- Diastolic heart failure refers to the heart's inability to relax between contractions (diastole) and allow enough blood to enter the ventricles. Symptoms are identical to systolic heart failure. Diastolic heart failure is often a precursor to systolic heart failure. Patients with diastolic heart failure may or may not have normal systolic function. Diastolic dysfunction causes about one-third of all heart failure in people over age sixty-five.

Picture the heart as a balloon. Systolic heart failure is when the heart muscle is weak and flabby, like an old, worn-out balloon. Diastolic heart failure is when the heart muscle is stiff and hard, like a brand-new, never-inflated balloon. Neither extreme allows the heart to function properly, leading to a buildup of blood in the lungs and shortness of breath (dyspnea). Heart failure tends to get progressively worse over time. The New York Heart Association classification describes four levels of heart failure, each more serious than the one before it. These levels are as follows (with approximate percentage of patients):

- **Class I**: No obvious symptoms, no limitations on patient physical activity (35 percent of heart failure patients).

- **Class II**: Some symptoms during or after normal activity, mild physical activity limitations (35 percent of heart failure patients).

- **Class III**: Symptoms with mild exertion, moderate to significant physical activity limitations (25 percent of heart failure patients).

- **Class IV**: Significant symptoms at rest, severe to total physical activity limitations (5 percent of heart failure patients).

The American Heart Association (AHA) and American College of Cardiology (ACC) have put forth another classification, which emphasizes the importance of treating the causes and risk factors for heart failure prior to the actual onset of symptoms. Aggressive treatment of high blood pressure, diabetes mellitus, and coronary artery disease could prevent development of symptomatic heart failure. The AHA/ACC stages are:

- **Stage A**: The patient is at high risk for heart failure, but has no heart abnormalities.

- **Stage B**: The patient has structural abnormalities of the heart, but no symptoms.

- **Stage C**: The patient has past or present symptoms associated with heart disease.

- **Stage D**: The patient has end-stage disease, requiring specialized treatment (e.g., continuous intravenous [IV] drug therapy, left ventricular assist device, heart transplant).

How do age, gender, and race affect heart failure risk?

The American Heart Association estimates that nearly five million Americans are currently living with heart failure. While heart failure occurs in every age, gender, and racial group, its development tends to show different patterns in some groups than in others, but is most commonly seen in the elderly.

Comparing the incidence and course of heart failure between Caucasian and African Americans is provocative. Studies have found that, in Caucasian patients, heart failure most often occurs as a result of coronary artery disease (CAD), such that CAD develops directly into systolic heart failure. African Americans, however, tend to progress more gradually from hypertension (high blood pressure), to heart wall thickening, to diastolic heart failure, and finally to systolic heart failure. Statistics also show African American heart failure patients to be younger and more likely female, as compared to Caucasian patients. In addition, African Americans with heart failure are more likely to be diagnosed with hypertension and diabetes. While some studies have shown that African Americans have higher heart failure mortality rates than whites, other studies have shown similar survival rates between the two racial groups. The reasons for these differences are still being investigated.

Research has uncovered a significant difference in the way heart failure appears in older patients, according to a study sponsored by the National Heart, Lung and Blood Institute. The Cardiovascular Health Study examined the rates and types of heart failure found in more than 5,800 individuals age sixty-five and over. Incidences of heart failure were greater among men in the trial than women and increased progressively with age. In addition, heart failure rates were higher among patients with a history of diabetes, atrial fibrillation (a heart rhythm disorder), or mild kidney failure.

What are the signs and symptoms of heart failure?

Symptoms of heart failure are related to "pooling" of fluid in the lungs or legs, or may be secondary to decreased blood flow to other organs. These symptoms may develop over a lengthy span of time, even over a period of years. Because they may not seem important on their own, people may not seek treatment until heart failure has caused significant damage. They include the following:

- Shortness of breath (dyspnea). This is one of the earliest symptoms of heart failure. The patient gets winded and fatigued more quickly than before, just by doing regular daily activities or even lying in bed. There is also decreased tolerance to exercise, and the muscles may feel weaker than before.
- Swelling (edema) of the legs is another common symptom in heart failure, though it could also be caused by unrelated conditions.
- Swollen neck veins.
- Abdominal discomfort such as swelling, pain, or nausea.
- Mental confusion.
- Galloping heartbeat (palpitations).
- Kidney malfunction or failure (in the later stages of heart failure).

In addition to the symptoms listed here, which the patient may notice, the physician may also be able to detect signs of congestive heart failure, which include the following:

- An abnormal heart murmur (a telltale sign of a valve-related disorder).
- A crackling sound of fluid in the lungs (rales), which is a sign of pulmonary congestion.
- A rapid heartbeat (tachycardia) or abnormal heart rhythm (arrhythmias).
- Swelling and fluid retention (edema) in the liver or gastrointestinal tract (in advanced stages of heart failure).
- Hypertrophy or enlargement of the heart.
- Liver malfunction.

How is heart failure diagnosed?

Heart failure is typically diagnosed based on a medical history and complete physical examination, which includes a blood pressure check, listening to the patient's heart through a stethoscope, and taking the patient's pulse. A chest x-ray may also be taken to evaluate the size and shape of the heart, as well as to view the lung and any fluid that may have built up. A blood test that measures levels of B-type natriuretic peptide (BNP), a protein that is produced by the heart as it fails, may also be drawn. Additional tests that a physician may use to determine the cause and severity of heart failure include:

- **Blood tests**. Traditional tests evaluate potential causes of heart failure, such as anemia and thyroid function, and electrolytes and kidney function. However, a new test may be effective in diagnosing heart failure. The blood test measures levels of B-type natriuretic peptide (BNP), a protein that is produced by the heart as it fails.

- **Echocardiogram** of the heart and major arteries. This test uses ultrasound technology to closely examine the overall muscle function of the heart, allowing the physician to evaluate the size, thickness, and pumping action of the heart, and how well the heart valves are functioning. A stress echocardiogram may also be useful in assessing how well the heart is functioning at rest and during exercise. An echocardiogram is the single most important test for the diagnosis of heart failure.

- **Electrocardiogram** (EKG). A test that measures the heart's electrical activity. It is designed to detect any abnormal heart rhythms, heart enlargement, cardiac ischemia, or heart attack.

- **Exercise stress test**. A test in which an EKG is performed at rest and then under the physical stress of exercise, to compare the heart's performance at rest and during times of physical exertion.

- **Radionuclide imaging** tests, such as a radionuclide stress test or ventriculogram. These provide contrast images of the heart, which can pinpoint areas of damage and dysfunction and determine how well the heart is pumping.

- **Chest roentgenography** (x-ray) to evaluate the size and shape of the heart, as well as to view the lungs and any fluid that may have built up.

More invasive exploratory tests may be ordered in conjunction with, or instead of, the preceding. These tests include a coronary angiogram, in which a contrast dye is delivered by catheter to the coronary arteries to visualize the blood vessels and identify heart damage or dysfunction.

How is heart failure treated?

Heart failure is the result of what may have been years of prolonged damage and overwork. The earlier it is detected and treated, the better a patient's long-term chances for survival. Treatment is also directed to patients at risk for heart failure prior to the development of disease.

Most patients are advised to make lifestyle changes, regardless of the severity of their condition. These may include modifying their diet, limiting salt intake, achieving and maintaining a healthy weight, learning and practicing stress management skills, quitting smoking, and getting regular exercise, depending on the severity of the illness.

Lifestyle choices that are more specific to heart failure may include the following:

- Limiting physical activity until approved by one's physician, and then staying as active as possible. Heart failure patients who exercise regularly typically show significant improvement, whereas heart failure patients who were inactive showed a clear decline. In studies, Tai Chi (an ancient Chinese workout involving slow relaxing movements) has been shown to benefit patients living with heart failure. However, exercise in any form is beneficial. Patients should consult their physician before beginning an exercise program.

- Scheduling relaxation and rest periods throughout the day.

- Avoiding excessive fluid intake.

- Keeping a diary of one's daily weight, and notifying one's physician if there is a weight gain of three or more pounds in a single week (which may indicate fluid retention and the need for an immediate change in treatment). Patients experiencing weight loss in spite of what appears to be adequate calorie intake should also discuss their situation with their physician. A study has found that some patients with heart failure may need to adjust their diet to meet increased energy needs.

Patients with heart failure should always consult their physician before taking any over-the-counter medicines, vitamins, or herbal supplements.

Depending upon the nature of the underlying damage or malfunction that leads to heart failure, medications may be prescribed to reduce the heart's workload, affect remodeling, counter abnormal hormonal levels, increase blood flow, widen vessels, or eliminate excess water from the body. Medications used to treat heart failure and related conditions include the following:

- **ACE inhibitors**. A type of vasodilator that expands blood vessels to allow blood to flow easier and more freely, allowing the heart to pump more efficiently. ACE inhibitors act by preventing the production of a chemical that causes blood vessels to tighten and narrow. ACE inhibitors lower blood pressure so that the heart does not have to work as hard to pump blood. Reports from the National Institutes of Health indicate that the use of ACE inhibitors has been the most significant factor in heart failure survival rate improvement over recent years. They also have a favorable impact on the heart itself (e.g., affecting remodeling).

- **Angiotensin II receptor blockers** may also be used in conjunction with ACE inhibitors. They can also be used in patients who cannot take ACE inhibitors or beta blockers.

- **Beta blockers**. May prevent progression of the disease and improve symptoms by slowing the heart's contraction rate and reducing its pumping action, thus lessening the heart's workload. For many years beta blockers were considered inappropriate for people with heart failure because they can potentially weaken the heart muscle and cannot be used when the patient's health is unstable. Recent studies have shown that selected beta blockers may be very helpful in treating heart failure. They have been shown to decrease mortality and improve left ventricular function in these patients. Beta blockers also reduce the likelihood that these patients will suffer from significant heart rhythm problems.

- **Diuretics**. Often referred to as water pills, these reduce the symptoms of congestion by helping to flush away excess salt and fluids from the body. They are very useful in treating people with heart failure and fluid retention. Spironolactone, a "potassium-sparing" diuretic, has been found to be effective therapy in patients with severe heart failure.

- **Inotropes**. Intravenous drugs that increase the force of the heart's contractions, allowing the heart to beat less frequently and more effectively. Individuals with severe heart failure often benefit from being hospitalized and being given these powerful medicines intravenously for twenty-four to forty-eight hours.

- **Digoxin.** A weak inotrope, digoxin appears to have an effect on hormones that make heart failure worse. It helps the heart contract more vigorously and effectively, and helps to reduce the symptoms of heart failure. It is most often used to control the fast heart rate of atrial fibrillation. It may be ineffective in women with heart failure and abnormal rhythm.

It is important to note that when heart failure is a result of underlying damage or decreased blood flow due to blocked arteries or high blood pressure (hypertension), the goal of treatment is usually to relieve the symptoms of these conditions. In some cases (e.g., heart failure caused by acute ischemia), heart failure can be reversed once the underlying condition has been treated. For most people, however, heart failure is a chronic and progressive condition that can be managed but rarely cured.

Depending upon the severity of the damage and dysfunction, interventional procedures may be necessary. These procedures include the following:

- **Balloon angioplasty.** A catheter-based procedure in which plaque is pressed back against artery walls to make more room for blood to flow through the artery.

- **Coronary stenting.** The insertion of a wire mesh metal tube called a stent into a clogged vessel in order to help keep it open.

In the most serious cases, surgery may be necessary. These procedures include:

- **Coronary artery bypass surgery**, for patients with severe or total artery blockage.

- **Heart valve surgery**, in patients with severe valvular regurgitation or valvular stenosis

- **Pacemaker** insertion to correct the slow heart rhythm (bradycardia) that can worsen heart failure.

- **Cardiac resynchronization** (e.g., biventricular pacemaker) to coordinate the contraction of the right and left ventricles in patients with heart failure.

- **Implantable cardioverter defibrillator** (ICDs) to monitor for and, if necessary, correct episodes of life-threatening (arrhythmias). ICDs are sometimes used in combination with a biventricular pacemaker.

- **Aneurysm surgery** in selected patients.

- **Heart transplant surgery**, in the most severe cases.

- Insertion of a **left ventricular assist device** prior to transplant surgery.

What heart failure treatment options are on the horizon?

A variety of new therapies are currently being studied for use in treating heart failure. They include:

- **Total artificial heart**. The Food and Drug Administration (FDA) has approved clinical trials for a fully implantable total artificial heart. The grapefruit-sized device is powered by a battery that can be recharged from outside the body without the need for tubes to remain connected through the skin. Subjects of the study are end-stage heart failure patients who are not eligible for a heart transplant, cannot be helped by other available therapies, and are at imminent risk of death.

- **Vascular endothelial growth factor (VEGF)**. A form of therapeutic angiogenesis currently being studied in a trial named VIVA (VEGF for Ischemia in Vascular Angiogenesis). Phase I clinical trials of intracoronary (directly into the heart) and intravenous (IV) injection of VEGF have shown promising results. Researchers found that patients experienced significant improvement in angina and quality of life by day 120 of the trial. Research is still ongoing.

- **Heart jacket**. A synthetic, elastic material that is surgically attached and wrapped around the heart surface. The mesh-like fabric supports the ventricles (the heart's lower chambers), providing a snug fit but without constricting the heart. The goal is to reverse remodeling of the left ventricle. Remodeling was assumed to be irreversible, but recent successes with beta blockers and ventricular assist devices show that remodeling can be improved. In earlier animal and now human studies, the heart jacket support device demonstrated that it does more than keep the left ventricle from enlarging. It can actually re-shape and restore it to a more normal form. This led to a significant decrease in the process of self-destruction of heart muscle cells—another hallmark of heart failure. There was a rise in cardiac output as well as improved ejection fraction. Even with the success of the device so far, it is expected that patients receiving heart jackets will continue their medications (e.g., beta blockers).

- **Heart valve repair**. When a heart becomes enlarged it often prevents the heart's valves from properly closing, allowing blood to leak back in the wrong direction (regurgitation). Certain heart valve surgeries can implant an annuloplasty ring to restore the normal dimensions of the valve, allowing it to come together properly. These surgeries are common as treatments for valvular heart disease, and have recently been shown to be successful in treating heart failure.

What are the prospects for recovery from heart failure?

Many patients who are hospitalized for heart failure—almost one million each year in the United States alone—can return to a modified version of their everyday routine within weeks or months, depending upon the severity of their condition. Regardless of the nature and severity of heart failure, each patient is encouraged to avoid physical and emotional stress as much as possible, rest often (although supervised exercise can be beneficial to certain patients), avoid extreme temperatures, and report to a physician any symptom changes (e.g., weight gain) that may be a sign of fluid retention.

Fifty percent of heart failure patients survive past the five-year mark, but the condition is responsible for about 50 percent of all heart-related deaths. While heart failure is most prevalent in older populations (about ten out of every one thousand people over age sixty-five are diagnosed with heart failure), it can affect people of all ages. Chances of survival are based on the cause and severity of heart failure, as well as lifestyle changes that the patient chooses to make (e.g., taking all medications as instructed, eating a heart-healthy diet, and quitting smoking).

The earlier the condition is diagnosed and treatment begins, the better a patient's prospects for an improved quality of life down the road.

About HeartCenterOnline

HeartCenterOnline is a cardiovascular specialized health care website providing tools to help patients and their families better understand the complex nature of heart-related conditions, treatments, and preventive care. The website includes a library of physician-edited patient education information, interactive health-tracking tools, and an online cardiovascular community for patients, their families and other site visitors.

HeartCenterOnline
One South Ocean Boulevard, Suite 201
Boca Raton, FL 33432
http://www.heartcenteronline.com

Chapter 33

Cardiomyopathy

What is cardiomyopathy?

Cardiomyopathy is a serious disease in which the heart muscle becomes inflamed and doesn't work as well as it should. There may be multiple causes including viral infections.

Cardiomyopathy can be classified as primary or secondary. Primary cardiomyopathy can't be attributed to a specific cause, such as high blood pressure, heart valve disease, artery diseases, or congenital heart defects. Secondary cardiomyopathy is due to specific causes. It's often associated with diseases involving other organs as well as the heart.

There are three main types of cardiomyopathy—dilated, hypertrophic, and restrictive.

What is dilated (congestive) cardiomyopathy?

This is the most common form. In it, the heart cavity is enlarged and stretched (cardiac dilation). The heart is weak and doesn't pump normally, and most patients develop congestive heart failure. Abnormal heart rhythms called arrhythmias and disturbances in the heart's electrical conduction also may occur.

Blood flows more slowly through an enlarged heart, so blood clots easily form. A blood clot that forms in an artery or the heart is called a thrombus. A clot that breaks free, circulates in the bloodstream, and blocks a small blood vessel is called an embolus.

- Clots that stick to the inner lining of the heart are called mural thrombi.

- If the clot breaks off the right ventricle (pumping chamber), it can be carried into the pulmonary circulation in the lung, forming pulmonary emboli.

- Blood clots that form in the heart's left side may be dislodged and carried into the body's circulation to form cerebral emboli in the brain, renal emboli in the kidney, peripheral emboli, or even coronary artery emboli.

A condition known as Barth syndrome, a rare and relatively unknown genetically linked cardiac disease, can cause dilated cardiomyopathy. This syndrome affects male children, usually during their first year of life. It can also be diagnosed later. (For more information on Barth syndrome, visit the Barth Syndrome Foundation at http://www.barthsyndrome.org.)

In these young patients the heart condition is often associated with changes in the skeletal muscles, short stature, and an increased likelihood of catching bacterial infections. They also have neutropenia, which is a decrease in the number of white blood cells known as neutrophils. There are clinical signs of the cardiomyopathy in the newborn child or within the first months of life. These children also have metabolic and mitochondrial abnormalities.

How is dilated (congestive) cardiomyopathy treated?

A person with cardiomyopathy may suffer an embolus before any other symptom of cardiomyopathy appears. That's why anti-clotting (anticoagulant) drug therapy may be needed. Arrhythmias may require anti-arrhythmic drugs. More rarely, "heart block" may develop, requiring an artificial pacemaker. Therapy for dilated cardiomyopathy is sometimes disappointing, however. If the person is young and otherwise healthy, and if the disease gets worse and worse, a heart transplant may be considered.

When cardiomyopathy results in a significantly enlarged heart, the mitral and tricuspid valves may not be able to close properly, resulting in murmurs. Blood pressure may increase because of increased sympathetic nerve activity. These nerves can also cause arteries to narrow. This mimics hypertensive heart disease (high blood pressure). That's why some people have high blood pressure readings. Because the blood pressure determines the heart's workload and oxygen needs, one treatment approach is to use vasodilators (drugs that "relax" the arteries). They lower blood pressure and thus the left ventricle's workload.

What is hypertrophic cardiomyopathy?

In this condition, the muscle mass of the left ventricle enlarges or "hypertrophies."

In one form of the disease, the wall (septum) between the two ventricles (pumping chamber) becomes enlarged and obstructs the blood flow from the left ventricle. The syndrome is known as hypertrophic obstructive cardiomyopathy (H.O.C.M.) or asymmetric septal hypertrophy (A.S.H.). It's also called idiopathic hypertrophic subaortic stenosis (I.H.S.S.).

Besides obstructing blood flow, the thickened wall sometimes distorts one leaflet of the mitral valve, causing it to leak. In over half the cases, the disease is hereditary. Close blood relatives (parents, children, or siblings) of such persons often have enlarged septums, although they may have no symptoms. This disease is most common in young adults.

In the other form of the disease, nonobstructive hypertrophic cardiomyopathy, the enlarged muscle doesn't obstruct blood flow.

The symptoms of hypertrophic cardiomyopathy include shortness of breath on exertion, dizziness, fainting, and angina pectoris. (Angina is chest pain or discomfort caused by reduced blood supply to the heart muscle.) Some people have cardiac arrhythmias. These are abnormal heart rhythms that in some cases can lead to sudden death. The obstruction to blood flow from the left ventricle increases the ventricle's work, and a heart murmur may be heard.

How is hypertrophic cardiomyopathy treated?

The usual treatment involves taking a drug known as a beta blocker (such as propranolol) or a calcium channel blocker. If a person has an arrhythmia, an anti-arrhythmic drug may also be used. Surgical treatment of the obstructive form is possible in some cases if the drug treatment fails.

Alcohol ablation is another nonsurgical treatment being developed for hypertrophic obstructive cardiomyopathy. It involves injecting alcohol down a small branch of one of the heart arteries to the extra heart muscle. This destroys the extra heart muscle without having to cut it out surgically.

People undergoing this procedure usually suffer chest pain during the alcohol injection. The alcohol can also disrupt normal heart rhythms and require the insertion of a pacemaker. Alcohol ablation is a relatively new procedure being performed at only a few specialized centers in the United States. It's too soon to know whether this treatment will result in long-term benefit. It's still considered experimental.

What is restrictive cardiomyopathy?

This is the least common type in the United States. The myocardium (heart muscle) of the ventricles becomes excessively "rigid," so it's harder for the ventricles to fill with blood between heartbeats. A person with restrictive cardiomyopathy often complains of being tired, may have swollen hands and feet, and may have difficulty breathing on exertion. This type of cardiomyopathy is usually due to another disease process.

Chapter 34

Valvular Disease

Valvular Disease Overview

Heart valve abnormalities are quite common and most often are not severe.

However, left undiagnosed and untreated, some can cause progressive deterioration in heart function, which can result in heart failure and premature death.

Valves are the doors to a healthy heart. Understanding how valves work clearly illustrates the essential role they play in efficient heart action.

Heart failure is the second most common cause of cardiac death, and valve diseases are among the most important causes of heart failure. Heart failure occurs when the heart fails to pump sufficient blood to enable the body to carry out its normal functions.

Even mild valvular heart disease is important to catch, because it can progress and become severe. Also, it can cause susceptibility to heart valve infection and, less frequently, stroke. However, if valve disease is diagnosed, these problems can be prevented.

The information on valvular disease is reprinted from "Valvular Disease," Howard Gilman Institute for Valvular Heart Diseases, © 2004. The website material is the property of The Howard Gilman Institute for Valvular Heart Diseases, Weill Medical College of Cornell University. Any reproduction without express permission of Weill Medical College is prohibited. Additional information on mitral-valve prolapse is reprinted from "Facts about Mitral-Valve Prolapse," National Heart, Lung, and Blood Institute, National Institutes of Health, NIH Publication No. 00-865, March 2000.

When valve disease is severe, symptoms frequently are absent until heart damage is well advanced. Therefore, too often, the patient is unaware that the disease is progressing. By the time it is caught, it can be too late—the patient may have irreversible heart damage and congestive heart failure or may suddenly die.

Usually, there is a long lag time between the onset of valvular heart disease and clinical problems. Heart valve abnormalities can be picked up through a careful physical examination. Even if a patient has no symptoms, the signs of disease will still be there.

Regular evaluation is the key to preventing serious heart disease caused by valve problems.

How Valves Work

The heart is a muscular pump divided into two separate but physically joined organs—the right heart and the left heart.

The left heart pumps blood via the aorta artery into the systemic arteries, bringing necessary oxygen and nutrients to all parts of the body. The right heart sends blood via the pulmonary artery into the smaller blood vessels of the lungs, allowing the lungs to extract oxygen efficiently and eliminate carbon dioxide.

The right and left hearts each have two chambers. The upper chambers are atria; the lower chambers are ventricles.

There are four heart valves—doors that keep the blood moving in a single direction through the heart. They are the:

- tricuspid valve, regulating blood flow between the right atrium and right ventricle

- pulmonic valve, managing blood flow between the right ventricle and pulmonary artery

- mitral valve, controlling blood flow between the left atrium and left ventricle

- aortic valve, regulating blood flow between the left ventricle and the aorta

Blood enters the heart through the right atrium, which then contracts and sends it to the right ventricle. The right ventricle contracts and propels the blood into the blood vessels of the lungs.

Full of oxygen, the blood leaves the lungs and reenters the heart through the pulmonary veins, which empty into the left atrium. The left atrium contracts and thrusts the blood into the left ventricle. The left ventricle contracts and sends the blood to the body and brain via the aorta and its branches.

During each heartbeat, valves open and close in a complex sequence that ensures efficient forward movement of blood.

The tricuspid and mitral valves open to allow blood to flow into the ventricles from the atria. During this time, the pulmonic and aortic valves are closed, preventing leakage back into the ventricles of the blood ejected during the previous beat.

As the newly filled ventricles contract, the pulmonic and aortic valves open, enabling blood to leave the heart. During this time, the mitral and tricuspid valves are closed, preventing blood from flowing back into the atria.

Valves are essential to the efficient movement of blood throughout the heart and into the body.

Each valve has a set of flaps known as leaflets or cusps. When the valves are in good working order the flaps open and close completely. If the valves are not working properly, the heart has to work harder than normal to pump blood.

Valve Diseases

Valvular heart disease occurs when one or more valves do not open or close properly, robbing the heart of its normal efficiency.

Types of Valvular Disease

Stenosis: When valves don't open completely, the condition is known as stenosis. When a valve is stenotic, blood has to flow through a smaller opening than normal, forcing the chamber behind the valve to pump blood more forcefully than usual. Stenosis results from progressive hardening or stiffening of valve leaflets from calcium deposits or scarring. This causes abnormal stress and strain on the heart muscle, which can become irreversibly weakened.

Regurgitation: When valves don't close completely, the condition is known as regurgitation or insufficiency. The valves, themselves, or supporting structures below, may be loose, torn, or distorted, allowing a gap to develop between the valve leaflets. If the valve doesn't close completely, blood leaks backward into the cardiac chamber at the same time it is receiving blood from the preceding chamber. This results in overstretching of the heart muscle, which, if sufficiently severe and prolonged, can permanently damage the heart muscle.

Causes of Valvular Diseases

Valvular heart diseases are caused by:

- hereditary (genetic) factors
  - congenital/structural heart malformations
  - abnormalities of the inner working of heart muscle cells in structurally normal hearts
- rheumatic fever
- bacterial infections such as infective endocarditis
- changes resulting from the aging process

Currently, most valve diseases result from genetically determined factors.

Who's at Risk

The real incidence of valve abnormalities among Americans is difficult to determine. However, a recent six-year survey indicates that the number of hospital discharges resulting from heart valve diseases has grown substantially throughout the nation. It is estimated that at least ten million Americans have some type of heart valve abnormality, while three to four million have disease severe enough to require surgery, at some time in their lives.

A recent survey used echocardiography to detect valvular regurgitation (valves with closing problems) among three thousand healthy people, ages eighteen through thirty-five, who were not known to have valvular disease.

Among those tested, 3.5 percent had leaking heart valves. If this percentage were applied to the total number of Americans between the ages of eighteen and thirty-five, it would mean that 8.5 million people in this age range have valvular insufficiency.

This number does not take into account Americans with severe or diagnosed disease. It does not factor in that valvular heart disease increases with age. Nor does it take into account patients with stenotic disease (valves that don't open completely).

Aortic stenosis is the most prevalent stenotic disease. Although some children have severe aortic stenosis, the disease usually develops between the ages of fifty and eighty, worsening progressively with age.

As the baby boom generation gets older, aortic stenosis will become a more prevalent heart problem.

Facts about Mitral-Valve Prolapse

The mitral valve is the heart valve between the left atrium and left ventricle. It has two flaps, called leaflets or cusps, which open and close when the heart contracts (beats) and rests.

Mitral-valve prolapse (MVP) is frequently diagnosed in healthy people and is, for the most part, harmless. Most people suffer no symptoms at all. New estimates are that about 2 percent of the adult population has the condition. MVP is also called floppy valve syndrome, Barlow's or Reid-Barlow's syndrome, ballooning mitral valve, midsystolic-click-late systolic murmur syndrome, or click murmur syndrome. MVP can be present from birth or develop at any age and occurs equally in both men and women. MVP is one of the most frequently made cardiac diagnoses in the United States.

What Is Mitral-Valve Prolapse?

The heart's valves work to maintain the flow of blood in one direction, ensuring proper circulation. The mitral valve controls the flow of blood into the left ventricle. Normally, when the left ventricle contracts, the mitral valve closes and blood flows out of the heart through the aortic valve and into the aorta to start its journey to all other parts of the body.

In MVP, the shape or dimensions of the leaflets of the valve are not ideal; they may be too large and fail to close properly or they balloon out, hence the term "prolapse." When the valve leaflets flap, a clicking sound may be heard. Sometimes the prolapsing of the mitral valve allows a slight flow of blood back into the left atrium. This is called "mitral regurgitation," and may cause a sound called a murmur. Some people with MVP have both a click and a murmur and some have only a click. Many have no unusual heart sounds at all; those who do may have clicks and murmurs that come and go.

Diagnosis

Sometimes, once a physician has heard the characteristic sounds of MVP through a stethoscope, other tests may be ordered. Echocardiography is a common and painless test that uses very high frequency sound waves. The sound waves travel through the layers of the skin and muscle to produce an image of the heart that can be seen on a screen. In this sense, it is similar to radar or sonar imaging.

Initially, "M-mode" echocardiography was used. This technology provides a single-plane view of the mitral valve and often resulted in

261

overdiagnosis of MVP in the 1970s and 1980s. A study from the National Heart, Lung, and Blood Institute's (NHLBI) Framingham Heart Study, reported in the July 1, 1999, issue of the *New England Journal of Medicine*, indicated that MVP is less common and less serious than previously thought.

The investigators used standard echocardiography equipment along with new, more accurate criteria that minimize false positive and false negative diagnoses. Whereas earlier estimates put the number of people with MVP at 5 to 35 percent of the population, the new NHLBI study showed the number is closer to 2 percent. In addition,

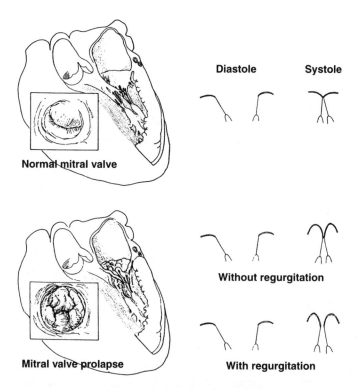

Figure 34.1. *The heart is shown with a normal mitral valve and a prolapsed mitral valve. The line drawings show the valves in diastole, the period of relaxation, and systole, the period of contraction. Regurgitation, if it occurs, occurs during systole. The illustration is by Howard Bartner based upon photographs from the Laboratory of Dr. William C. Roberts. National Heart, Lung, and Blood Institute.*

MVP has long been thought to be more prevalent in women than men but the new study reported that the condition appears with similar frequency in both men and women.

In light of this new information, NHLBI suggests that people who have been diagnosed with MVP since the 1970s discuss their current health status with their health care provider to determine if a new diagnostic test is warranted.

Symptoms

The vast majority of people with MVP have no discomfort at all. Most are surprised to learn that their heart is functioning in any way abnormally. Some individuals report mild and common symptoms such as shortness of breath, dizziness, and either "skipping" or "racing" of the heart. More rarely, chest pain is reported. However, these are symptoms that may or may not be related to the MVP.

Treatment

In most cases, no treatment is needed. For a small proportion of individuals with MVP, beta-blockers or other drugs are used to control specific symptoms and some blood pressure lowering drugs may be used to treat mitral regurgitation. Serious problems are rare, and can easily be diagnosed and, if necessary, treated surgically.

Preventing Complications

The overwhelming majority of people with MVP are free of symptoms and never develop any noteworthy problems. However, it is important to understand that in some cases mitral regurgitation, the flow of blood back into the left atrium, can occur. Where mitral regurgitation has been diagnosed, there is an increased risk of acquiring bacterial endocarditis, an infection in the lining of the heart. To prevent bacterial endocarditis, many physicians and dentists prescribe antibiotics before certain surgical or dental procedures. Patients with significant mitral regurgitation should be followed more closely by their physician so that medical therapy and, if necessary, surgery, can be pursued at the appropriate time.

Clinical Significance

As stated, people with MVP have no symptoms and never develop any notable problems. Whether or not there is any discomfort, however, patients should notify their health care providers of the existence of MVP. This will allow decisions and recommendations to be made about the advisability of using antibiotics to protect against bacterial endocarditis.

Chapter 35

Congenital Heart Defects

Signs and Symptoms of Heart Defects

Parents should be alert to the following symptoms in infancy:

- Tires easily during feeding (i.e., falls asleep before feeding finishes)
- Sweating around the head, especially during feeding
- Fast breathing when at rest or sleeping
- Pale or bluish skin color
- Poor weight gain
- Sleeps a lot—not playful or curious for any length of time
- Puffy face, hands, or feet
- Often irritable, difficult to console

Some children with congenital heart defects may not have any symptoms until later in childhood. Things to look for include:

"Signs and Symptoms of Heart Defects" is reprinted with permission from The Congenital Heart Information Network, http://www.tchin.org. © 2003. All rights reserved. "Facts about Congenital Heart Defects" is reprinted from "Congenital Heart Defects," © 2004 March of Dimes Birth Defects Foundation. All rights reserved. For additional information, contact the March of Dimes at their website, http://www.marchofdimes.com. To purchase a copy of this article from the March of Dimes, call 800-367-6630.

- Gets out of breath during play
- Difficulty "keeping up" with playmates
- Tires easily/sleeps a lot
- Change in color during active play or sports (looks pale or has a bluish tint around mouth and nose)
- Frequent colds and respiratory illnesses
- Slow growth and weight gain/poor appetite
- Complains of chest pain or heart pounding

If your child has two or more of these symptoms, talk to your pediatrician about a referral to a pediatric cardiologist.

Facts about Congenital Heart Defects

More than 32,000 infants (one out of every 125 to 150) are born with heart defects each year in the United States. The defect may be so slight that the baby appears healthy for many years after birth, or so severe that its life is in immediate danger.

Heart defects are among the most common birth defects, and are the leading cause of birth defect-related deaths. However, advances in diagnosis and surgical treatment over the past forty years have led to dramatic increases in survival for children with serious heart defects. Between 1987 and 1997, the death rates from congenital heart defects dropped 23 percent.

What is a congenital heart defect?

A condition is called congenital when it is present at birth. Heart defects originate in the early part of pregnancy when the heart is forming. Congenital heart defects can affect any of the different parts or functions of the heart.

How does the heart work?

The heart is a muscle that pumps blood to the body. It is divided into four hollow parts called chambers. Two chambers are located on the right side of the heart, and two are on the left.

Within the heart are four valves (one-way openings) that let the blood go forward and keep it from going back. Blood goes from the heart to the lungs where it picks up oxygen. The blood carrying oxygen, which appears bright red, goes back to the heart. The heart then pumps the oxygen-rich blood through the body by way of arteries. As the oxygen is used up by the body's tissues and organs, the blood becomes dark and returns by way of veins to the heart, where the process starts over again.

How do heart defects affect a child?

Some babies and children with heart defects experience no symptoms. The heart defect may be diagnosed if the doctor hears an abnormal sound, referred to as a murmur. Children with normal hearts also can have heart murmurs. These are called "innocent" or "functional" murmurs. A physician may suggest tests to rule out a heart defect.

Certain heart defects prevent the heart from pumping adequate blood to the lungs or other parts of the body. This can cause congestive heart failure. An affected child may experience a rapid heartbeat and breathing difficulties, especially during exercise (or in infants, during feeding—sometimes resulting in inadequate weight gain). Swelling of the legs or abdomen or around the eyes also may occur.

Some heart defects result in a pale grayish or bluish coloring of the skin (called cyanosis), usually appearing soon after birth or during infancy. On occasion, it may be delayed until later in childhood. It is a sign of defects that prevent the blood from getting enough oxygen. Children with cyanosis may tire easily. Symptoms such as shortness of breath and fainting often worsen when the child exerts himself. Some youngsters may squat frequently to ease their shortness of breath.

What causes congenital heart defects?

In most cases, scientists do not know what makes a baby's heart develop abnormally. Both genetic and environmental factors appear to play roles.

Among the few environmental factors known to contribute to congenital heart defects are a virus and certain drugs. Women who contract rubella (German measles) during the first three months of pregnancy have a high risk of having a baby with a heart defect. Other viral infections also may contribute.

Certain medications also increase the risk. These include the acne medication Accutane, lithium (used to treat certain forms of mental illness), and, possibly, certain anti-seizure medications. Drinking alcohol in pregnancy also can increase the risk of heart defects—babies with fetal alcohol syndrome (FAS) often have them. Studies also suggest that use of cocaine in pregnancy increases the risk of these birth defects.

Certain chronic illnesses in the mother also can increase the risk of heart defects. For example, women with diabetes are at increased risk of having a baby with a heart defect, although this risk can be reduced or eliminated if the diabetes is closely controlled, starting before pregnancy. Women with an inborn error of body chemistry called phenylketonuria (PKU) also are at high risk of having a baby with a heart defect, unless they follow a special diet before pregnancy and during the first trimester. Several studies suggest that women who do not consume enough of the B vitamin folic acid before and during the early weeks of pregnancy are at increased risk of having a baby with a heart defect.

While most families have no more than one child with a heart defect, these malformations are more likely to occur in siblings or offspring of people who have heart defects than in unaffected families. This fact has long suggested that genetics plays a role in heart defects, at least in those families. In fact, scientists have recently discovered more than one hundred mutations (changes) in more than a dozen genes that directly impair the heart. Many of these mutations cause cardiomyopathy (enlargement of the heart) or heart rhythm disturbances that can be fatal in childhood, adolescence, or adulthood.

However, scientists also have pinpointed several mutations that affect the formation of the heart, leading to congenital heart malformations. For example, in 1999 a March of Dimes grantee at the University of Texas Southwestern Medical Center in Dallas discovered a gene that appears to contribute to a common, important group of malformations affecting the heart's outflow tract and the blood vessels arising from it. Researchers at Harvard Medical School identified a gene responsible for the heart defect called atrial septal defect (a hole between the upper chambers of the heart) in four families with multiple members affected by heart disease. The same researchers also identified another gene mutation that causes atrial septal defects accompanied by arm and hand malformations (Holt-Oram syndrome).

Researchers appear to be on the brink of discovering the genes that underlie numerous heart defects. They have recently identified several genes that direct development of the embryonic heart in mice. This should greatly improve our understanding of these genes' human counterparts—and possibly lead to ways to prevent the various heart defects that mutations of those genes may cause.

Heart defects also can be part of a wider pattern of birth defects. For example, more than one-third of children with the chromosomal abnormality Down syndrome (characterized by mental retardation and physical birth defects) have heart defects, as do about a quarter of girls with another chromosomal abnormality called Turner syndrome (short stature, lack of sexual development, and other problems). In fact, approximately 10 percent of children with heart defects have a chromosomal abnormality. Children with Down, Turner, and certain other chromosomal abnormalities should be routinely evaluated for heart defects. Heart defects also are common in children with a variety of inherited disorders, including: Noonan (short stature, learning disabilities), Alagille (liver and other problems), Marfan (skeletal and eye defects), and Williams (mental retardation) syndromes.

How are congenital heart defects treated?

The outlook has never been brighter for babies and children with congenital heart defects. Today, most heart defects can be corrected, or at least helped, by surgery, medicine, or devices such as artificial valves and pacemakers. In the last thirty years, advances in treatment of heart defects have enabled nearly one million U.S. children with significant heart defects to survive into adulthood. Half the children who require surgical repair of a heart defect now undergo surgery before age two. Until fairly recently, it was often necessary to make temporary repairs and postpone corrective surgery until later in childhood. Early corrective surgery often prevents development of additional complications and allows the child to live a more normal life sooner. Some of the most common defects include:

- **Patent ductus arteriosus.** Before birth, much of a fetus's blood goes through a passageway (ductus arteriosus) from one blood vessel to another instead of through the lungs, because the lungs are not yet in use. The passageway should close soon after birth, so the blood can take the normal route from heart to lungs and back. If it doesn't close, blood doesn't flow correctly. This problem occurs most frequently in premature babies. In some cases, drug treatment can help close the passageway. If that doesn't work, surgery can close it.

- **Septal defects.** If the defect is a hole in the wall (septum) that divides the two upper or two lower chambers, the blood can't circulate as it should and the heart has to work too hard. A surgeon can close the hole by sewing or patching it. Small holes may heal by themselves or not need repair at all.

- **Coarctation of the aorta.** Part of the aorta, the large artery that sends blood from the heart to the rest of the body, may be too narrow for the blood to flow evenly. A surgeon can cut away the narrow part and sew the open ends together, replace the constricted section with man-made material, or patch it with part of a blood vessel taken from elsewhere in the body. Sometimes, this narrowed area can be widened by inflating a balloon on the tip of a catheter inserted through an artery.

- **Heart valve abnormalities.** Some babies are born with heart valves that do not close normally or are narrowed, closed, or blocked and prevent blood from flowing smoothly. Surgeons usually can repair the valves or replace them with man-made ones. Balloons on catheters also are frequently used to fix faulty valves.

- **Tetralogy of Fallot.** A combination of four heart defects keeps some blood from getting to the lungs, so that a baby has episodes of cyanosis and may grow poorly. New surgical techniques allow early repair of this complex heart defect, so that most affected children live normal or near-normal lives.

- **Transposition of the great arteries.** Here, the positions of the two major arteries leaving the heart are reversed, so that each arises from the wrong pumping chamber. Recent surgical advances have enabled correction of this otherwise lethal defect in the early newborn period.

- **Hypoplastic left heart syndrome.** A combination of defects results in a left ventricle (the heart's main pumping chamber) that is too small to support life. This defect is the most common cause of death from congenital heart disease. New surgical procedures and heart transplants have begun to save some of these babies, but the long-term outlook for these babies remains uncertain.

Children and adults with certain heart defects, even after surgical repair, remain at increased risk of infection involving the heart and its valves. Parents of children with heart defects and adults with repaired heart defects should discuss with their doctor whether they need to take antibiotics before certain dental and surgical procedures in order to prevent these infections.

Is there a prenatal test for congenital heart defects?

A special form of sonography (looking at the fetus by means of sound waves) called echocardiography can accurately identify many heart defects. If certain heart problems, such as a heart that is beating too fast or too slowly, are diagnosed before birth, medications may restore a normal heart rhythm before the fetal heart starts to fail. In other cases, where the heart defect can't be treated before birth, knowing that it exists enables doctors to be ready to give the baby the treatment it needs as soon as it is born.

Can congenital heart defects be prevented?

While most congenital heart defects cannot yet be prevented, there are some steps a woman can take that may help reduce her risk of having a baby with a heart defect. A woman should be tested prior to pregnancy for immunity to rubella, and vaccinated if she is not immune. Pregnant women should avoid alcohol and unprescribed drugs. Those with chronic health conditions such as diabetes, seizure disorders, and PKU should consult their doctors before they attempt to conceive so that their medications or diets can be adjusted. Any woman who could become pregnant should take a multivitamin containing 400 micrograms of folic acid daily to reduce the risk of serious birth defects of the brain and spinal cord and, possibly, other birth defects including heart defects.

Genetic counselors can tell parents of affected children roughly what the chances are that any future child of theirs will have a heart defect. Siblings of an affected child are slightly more likely than other children to have the same kind of heart defect as their brother or sister. In some cases, if the affected child's heart defect is part of a syndrome of other defects, the recurrence risk may be higher. Parents who themselves have a heart defect also are at increased risk of having a child with a heart defect.

What research is under way on congenital heart defects?

Scientists funded by the March of Dimes are among many who are trying to learn more about the causes of heart defects, so that they can develop better ways of preventing and treating them. For example, several March of Dimes grantees are studying genes that may underlie specific heart defects. While nearly all heart defects are attributed to interactions of unknown genes with usually unknown environmental factors, few causal genes have yet been linked with specific heart defects. Grantees also are seeking to develop better ways to treat babies with serious heart defects.

References

American Heart Association. "Congenital Cardiovascular Disease." *Heart and Stroke A–Z Guide*. American Heart Association, 2000.

Brickner, M. E., et al. "Congenital Heart Disease in Adults, Part 1." *New England Journal of Medicine* 342, no. 4 (January 27, 2000): 256–63.

Brickner, M. E., et al. "Congenital Heart Disease in Adults, Part 2." *New England Journal of Medicine* 342, no. 5 (February 3, 2000): 334–42.

Lewin, M. B. "The Genetic Basis of Congenital Heart Disease." *Pediatric Annals* 29, no. 8 (August 2000): 469–80.

Morris, C. D., et al. "Thirty-Year Incidence of Infective Endocarditis after Surgery for Congenital Heart Defect." *Journal of the American Medical Association* 279, no. 8 (February 25, 1998): 599–603.

Chapter 36

Patent Foramen Ovale (PFO)

Have you or someone you know had a stroke or TIA (transient is-chemic attack or mini-stroke) "out of the blue" with no obvious risk factors? Did doctors check to see if the stroke or TIA might have been caused by a "hole" in the heart called a patent foramen ovale (PFO)?

About one in five Americans has a PFO. Many don't know it until a medical condition like a stroke or TIA occurs. PFOs often have no symptoms but they may increase your risk for stroke and TIA. Many PFO-related strokes are called cryptogenic, meaning they have no apparent cause.

What is a PFO?

All people are born with flaplike openings in their hearts. But, for most, the opening closes by itself shortly after birth. In some people, an open flap remains between the two upper chambers of the heart (the left and right atria). This opening can allow a blood clot from one part of the body to travel through the flap and up to the brain, caus-ing a stroke.

What can you do about it?

The first step is to get a diagnosis. An ultrasound of the heart, called an echocardiogram, can show doctors if a PFO is present. The

---

Reprinted with permission from the National Stroke Association, http://www.stroke.org. © 2002 National Stroke Association. All rights reserved.

second step is to discuss with your doctor the treatment options. Currently, there are two main treatment methods for PFO: medications or PFO closure, which can include open-heart surgery or a newer procedure that closes the flap without major surgery.

The medications don't treat the actual PFO. They can control clotting factors in the blood so stroke-causing blood clots are less likely to form in the first place. Open-heart surgery is rarely used for people who don't respond to the medications. With any major surgery, patients and their doctors need to weigh the risks of the surgery with the benefits before moving ahead with this treatment option. In recent years, a new approach has been developed enabling doctors to seal the PFO without major surgery.

An implanted closure device, which can resemble a tiny two-ended umbrella, is delivered to the PFO using a small tube threaded to the heart from a vein in the thigh. The implant is inserted through the flap and released from the tube. It expands and tissue grows in and around the implant to seal the PFO from both sides. This procedure requires minimal recovery time. Currently, the U.S. Food and Drug Administration allows this treatment method only for "humanitarian" uses, meaning that the procedure is used only for people who don't respond to medications and have already had a second stroke.

What research is being done?

Which is the better treatment option: medication or PFO closure? That question still needs to be answered. The good news is that research now is being conducted to see if PFO-closure implant procedures are better than medications at helping reduce the risk of recurrent stroke in stroke and TIA survivors. However, the only way scientists will have meaningful research studies is if they have enough people participating.

If you or someone you know has had a PFO-related stroke or TIA, you may want to consider participating in a clinical trial. As a participant in a clinical trial, you will be carefully evaluated by doctors and receive extensive follow-up care. During your treatment, you may also receive the latest version of a current PFO closure device. The FDA has approved a prior version of this device, and more than fifteen thousand people around the world have been treated with this procedure. You will also be helping medical science find the most effective treatment to lower the number of PFO-related strokes and TIAs.

Chapter 37

Rheumatic Heart Disease

Rheumatic Heart Disease/Rheumatic Fever

What Are Rheumatic Heart Disease and Rheumatic Fever?

Rheumatic heart disease is a condition in which the heart valves are damaged by rheumatic fever.

Rheumatic fever begins with a strep throat from streptococcal infection.

Rheumatic fever is an inflammatory disease. It can affect many of the body's connective tissues—especially those of the heart, joints, brain or skin. Anyone can get acute rheumatic fever, but it usually occurs in children five to fifteen years old. The rheumatic heart disease that results can last for life.

What Are the Symptoms of Rheumatic Heart Disease?

Symptoms vary greatly. Often the damage to heart valves isn't immediately noticeable. A damaged heart valve either doesn't fully close or doesn't fully open.

Eventually, damaged heart valves can cause serious, even disabling, problems. These problems depend on how bad the damage is and which heart valve is affected. The most advanced condition is congestive heart failure. This is a heart disease in which the heart enlarges and can't pump out all its blood.

How Can I Prevent Rheumatic Heart Disease?

The best defense against rheumatic heart disease is to prevent rheumatic fever from ever occurring. By treating strep throat with penicillin or other antibiotics, doctors can usually stop acute rheumatic fever from developing.

People who've already had rheumatic fever are more susceptible to attacks and heart damage. That's why they're given continuous monthly or daily antibiotic treatment, maybe for life. If their heart has been damaged by rheumatic fever, they're also given a different antibiotic when they undergo dental or surgical procedures. This helps prevent bacterial endocarditis, a dangerous infection of the heart's lining or valves.

Additional Information about Rheumatic Fever

Definition

Rheumatic fever is an inflammatory disease which may develop after an infection with streptococcus bacteria (such as strep throat or scarlet fever) and can involve the heart, joints, skin, and brain.

Causes, Incidence, and Risk Factors

Rheumatic fever is common worldwide and is responsible for many cases of damaged heart valves. While it is far less common in the United States since the beginning of the twentieth century, there have been a few outbreaks since the 1980s.

Rheumatic fever primarily affects children between ages six and fifteen and occurs approximately twenty days after strep throat or scarlet fever. In up to a third of cases, the underlying strep infection may not have caused any symptoms.

The rate of development of rheumatic fever in individuals with untreated strep infection is estimated to be 3 percent. Persons who have suffered a case of rheumatic fever have a tendency to develop flare-ups with repeated strep infections.

Symptoms

- Fever
- Joint pain, migratory arthritis—involving primarily knees, elbows, ankles, and wrists

- Joint swelling; redness, or warmth
- Abdominal pain
- Skin rash (erythema marginatum)
  - Skin eruption on the trunk and upper part of arms or legs
  - Eruptions that are ring-shaped or snakelike in appearance
- Skin nodules
- Sydenham's chorea—emotional instability, muscular weakness, and rapid, uncoordinated jerky movements affecting primarily the face, feet, and hands
- Epistaxis (nosebleeds)
- Cardiac (heart) involvement which may be asymptomatic or may result in shortness of breath, chest pain

Signs and Tests

Given the different manifestations of this disease, there is no specific test that can definitively establish a diagnosis. In addition to a careful physical examination of heart sounds, skin, and joints, blood samples may be taken as part of the evaluation. These include tests for recurrent strep infection (ASO [antistreptolysin O] or anti-DNase-B), complete blood counts, and [erythrocyte] sedimentation rate (ESR). As part of the cardiac evaluation, an electrocardiogram may also be done.

In order to standardize the diagnosis of rheumatic fever, several minor and major criteria have been developed. These criteria, in conjunction with evidence of recent streptococcal infection, establish a diagnosis of rheumatic fever.

The major diagnostic criteria include:

- Carditis (heart inflammation)
- Polyarthritis
- Subcutaneous skin nodules
- Chorea (Sydenham's chorea)
- Erythema marginatum.

The minor criteria include fever, arthralgia (joint pain), elevated erythrocyte sedimentation rate, and other laboratory findings.

Two major criteria, or one major and two minor criteria, when there is also evidence of a previous strep infection (positive culture or rising antibody level—ASO or anti-DNAse-B) support the diagnosis of rheumatic fever.

Treatment

The management of acute rheumatic fever is geared toward the reduction of inflammation with anti-inflammatory medications such as aspirin or corticosteroids. Individuals with positive cultures for strep throat should also be treated with antibiotics. Another important cornerstone in treating rheumatic fever includes the continuous use of low-dose antibiotics (such as penicillin, sulfadiazine, or erythromycin) to prevent recurrence.

Expectations

The recurrence of rheumatic fever is relatively common in the absence of maintenance of low-dose antibiotics, especially during the first three to five years after the first episode of rheumatic fever. Heart complications may be long-term and severe, particularly if the heart valves are involved.

Complications

- Damage to heart valves (in particular, mitral stenosis and aortic stenosis)
- Endocarditis
- Heart failure
- Arrhythmias
- Pericarditis
- Sydenham's chorea

Calling Your Health Care Provider

Call your health care provider if you develop symptoms of rheumatic fever. There are numerous conditions that may have similar symptoms; therefore you will require careful medical evaluation.

If you have symptoms of strep throat, notify your health care provider. You will need to be evaluated and treated if strep throat is confirmed, to decrease your risk of developing rheumatic fever.

Prevention

The most important way to prevent rheumatic fever is by proper and prompt treatment of strep throat and scarlet fever.

Chapter 38

Bacterial Endocarditis

What is bacterial endocarditis?

Bacterial endocarditis (BE) is an infection of the valves and inner lining of the heart (called the endocardium). It happens when bacteria from the skin, mouth, or intestines enter the bloodstream and infect the heart valves and lining.

Who gets bacterial endocarditis?

Although BE can occur in anyone, people with a heart valve problem, an artificial valve, or a heart defect are at greatest risk. Having a heart murmur sometimes increases the chances of getting BE. Your doctor can usually determine whether you have a type of heart murmur that increases your risk of BE.

Do medical and dental procedures increase the risk of BE?

Dental work (including professional teeth cleaning) and some medical procedures (such as colonoscopy, cystoscopy, and sigmoidoscopy) increase the risk of bacteria entering the bloodstream. If you have an abnormal heart valve or another heart defect, you are at risk of BE any time bacteria gets into your bloodstream.

Can BE be prevented?

If you have a heart defect or valve problem, make sure your doctor or dentist knows about it. If you have your teeth cleaned or have another one of the procedures mentioned previously, you need to take antibiotics. The antibiotics can help keep bacteria from surviving in your bloodstream.

BE can't always be prevented, because doctors don't always know when bacteria might get into your bloodstream. That's why you need to keep a close eye on your health if you have a heart defect or a valve problem.

How can you tell if you have BE?

Fever, chills, and other flu-like symptoms may be the only signs of BE. Other symptoms are unexplained weight loss and weakness. Your doctor may suspect you have BE if he or she hears abnormal heart sounds with a stethoscope. Your doctor will then need to do more tests, such as blood tests and echocardiography (looking at the heart by using an ultrasound) to find out if you have BE.

How is BE treated?

BE is treated with antibiotics. Antibiotics are usually started intravenously (through an IV) in the hospital, but many people can finish their treatment at home. For more complicated infections, heart surgery may be needed.

Are there complications of BE?

Once infected, your heart may not pump blood as well as it did before. This is called heart failure. Other problems include irregularities of the heartbeat, damage to the heart muscle, and blood clots. If BE isn't treated, it can lead to death.

Chapter 39

Pericarditis

The pericardium is a sac of tough fibrous tissue that envelops the heart and the roots of the blood vessels that enter and leave the heart. The small amount of lubricating fluid (approximately 30 ml) contained in the sac and the sac's incomplete attachment to the heart allow the heart to move within it.

Pericarditis is the name given to a variety of diseases, all of which have the major characteristics of inflammation of the pericardium and an increase in volume of the pericardial fluid.

Pericarditis may be acute or chronic. It may be completely cured or may recur. Pericarditis is a progressive disease that can be life-threatening if not treated in a timely manner.

Most people do not have any symptoms or merely have the symptoms of an underlying disease. If you have pericarditis, you may experience chest pain. The pain may come on suddenly.

What causes pericarditis?

Usually, pericarditis is the consequence of another disease, often an infection. The infection may be bacterial, viral, or occasionally, fungal. Some other diseases that cause pericarditis are: kidney failure, tuberculosis, cancer, rheumatoid arthritis, rheumatic fever, lupus, and scleroderma.

Pericarditis may develop as a complication of myocardial infarction (heart attack). Radiation treatment or surgical complications may also cause pericarditis. On rare occasions, pericarditis may develop as a reaction to certain medications.

Pericarditis is sometimes caused by injury or trauma such as gunshot or stab wounds, even if there is no penetration.

What is acute pericarditis?

Typically, acute pericarditis is accompanied by symptoms of sharp, stabbing chest pain, shortness of breath, fever, perspiration, chills, and the symptoms of the underlying illness. The chest pain may radiate to your neck, back, left shoulder, and upper arm. The pain may intensify during respiration, coughing, swallowing, or when you are lying supine or turning.

If you have acute pericarditis, expect it to last two to three weeks. You may experience one or more recurrences in the six- to twelve-month period following your convalescence.

What is chronic pericarditis?

If your pericarditis persists for six to twelve months following the acute episode, it is considered chronic.

What is constrictive pericarditis?

Constrictive pericarditis is a serious form of pericarditis in which the pericardium becomes so thickened and scarred that it loses some of its elasticity. It compresses the heart, interferes with the ability of the heart to fill up with blood, and reduces the amount of blood pumped out to the body. Constrictive pericarditis may cause heart failure and lead to kidney disease.

If you have constrictive pericarditis, you may experience chest pain, difficulty in breathing, swelling of your feet and ankles, fatigue, and weakness.

You may be given a low dose of diuretics (water pills) to gradually decrease excess fluid. You may be given painkillers and put on a low-sodium diet.

If you have severe symptoms that are not alleviated by other means, surgery may be recommended. The surgery involves a high-risk procedure called a "pericardiectomy." This procedure entails the removal of a portion or all of the pericardium to relieve the constriction.

Constrictive pericarditis may be life threatening if untreated.

What is adhesive pericarditis?

Adhesions may be present between the layers of the pericardium or between the pericardium and other parts of the chest area. This is not a serious condition, but if untreated, it may develop into constrictive pericarditis.

What should I know about viral pericarditis?

If you have viral pericarditis, you may have chest discomfort or pain and fever. You probably have had a recent upper respiratory infection.

The viruses most likely to cause pericarditis are: Coxsackie B, mumps, infectious mononucleosis, influenza, poliomyelitis, and occasionally chickenpox.

You can expect the illness to last one to two weeks. Most likely you will not have a recurrence.

What should I know about bacterial pericarditis?

Bacterial pericarditis is rare. It generally occurs in debilitated, chronically ill people who have other underlying diseases. Bacterial pericarditis very rarely occurs as an isolated illness.

If you have bacterial pericarditis, you may experience the following symptoms: shortness of breath, night sweats, cough, a high, spiking fever, an elevated pulse, the symptoms of the bacterial infection, and the symptoms of the underlying disease. The symptoms of the underlying disease vary.

Bacterial pericarditis is treated with antibiotic medication, by drainage of excess fluids, and sometimes by early pericardiectomy surgery to prevent constrictive pericarditis.

The incidence of bacterial pericarditis has declined sharply with the advent of penicillin and other antibiotics.

What is fungal pericarditis?

If you have fungal pericarditis, you are probably already severely ill with another disease such as lymphoma, leukemia, or endocarditis. Fungal pericarditis is often a complication of a pulmonary (lung) infection or may be a complication of cardiac surgery. The symptoms are usually the same as those of the underlying disease. If left untreated, fungal pericarditis will progress to pericardial constriction. The treatment includes medication for the underlying infection.

What is uremic pericarditis?

Uremic pericarditis is caused by kidney failure and may be treated by dialysis, which is a procedure that filters and cleanses the blood. This procedure may be necessary to reduce the severity of your symptoms. In rare but serious situations, a pericardiectomy will be performed. If you have uremic pericarditis, your symptoms may include chest pain and a fever.

How is pericarditis diagnosed?

Your doctor will take your medical history and perform a complete physical examination. He will order diagnostic tests. These may include blood tests, chest x-rays, electrocardiograms (ECGs), and echocardiograms. He may order computed tomography (CT) and magnetic resonance imaging (MRI) scans to determine if there has been a thickening of the pericardium. He may order a diagnostic biopsy.

How is pericarditis treated?

Most people are treated for pericarditis outside the hospital setting. Treatment may include: painkillers, antibiotics, antituberculous agents, fungicidal drugs, dialysis, and chemotherapy, depending upon the type and basis of the disease.

Sometimes pericarditis is treated in the hospital. If you need to be hospitalized, you will be given strict bed rest until your symptoms abate. In the hospital, you will receive painkillers. You may be given corticosteroids to hasten the healing. You may undergo a process called "pericardiocentesis" in which the fluid in your pericardium will be drained through a catheter which is placed into your pericardial cavity. The drainage may take many hours to overnight. Finally, you may have to undergo surgery.

Part Four

Facts about Vascular Diseases and Disorders

Chapter 40

Atherosclerosis

What is atherosclerosis?

Atherosclerosis is the buildup of fatty deposits called plaque on the inside walls of arteries. Arteries are blood vessels that carry oxygen and blood to the heart, brain, and other parts of the body. As plaque builds up in an artery, the artery gradually narrows and can become clogged. As an artery becomes more and more narrowed, less blood can flow through. The artery may also become less elastic (called "hardening of the arteries"). Atherosclerosis is the main cause of a group of diseases called cardiovascular diseases—diseases of the heart and blood vessels.

Atherosclerosis can lead to clogged arteries in any part of the body. When the arteries to the heart are affected, angina (chest pain) or a heart attack may result. If arteries in the leg are affected, leg pain may occur. Atherosclerosis of the arteries to the brain can cause strokes.

Atherosclerosis is common in the United States. It often starts in childhood and the arteries become narrowed or clogged over many years.

What is plaque?

Plaque is a combination of cholesterol, other fatty materials, calcium, and blood components that stick to the artery wall lining. A hard

Reprinted from "Atherosclerosis," National Women's Health Information Center (www.4woman.gov), October 2002.

shell or scar covers the plaque. Plaques have various sizes and shapes. Some plaques are unstable and can rupture or burst. When this happens, it causes blood clotting inside the artery. If a blood clot totally blocks the artery, it stops blood flow completely. This is what happens in most heart attacks and strokes.

What causes plaque to form in arteries?

Although many risk factors are well known, the exact causes of atherosclerosis are not clear. Too much cholesterol in the blood, damage to the artery wall, and inflammation appear to play important roles in plaque buildup. Researchers are studying why and how the arteries become damaged, how plaque develops and changes over time, and why plaque can break open and lead to blood clots. There may be other factors that prove to be important in causing atherosclerosis.

What are the symptoms of atherosclerosis?

There are usually no symptoms until one or more arteries are so clogged with plaque that blood flow is severely reduced. This reduced flow of blood and oxygen to some part of the body (such as the heart) is called ischemia and may cause pain or discomfort. Some people have no symptoms until a blood clot forms, completely blocks an already narrowed artery, and causes a heart attack or stroke.

The symptoms you have depend on which arteries are badly clogged and what part of the body is affected by the reduced flow of blood.

- If arteries taking blood to your heart muscle are affected, you have coronary artery disease (CAD). You may have chest pain called angina that happens when you exert yourself and goes away when you rest. You could also have a heart attack.

- If arteries taking blood to your brain are affected, you have cerebrovascular disease. You could have a transient ischemic attack (TIA) or a stroke.

- If arteries taking blood to your legs are affected, you have peripheral arterial disease (PAD). You may have pain in the calf or thigh muscle called intermittent claudication that happens when you walk. This kind of pain goes away when you stop and rest.

All of these conditions are serious and should not be ignored. Arteries taking blood to the intestines, the kidneys, or other organs can also become clogged by plaque. This can sometimes lead to a medical emergency similar to a heart attack or stroke. Atherosclerosis can also cause erectile dysfunction in men.

What risk factors raise my chances of having atherosclerosis?

These risk factors raise your chances of having atherosclerosis:

- having high blood cholesterol, especially high LDL ("bad cholesterol") and low HDL ("good cholesterol") levels
- aging and being male (women are affected more after menopause)
- having close relatives who had heart disease or a stroke at a relatively young age
- having high blood pressure
- having diabetes
- smoking
- having trouble managing stress
- being obese
- being physically inactive

The more risk factors you have, the more likely it is that you have atherosclerosis. Talk with your health care provider about your risks for atherosclerosis and cardiovascular disease.

How is atherosclerosis diagnosed?

If you don't have any symptoms and have not been diagnosed with cardiovascular disease, it is not easy to tell if your arteries are becoming clogged with plaque. However, if you have high blood cholesterol, are overweight and get little exercise, smoke, or have other risk factors, there is a good chance that you have atherosclerosis. Eventually it can lead to heart disease, a stroke, or other problems.

There are a number of tests that doctors use in diagnosing cardiovascular diseases, including blood tests, electrocardiograms (ECGs), stress testing, coronary angiography, ultrasound, and computed tomography (CT). If you are at high risk for cardiovascular disease, your health care provider may suggest that you be tested.

Researchers are studying new tools to help find cardiovascular disease in earlier stages, before symptoms appear. For example, the National Heart, Lung, and Blood Institute is sponsoring a ten-year study called the Multi-Ethnic Study of Atherosclerosis (MESA). The MESA study will help show which risk factors are the best predictors of future heart disease in men and women and in certain ethnic groups.

How is atherosclerosis treated?

If your atherosclerosis leads to symptoms, the symptoms (such as angina) can be treated. Medicines are usually the first step in treating cardiovascular diseases. Other treatments include angioplasty procedures to open up clogged arteries and surgery, such as bypass surgery.

If you have high blood pressure, diabetes, or high blood cholesterol, these conditions can be treated as well. Lowering your blood cholesterol level can slow, stop, or even reverse the buildup of plaque. Cholesterol lowering can reduce the cholesterol content in unstable plaques to make them more stable and less prone to rupture.

One of the most important ways to have healthier arteries is to make lifestyle changes. Adopt a healthy diet, balance healthful eating with regular physical activity, don't smoke, and lose weight if you are overweight. If you have high blood cholesterol, high blood pressure, or diabetes, follow your treatment plan. Making lifestyle changes can also help control these health problems.

Can I prevent or reverse atherosclerosis?

Yes. You can't do anything about your genes, your gender, or your age, but you can adopt a healthy lifestyle.

- Maintain a healthy weight and avoid weight gain as you get older.
- Get plenty of regular exercise—at least thirty minutes a day, most days of the week.
- Eat a healthy diet low in saturated fat and rich in fruits and vegetables.
- If you have high blood cholesterol or high blood pressure, you may need medicine to help lower it. Stick to your treatment plan.
- If you have diabetes, follow your treatment plan.
- If you smoke, stop.
- If stress is a problem, find ways to reduce or control it.

Talk to your health care provider about what you can do to lower your risks for atherosclerosis and cardiovascular disease.

Chapter 41

Stroke

Signs of a Stroke

The National Institute of Neurological Disorders and Stroke notes these major signs of stroke:

- Sudden numbness or weakness of the face, arms, or legs
- Sudden confusion or trouble speaking or understanding others
- Sudden trouble seeing in one or both eyes
- Sudden trouble walking, dizziness, or loss of balance or coordination
- Sudden severe headache with no known cause

If you think someone is having a stroke, you should call 911 immediately.

Stroke Statistics

Stroke is the third leading cause of death in the United Sates. In 2001, stroke killed 163,538 people, accounting for about one of every

"Signs of a Stroke" is excerpted from "Know the Signs and Symptoms of a Stroke," Cardiovascular Health Section of the National Center for Chronic Disease Prevention and Health Promotion, Centers for Disease Control and Prevention (CDC), January 2004. "Facts about Stroke" is reprinted from "Stroke," National Women's Health Information Center, November 2002. "Types of Stroke" is reprinted with permission from the National Stroke Association, http://www.stroke.org. © 2002 National Stroke Association. All rights reserved.

fourteen deaths in the United States. According to the American Heart Association, about 700,000 people in the United States suffer a stroke each year (about 500,000 first attacks and 200,000 recurrent attacks). Four million Americans who have survived a stroke are living with impairments and 15 to 30 percent are permanently disabled. The American Heart Association also estimates that stroke cost about $51.2 billion in both direct and indirect costs in 2003 in the United States alone.

With timely treatment, the risk of death and disability from stroke can be lowered. It is very important to know the symptoms of a stroke and act in time.

References

American Heart Association. Heart Disease and Stroke Statistics—2004 Update. Dallas, TX: AHA, 2003. Available at http://www.american heart.org/presenter.jhtml?identifier=1200026. Accessed January 26, 2004.

National Center for Health Statistics. *Health, United States, 2003 Chartbook on the Health of Americans.* Hyattsville, MD: Department of Health and Human Services, 2003. Available at http://www.cdc.gov/ nchs/hus.htm. Accessed December 12, 2003

Facts about Stroke

What Is a Stroke?

A stroke is sometimes called a "brain attack." A stroke can injure the brain like a heart attack can injure the heart. Stroke is the result of cerebrovascular disease—disease of the blood vessels in the brain.

There are two types of stroke:

- *Ischemic stroke,* the most common type of stroke. This type of stroke happens when there is a sudden lack of blood flow to some part of the brain, usually due to a blood clot blocking an artery or blood vessel. Often the artery is already clogged with fatty deposits (atherosclerosis).

- *Hemorrhagic stroke.* Bleeding in the brain from a broken or leaking blood vessel causes this type of stroke. A hemorrhagic stroke may be due to an aneurysm—a thin or weak spot in an artery that balloons out and can burst.

Either type of stroke can cause brain cells to die. This brain damage may cause a person to lose control of certain functions, such as speech, movement, and memory. Like a heart attack, a stroke is an emergency and should be treated as quickly as possible.

What Is a "Mini-Stroke" or TIA?

A "mini-stroke" refers to a transient ischemic attack (TIA). In a TIA, there is a short-term reduction in blood flow to the brain. This causes temporary stroke symptoms (often just for a few minutes) such as weakness or tingling in an arm or leg. TIAs don't cause brain damage, but they are important warning signs that a person is at risk of having a stroke. If you have a TIA, you should seek medical care right away to prevent a full stroke.

What Are the Effects of Stroke?

A person who has a stroke may suffer little or no brain damage and disability, especially if the stroke is treated promptly. However, stroke can lead to severe brain damage and disability, or even death. The type of disability caused by a stroke depends on the extent of brain damage and what part of the brain is damaged.

Stroke may cause paralysis or weakness of one side of the body, memory problems, mood changes, trouble speaking or understanding speech, problems with eating and swallowing, pain, depression, and other problems. Rehabilitation and medical treatment can help a person recover from the effects of stroke and prevent another stroke from occurring.

Where Can Stroke Occur in the Brain and How Does That Affect the Body?

The brain is a complex organ. Each area of the brain is responsible for a particular function or ability. The brain is divided into four main parts: the right hemisphere (or half), the left hemisphere, the cerebellum, and the brain stem.

A stroke in the right hemisphere of the brain often causes paralysis in the left side of the body. This is known as left hemiplegia. In addition, a stroke in this part of the brain may cause:

- Problems with spatial and perceptual abilities. For example, the stroke survivor may misjudge distances and fall, or be unable to guide his or her hands to pick up an object.

- Impaired judgment and behavior. For example, the stroke survivor may try to do things that he or she should not attempt to do, such as trying to drive a car.

- Problems with short-term memory. Although he or she may be able to recount events from thirty years ago, the stroke survivor may be unable to remember what he or she ate for breakfast that morning.

Someone who has had a left hemisphere stroke may have right hemiplegia, paralysis of the right side of the body. He or she may also have:

- Aphasia—speech and language problems.

- Slow and cautious behavior, in contrast to the behavior of a right-hemisphere stroke survivor. He or she may need a lot of help to complete tasks.

- Memory problems similar to those of right-hemisphere stroke survivors. For example, he or she may have trouble learning new information and have poor short-term memory.

A stroke that takes place in the cerebellum can cause:

- Abnormal reflexes of the head and torso

- Coordination and balance problems

- Dizziness, nausea, and vomiting.

Strokes that occur in the brain stem are especially devastating. The brain stem is the area of the brain that controls all of our involuntary "life-support" functions, such as breathing rate, blood pressure, and heartbeat. The brain stem also controls abilities such as eye movements, hearing, speech, and swallowing. Since impulses generated in the brain's hemispheres must travel through the brain stem on their way to the arms and legs, patients with a brain stem stroke may also develop paralysis in one or both sides of the body.

Who Is at Risk for Stroke?

Stroke risks are higher in people who have a family or personal history of stroke and for African Americans. African Americans have a higher risk of disability and death from stroke than Caucasians do. This is partly because more African Americans have high blood pressure, a major stroke risk factor. Age is also a factor: the chance of having a stroke more than doubles for each decade of life after age fifty-five. Those who smoke or who have high blood pressure, heart disease, or diabetes are at greater risk of having a stroke. Hormonal changes with pregnancy, childbirth, and menopause are also linked to an increased risk of stroke.

How Is Stroke Prevented?

The more stroke risk factors you have, the greater the chance that you will have a stroke. You can't control some risk factors, such as aging, family health history, race, and gender. Yet you can change or treat most other risk factors to lower your risk.

Here are some of the best ways to prevent stroke:

- Eat a healthy diet low in saturated fat and rich in fruits, vegetables, and whole grains. Don't overeat, and keep your weight under control.

- Get regular exercise (thirty minutes a day, most days of the week, or more).

- Find ways to manage stress in your life.

- If you have high blood pressure, take your blood pressure medicine as prescribed by your health care provider.

- If your cholesterol level is too high, talk to your health care provider about ways to lower it.

- If you smoke, stop smoking. If it is hard to quit on your own, there are products like nicotine patches, support groups, and programs to help you stop smoking.

- If you have heart disease or diabetes, take good care of yourself. See your health care provider and take your medicine as prescribed.

- Get help if you have a TIA ("mini-stroke"). Talk to your health care provider to see if you need medicine or surgery.

- Aspirin therapy may be useful, but check with your health care provider before starting to take aspirin on a daily basis.

How Is Stroke Diagnosed?

Before a stroke can be treated, diagnostic tests must be performed. Health care providers must find out what kind of stroke it is to treat it correctly. A person thought to be having a stroke may have a neurological exam, blood tests, and an electrocardiogram.

Other kinds of tests used in diagnosing stroke include:

- Imaging tests that give a picture of the brain. These include CT (computed tomography) scanning, sometimes called CAT scans, and MRI (magnetic resonance imaging) scanning. CT scans are particularly useful for determining if a stroke is caused by a blockage or by bleeding in the brain.

- Electrical tests such as EEG (electroencephalogram) and an evoked response test to record the electrical impulses and sensory processes of the brain.

- Blood flow tests, such as Doppler ultrasound tests, to show any changes in the blood flow to the brain.

How Is Stroke Treated?

Strokes caused by blood clots can be treated with clot-busting drugs such as TPA (tissue plasminogen activator). TPA must be given within three hours of the start of a stroke to be effective, and tests must be done first. This is why it is so important for a person having a stroke to get to a hospital fast.

Other medicines are used to treat and to prevent stroke. Anticoagulants such as warfarin and antiplatelet agents such as aspirin interfere with the blood's ability to clot and can play an important role in preventing stroke.

Surgery is sometimes used to treat or prevent stroke. For example, carotid endarterectomy is the surgical removal of fatty deposits clogging the carotid artery in the neck that could lead to a stroke. For hemorrhagic stroke, surgical treatment may include placing a metal clip at the base of an aneurysm or removing abnormal blood vessels.

What about Stroke Rehabilitation?

Rehabilitation is a very important part of recovery for many stroke survivors. The effects of stroke may mean that you must change, relearn, or redefine how you live. Stroke rehabilitation is designed to help you return to independent living.

Rehabilitation doesn't reverse the effects of a stroke. Its goals are to build your strength, capability, and confidence so you can continue your daily activities despite the effects of your stroke. Rehabilitation services may include:

- physical therapy to restore movement, balance, and coordination

- occupational therapy to relearn basic skills such as bathing and dressing oneself

- speech therapy.

Types of Stroke

Ischemic Stroke

In everyday life, blood clotting is beneficial. When you are bleeding from a wound, blood clots work to slow and eventually stop the bleeding. In the case of stroke, however, blood clots are dangerous because they can block arteries and cut off blood flow, a process called ischemia. An ischemic stroke can occur in two ways: embolic and thrombotic strokes.

Embolic Stroke

In an embolic stroke, a blood clot forms somewhere in the body (usually the heart) and travels through the bloodstream to your brain. Once in your brain, the clot eventually travels to a blood vessel small enough to block its passage. The clot lodges there, blocking the blood vessel and causing a stroke. The medical word for this type of blood clot is *embolus*.

Thrombotic Stroke

In the second type of blood-clot stroke, blood flow is impaired because of a blockage to one or more of the arteries supplying blood to the brain. The process leading to this blockage is known as thrombosis. Strokes caused in this way are called thrombotic strokes. That's because the medical word for a clot that forms on a blood-vessel deposit is *thrombus*.

Blood-clot strokes can also happen as the result of unhealthy blood vessels clogged with a buildup of fatty deposits and cholesterol. Your body regards these buildups as multiple, tiny, and repeated injuries to the blood vessel wall. So your body reacts to these injuries just as it would if you were bleeding from a wound—it responds by forming clots. Two types of thrombosis can cause stroke: large-vessel thrombosis and small-vessel disease (or lacunar infarction).

Large-Vessel Thrombosis

Thrombotic stroke occurs most often in the large arteries, so large-vessel thrombosis is the most common and best understood type of thrombotic stroke. Most large-vessel thrombosis is caused by a combination of long-term atherosclerosis followed by rapid blood clot formation. Thrombotic stroke patients are also likely to have coronary artery disease, and heart attack is a frequent cause of death in patients who have suffered this type of brain attack.

Small-Vessel Disease (Lacunar Infarction)

Small-vessel disease, or lacunar infarction, occurs when blood flow is blocked to a very small arterial vessel. The term's origin is from the Latin word *lacuna*, which means hole, and describes the small cavity remaining after the products of deep infarct have been removed by other cells in the body. Little is known about the causes of small-vessel disease, but it is closely linked to hypertension.

Hemorrhagic Stroke

Strokes caused by the breakage or "blowout" of a blood vessel in the brain are called hemorrhagic strokes. The medical word for this type of breakage is *hemorrhage*. Hemorrhages can be caused by a number of disorders that affect the blood vessels, including longstanding high blood pressure and cerebral aneurysms. An aneurysm is a weak or thin spot on a blood vessel wall. These weak spots are usually present at birth. Aneurysms develop over a number of years and usually don't cause detectable problems until they break. There are two types of hemorrhagic stroke: subarachnoid and intracerebral.

In an intracerebral hemorrhage, bleeding occurs from vessels within the brain itself. Hypertension is the primary cause of this type of hemorrhage.

In a subarachnoid hemorrhage (SAH), an aneurysm bursts in a large artery on or near the thin, delicate membrane surrounding the brain. Blood spills into the area around the brain that is filled with a protective fluid, causing the brain to be surrounded by blood-contaminated fluid.

The U.S. Food and Drug Administration (FDA) recently issued a voluntary recall of nonprescription medications containing PPA (phenylpropanolamine) after they were linked to an increased risk of hemorrhagic stroke in women.

Chapter 42

Brain Aneurysms

What Is a Brain Aneurysm?

A brain aneurysm, also called a cerebral or intracranial aneurysm, is an abnormal bulging outward of one of the arteries in the brain. It is estimated that up to one in fifteen people in the United States will develop a brain aneurysm during their lifetime.

Brain aneurysms are often discovered when they rupture, causing bleeding into the brain or the space closely surrounding the brain called the subarachnoid space, causing a subarachnoid hemorrhage. Subarachnoid hemorrhage from a ruptured brain aneurysm can lead to a hemorrhagic stroke, brain damage, and death.

The main goals of treatment once an aneurysm has ruptured are to stop the bleeding and potential permanent damage to the brain and to reduce the risk of recurrence. Unruptured brain aneurysms are sometimes treated to prevent rupture.

Incidence Rates of Brain Aneurysms

- Approximately 0.2 to 3 percent of people with a brain aneurysm may suffer from bleeding per year.

This chapter includes text from "What Is a Brain Aneurysm?" "Symptoms of Brain Aneurysms," and "Treatment of Brain Aneurysms," reprinted with permission from the American Society of Interventional and Therapeutic Neuroradiology (ASITN). © 2004. All rights reserved. For additional information, visit the ASITN patient education website at http://www.brainaneurysm.com.

- The annual incidence of aneurysmal subarachnoid hemorrhage in the United States exceeds thirty thousand people. Ten to fifteen percent of these patients will die before reaching the hospital and over 50 percent will die within the first thirty days after rupture. Of those who survive, about half suffer some permanent neurological deficit.

- Brain aneurysms can occur in people of all ages, but are most commonly detected in those ages thirty-five to sixty.

- Women are actually more likely to get a brain aneurysm than men, with a ratio of 3:2.

Symptoms of Brain Aneurysms

Ruptured Cerebral Aneurysm Symptoms

Sometimes patients describing "the worst headache in my life" are actually experiencing one of the symptoms of brain aneurysms related to having a rupture. Other ruptured cerebral aneurysm symptoms include:

- Nausea and vomiting
- Stiff neck or neck pain
- Blurred vision or double vision
- Pain above and behind the eye
- Dilated pupils
- Sensitivity to light
- Loss of sensation

Unruptured Cerebral Aneurysm Symptoms

Before an aneurysm ruptures, patients often experience no symptoms of brain aneurysms. In about 40 percent of cases, people with unruptured aneurysms will experience some or all of the following cerebral aneurysm symptoms:

- Peripheral vision deficits
- Thinking or processing problems
- Speech complications
- Perceptual problems

- Sudden changes in behavior
- Loss of balance and coordination
- Decreased concentration
- Short-term memory difficulty
- Fatigue

Because the symptoms of brain aneurysms can also be associated with other medical conditions, diagnostic neuroradiology is regularly used to identify both ruptured and unruptured brain aneurysms.

Diagnosis of Brain Aneurysms

Diagnosis of a ruptured cerebral aneurysm is commonly made by finding signs of subarachnoid hemorrhage on a CT scan (Computerized Tomography, sometimes called a CAT scan). The CT scan is a computerized test that rapidly x-rays the body in cross-sections, or slices, as the body is moved through a large, circular machine. If the CT scan is negative but a ruptured aneurysm is still suspected, a lumbar puncture is performed to detect blood in the cerebrospinal fluid (CSF) that surrounds the brain and spinal cord.

To determine the exact location, size, and shape of an aneurysm (ruptured or unruptured), neuroradiologists will use either cerebral angiography or tomographic angiography.

Cerebral angiography, the traditional method, involves introducing a catheter (small plastic tube) into an artery (usually in the leg) and steering it through the blood vessels of the body to the artery involved by the aneurysm. A special dye, called a contract agent, is injected into the patient's artery and its distribution is shown on x-ray projections. This method may not detect some aneurysms due to overlapping structures or spasm.

Computed tomographic angiography (CTA) is an alternative to the traditional method and can be performed without the need for arterial catheterization. This test combines a regular CT scan with a contrast dye injected into a vein. Once the dye is injected into a vein, it travels to the brain arteries, and images are created using a CT scan. These images show exactly how blood flows into the brain arteries.

Treatment of Brain Aneurysms

Surgery or minimally invasive endovascular coiling techniques can be used in the treatment of brain aneurysms. It is important to note, however, that not all aneurysms are treated at the time of diagnosis or are amenable to both forms of treatment. Patients need to consult a neurovascular specialist to determine if they are candidates for either treatment.

Surgical Treatment

To get to the aneurysm, surgeons must first remove a section of the skull, a procedure called a craniotomy. The surgeon then spreads the brain tissue apart and places a tiny metal clip across the neck to stop blood flow into the aneurysm. After clipping the aneurysm, the bone is secured in its original place, and the wound is closed.

Minimally Invasive Treatment: Coil Embolization or Endovascular Coiling

Endovascular therapy is a minimally invasive procedure that accesses the treatment area from within the blood vessel. In the case of aneurysms, this treatment is called coil embolization, or "coiling." In contrast to surgery, endovascular coiling does not require open surgery. Instead, physicians use real-time x-ray technology, called fluoroscopic imaging, to visualize the patient's vascular system and treat the disease from inside the blood vessel.

Endovascular treatment of brain aneurysms involves insertion of a catheter (small plastic tube) into the femoral artery in the patient's leg and navigating it through the vascular system, into the head and into the aneurysm. Tiny platinum coils are threaded through the catheter and deployed into the aneurysm, blocking blood flow into the aneurysm and preventing rupture. The coils are made of platinum so that they can be visible via x-ray and be flexible enough to conform to the aneurysm shape. This endovascular coiling, or filling, of the aneurysm is called embolization and can be performed under general anesthesia or light sedation. More than 125,000 patients worldwide have been treated with detachable platinum coils.

Endovascular Coiling v. Surgical Clipping

Treatment of Ruptured Aneurysms

Until recently, most studies on surgical clipping and endovascular treatment of brain aneurysms were either small-scale studies or were retrospective studies that relied on analyzing historical case records.

The only multicenter prospective randomized clinical trial—considered the gold standard in study design—comparing surgical clipping and endovascular coiling of ruptured aneurysm is the International Subarachnoid Aneurysm Trial (ISAT)[1].

The study found that, in patients equally suited for both treatment options, endovascular coiling treatment produces substantially better patient outcomes than surgery in terms of survival free of disability at one year. The relative risk of death or significant disability at one year for patients treated with coils was 22.6 percent lower than in surgically treated patients.

The study results were so compelling that the trial was halted early after enrolling 2,143 of the planned 2,500 patients because the trial steering committee determined it was no longer ethical to randomize patients to neurosurgical clipping. Long-term follow-up will be essential to assess the durability of the substantial early advantage of endovascular coiling over conventional neurosurgical clipping for the treatment of brain aneurysms.

It is important to note that patients enrolled in the ISAT were evaluated by both a neurosurgeon and an endovascular coiling specialist, and both physicians had to agree that the aneurysm was treatable by either technique. This study provides compelling evidence that, if medically possible, all patients with ruptured brain aneurysms should receive an endovascular consultation as part of the protocol for the treatment of brain aneurysms.

Treatment of Unruptured Aneurysms

Although no multicenter randomized clinical trial comparing endovascular coiling and surgical treatment of unruptured aneurysms has yet been conducted, retrospective analyses have found that endovascular coiling is associated with less risk of bad outcomes, shorter hospital stays, and shorter recovery times compared with surgery. Studies have shown that:

- Average hospital stays are more than twice as long with surgery as compared to endovascular coiling treatment.[2]

- Four times as many surgical patients report new symptoms or disability after treatment as compared to coiled patients.[3]

- There can be a dramatic difference in recovery times. One study showed that surgically treated patients had an average recovery time of one year, compared to coiled patients, who recovered in twenty-seven days.[3]

References

1. Molyneux A, Kerr R, Stratton I, Sandercock P, Clarke M, Shrimpton J, Holman R. International Subarachnoid Aneurysm Trial (ISAT) of neurosurgical clipping versus endovascular coiling in 2143 patients with ruptured intracranial aneurysms: A randomised trial. *Lancet.* 2002: 360: 1267–74.

2. Johnston SC, et. al. Surgical and Endovascular Treatment of Unruptured Cerebral Aneurysms at University Hospitals. *Neurology.* 1999; 52:1799–1805.

3. Johnston SC, et. al. Endovascular and Surgical Treatment of Unruptured Cerebral Aneurysms: Comparison of Risks. *Ann Neurology.* 2000; 48:11–19.

Chapter 43

Abdominal Aortic Aneurysm

Overview

Abdominal aortic aneurysms (AAA) are caused by progressive weakening of the aortic wall that causes a "ballooning" of the vessel. The aneurysm will grow larger and eventually rupture if it is not diagnosed and treated. Aneurysms occur most often in the aorta, the main artery of the chest and abdomen. The aorta carries blood flow from the heart to all parts of the body, including the vital organs and the legs and feet.

There are approximately fifteen thousand deaths per year related to the rupture of an aneurysm. Ruptured aneurysms are the tenth leading cause of death in men over fifty in the country. A ruptured aneurysm is an emergency and procedures must take place immediately to save one's life and avoid serious complications.

Causes of Abdominal Aortic Aneurysm

Proteins in the wall of the aorta, called elastin and collagen, provide strength and flexibility to this large artery. This is similar to muscles and tendons providing strength to the arms and legs. Aneurysms are caused by a progressive breakdown of these proteins that leads to a weakness of the wall of the aorta, which can steadily expand like a balloon. These proteins, collagen and elastin, may gradually deteriorate

Reprinted with permission from the Vascular Disease Foundation, http://www.vdf.org. Copyright 2004 Vascular Disease Foundation.

with age. Inflammation that is associated with atherosclerosis (hardening of the arteries) helps to accelerate this degenerative process even in younger people. Some of the body's naturally occurring enzymes may also cause the breakdown of collagen and elastin in the wall of the aorta. An excess of these enzymes or conditions that activate the enzymes may cause the formation of an aneurysm, or lead to its sudden growth. In rare cases an aneurysm may be caused by infection. There is still much to be learned about the cause of aneurysms and their growth.

Symptoms of Abdominal Aortic Aneurysm

In most cases, there are no major symptoms for AAA. Occasionally, patients may feel abdominal, back or side pain. Seventy-five percent of the aneurysms that are discovered are detected from diagnostic tests (such as x-rays) that were given for other health problems.

Risk Factors for Abdominal Aortic Aneurysm

- Age over sixty years
- A family history of AAA
- Tobacco use
- History of heart disease or peripheral arterial disease (PAD)
- High blood pressure

The risk of AAA increases with age, and AAAs are five to ten times more common in men than in women. Tobacco users are eight times more likely to be affected than non-users.

Diagnosis of Abdominal Aortic Aneurysm

Although AAA can be detected by physical examination, most are diagnosed today using an ultrasound scan or CAT scan. These are simple, non-invasive exams conducted on an outpatient basis. These exams also measure the size of AAA—a key element in determining the best treatment.

When aortic aneurysms are diagnosed early, treatment is safe and effective and the aneurysm can be cured. Aneurysms are often detected while performing tests for entirely different reasons. Most patients have no symptoms, so if you are at risk, it is important to have a discussion about AAA with your doctor.

Treatment Options

Surgical Treatment

If the AAA is larger than 5–6 centimeters in diameter (about the size of a lemon), it will require treatment. Your physician's decision to repair will be based on the risk of the aneurysm rupturing, along with surgical or procedure risks and risks associated with other pre-existing conditions. Smaller aneurysms that cause back or abdominal pain may also need treatment, especially for those that are enlarging rapidly.

Surgical treatment of AAA has been performed routinely in this country for about fifty years. It is a very successful and durable procedure. During the surgery, the surgeon makes an abdominal incision, then replaces the diseased part of the aorta with a Dacron or Teflon graft that is carefully matched to the normal aorta. This graft is sewn in place by the surgeon. Most patients stay in the hospital for five to ten days if no complications occur. Complete recovery from the operation may take one to two months before returning to a full and normal life.

After fifty years of experience with these procedures, the facts show that more than 90 percent of patients make a full recovery from surgery. Once patients have recovered, their aneurysms are permanently cured!

Less Invasive Treatments of AAA

Recent advances in catheter-based technologies have led to exciting new treatments for aortic aneurysms. Now, endovascular grafting technology allows the repair of the AAA by inserting a graft through a small incision in the groin. The endovascular method allows the graft to be delivered through a catheter or tube inserted in a groin artery. X-ray guidance is then used to accurately position the graft in the AAA. The graft is then expanded inside the aorta and held in place with metallic hooks rather than sutures. The hospital stay is usually only one or two days, and most patients can return to work or normal daily activities in about a week. Patients with other medical problems or those that could not withstand major surgery can be considered for repair by an endovascular graft.

Endovascular grafting may not be possible in every case. Endovascular grafts are specially manufactured and don't "fit" everyone's anatomical situation. Standard surgery may still be the best option for many. As a fairly new procedure, endografts do not yet have a fifty-year track record to compare to that of surgery for AAA. Speak with your physician about the best option for you.

The combination of earlier diagnosis with safer, simpler, and ever more successful treatments can prevent needless deaths due to ruptured abdominal aortic aneurysms.

Chapter 44

Peripheral Arterial Disease and Claudication

What is peripheral arterial disease?

Peripheral arterial disease (PAD) is a problem with blood flow in the arteries. Arteries carry blood to the muscles and organs in your body. When you have diseased arteries, they become narrow or blocked. The most common cause of narrow or blocked arteries is fatty deposits (also called atherosclerosis). The most common complaint of people with PAD is claudication. If you notice pain in your legs after you walk a block or more, ask your doctor about claudication and PAD.

What is claudication?

Claudication is pain in the calf or thigh muscle that occurs after you have walked a certain distance, such as a block or two. The pain stops after you rest for a while.

Each time the pain occurs, it takes about the same amount of time for the pain to go away after you stop walking.

How exactly are PAD and claudication related?

Claudication occurs because not enough blood is flowing to a muscle (PAD). The artery that normally supplies blood to the muscle gets narrow, and less blood can flow through the artery. When you're resting, enough blood flows to the muscle to meet the needs of the muscle. When you exercise (walk), the working muscle needs more blood, and the narrowed artery may not let enough through.

Who is at risk of getting PAD or claudication?

Risk factors for claudication and PAD include high blood pressure, diabetes, high cholesterol, cigarette smoking, and older age. Claudication is also more likely in people who already have atherosclerosis in other arteries, such as the arteries in the heart or brain. People with claudication may have had heart attacks or strokes.

How can my doctor be sure I have PAD or claudication?

Your doctor may suspect that your arteries have narrowed by listening to the blood flow in them, using a stethoscope. Then he or she may do some tests to see if you have PAD. Your doctor may also do tests to see if arteries in other parts of your body have atherosclerosis.

To check for claudication your doctor will check the pulses in the arteries in your legs. He or she may use a stethoscope to listen to the sound of your blood going through your arteries. Your doctor may hear a noise, called a bruit (say "brew-ee"), which may be a warning to your doctor that there is a narrow area in the artery.

What other tests might be done?

Your doctor may order a test to check the blood flow in your leg. This test is often performed in a hospital lab.

The test for checking the blood flow in your legs is called a Doppler study. With this test, blood pressure cuffs are wrapped around your arm and your leg on the same side. The kind of cuff put on your leg is the same kind of cuff that's wrapped around your arm to measure blood pressure. Four cuffs are wrapped around your leg—one at the upper thigh, one at the lower thigh, one at the upper calf, and one at the ankle—to measure the blood pressure from the top of your leg to your ankle. A cuff is also wrapped around your upper arm to measure the blood pressure in your arm. The blood pressure in your arm is compared with the blood pressure in your leg. A drop in the blood pressure in your leg may indicate narrowing of an artery.

If surgery might help treat the symptoms of claudication, your doctor may recommend an arteriography. This is an x-ray taken after dye is injected into an artery. The dye study may show narrowing in an artery and provides a "map" for the surgeon who will do the surgery.

Can PAD and claudication be treated?

Yes. PAD and claudication are often treated with diet and exercise, and sometimes medicine. People with PAD or claudication should not smoke. It is important for these people to bring down high cholesterol, high blood pressure, and high blood sugar levels.

A walking program is very helpful. You should walk at least three times a week for thirty to forty-five minutes each time. Walk until the pain is too uncomfortable to continue. Stop and rest until the pain goes away. Then start walking again. If you prefer to begin an exercise program, such as walking or stair climbing, begin exercising slowly and gradually increase the time you spend exercising. You may see improvement in your symptoms within two months. To begin an exercise program, exercise each day for thirty to sixty minutes.

Medicine can help some people with PAD and claudication. Pentoxifylline (brand name: Trental or Pentoxil) or cilostazol (brand name: Pletal) may help your claudication. Ask your doctor if medicine is right for you. If your arteries are badly blocked, you may need surgery to open them up.

Chapter 45

Critical Limb Ischemia

What is critical limb ischemia?

Critical limb ischemia, or CLI, is a severe obstruction of the arteries that seriously decreases blood flow to the extremities (hands, feet, and legs) and has progressed to the point of severe pain and even skin ulcers or sores. Critical limb ischemia (CLI) is often present in individuals with severe peripheral arterial disease (PAD). The pain caused by CLI can wake up an individual at night. This pain, also called "rest pain," can be relieved temporarily by hanging the leg over the edge of the bed or getting up to walk around.

CLI is a very severe condition of (PAD) and needs comprehensive treatment by a vascular surgeon or vascular specialist. This condition will not improve on its own!

How is it diagnosed?

The vascular specialist will assess the status of the disease by conducting a physical exam. He or she will want to ascertain what procedures or treatments have occurred in the past and what other conditions you have, such as diabetes, or heart disease. In addition, diagnostic tests will be performed to determine the severity of the disease and to identify the best treatment plan.

What are the treatment options?

Treatment for CLI can be quite complex and individualized, but the overall goal should always be to reduce the pain and improve blood flow to save the leg. A treatment plan will likely include medications, smoking cessation, ulcer care, and surgery or endovascular procedures.

Medications: Several medications may be prescribed to prevent further progression of the disease, to reduce the effect of contributing factors such as high blood pressure, high cholesterol, and diabetes, and most certainly to reduce the pain. Medications that prevent clotting or fight infections may also be prescribed.

Smoking Cessation: If you smoke, stop! It may save your leg and your life!

Ulcer Care: Treatment will likely include medications and dressings for ulcers.

Surgery or Endovascular Procedures: Surgical or endovascular procedures can be highly successful methods that restore oxygenated blood flow to the areas of skin breakdown. An endovascular procedure consists of a small incision through which a catheter is inserted to where the blockages occur. A balloon may be inflated (angioplasty), the plaque may be scraped off the artery, or the clot may be removed or broken up (thrombolysis). A wire-reinforced stent may be left in the artery to keep it open.

A bypass graft may be performed in more serious cases. This surgical procedure uses either an artificial tube or one of your veins as a new artery to bring improved blood flow to the area. Thus the place where the blood flow is constricted is bypassed. In a few cases, the surgeon may cut open the artery and scrape out the plaque, keeping the artery usable. The last recourse would be amputation of a toe, part of the foot, or leg. Amputation occurs in about 25 percent of all CLI patients.

Since treatment depends on the severity of the disease and many individual parameters, it is essential that someone with ulcers or pain in the legs or feet when walking or at rest see a vascular specialist as soon as possible. The earlier a diagnosis can be made, the earlier treatment can be started, with less serious consequences.

Chapter 46

Raynaud's Phenomenon

What is Raynaud's phenomenon?

Raynaud's phenomenon is a disorder that affects the blood vessels in the fingers, toes, ears, and nose. This disorder is characterized by episodic attacks, called vasospastic attacks, which cause the blood vessels in the digits (fingers and toes) to constrict (tighten or close). Raynaud's phenomenon can occur on its own, or it can occur with another condition such as scleroderma or lupus.

Although estimates vary, recent surveys show that Raynaud's phenomenon may affect 5 to 10 percent of the general population in the United States. Women are more likely than men to have the disorder. An attack of Raynaud's is usually triggered by exposure to cold or emotional stress. Along with the fingers and toes, the nose, lips, or earlobes can also be affected.

Under normal circumstances, when a person is exposed to cold, his or her body's response is to slow the loss of heat. The body does this by causing the blood vessels that control the blood flow to the skin's surface to move blood from the surface arteries to vessels deeper in the body.

For people who have Raynaud's, however, this normal body response is intensified by contractions of the small blood vessels that

"Raynaud's Phenomenon," © 2004 The Cleveland Clinic Foundation, 9500 Euclid Avenue, Cleveland, OH 44195. Additional information is available from the Cleveland Clinic Health Information Center, 216-444-3771, toll-free at 800-223-2273 ext. 43771, or www.clevelandclinic.org/health.

supply blood to the fingers and toes. In some cases, this causes the arteries of the fingers and toes to collapse. The result is a greatly decreased supply of blood to the affected body areas, causing skin discoloration.

A person with Raynaud's phenomenon can experience three phases of skin color changes. Pallor (whiteness) may occur in response to the collapse of the arteries in an affected body part. Cyanosis (blueness) appears because the fingers or toes are not getting enough oxygen-rich blood. Other symptoms that occur during cyanosis are feeling cold and numbness. Rubor (redness) occurs as the blood returns to the affected areas. After an attack is over, throbbing and tingling may occur in the fingers and toes. Attacks of Raynaud's phenomenon can last from less than a minute to several hours.

Doctors classify Raynaud's phenomenon as either primary or secondary.

Primary Raynaud's Phenomenon

Also known as Raynaud's disease, this form is the more common and the milder of the two types. A person who has primary Raynaud's has no other diseases that may causes Raynaud's symptoms or associated medical problems. About 75 percent of all cases of primary Raynaud's phenomenon are diagnosed in women between ages fifteen and forty. People with the primary form rarely develop other diseases related with Raynaud's such as lupus or scleroderma.

Secondary Raynaud's Phenomenon

Secondary Raynaud's phenomenon is less common than the primary form; however, it is often a more serious disorder. For patients with a secondary form of Raynaud's, the disorder is caused by an underlying disease or condition. It is especially common in people with connective tissue diseases. Some of these diseases reduce blood flow to the fingers and toes by causing the blood vessel walls to thicken and the vessels to constrict too easily. Raynaud's phenomenon occurs in about 85 to 95 percent of patients with scleroderma and it is present in about one-third of patients with systemic lupus erythematosus (lupus). Raynaud's also can occur in patients who have other connective tissue diseases, including Sjögren's syndrome, dermatomyositis, and polymyositis.

How is Raynaud's phenomenon diagnosed?

It is often fairly easy to diagnose Raynaud's but more difficult to identify the form of the disorder.

One diagnostic test useful in helping doctors determine the correct form of Raynaud's is known as nailfold capillaroscopy, in which capillaries are studied under strong magnification. For people with primary Raynaud's phenomenon, the results of this test will be normal; however, the results are abnormal for those who have the secondary form. During this test, the doctor places a drop of oil on the patient's nailfolds, which is the skin at the base of the fingernail. The doctor then examines the nailfolds under a microscope to look for abnormalities of the capillaries. If the capillaries are enlarged or abnormal, this may indicate that the patient has a connective tissue disease.

Two other tests that the doctor may order to help distinguish between the two forms of Raynaud's are the antinuclear antibody test (ANA) and the erythrocyte sedimentation rate (ESR).

The ANA test determines whether the body is producing special proteins (antibodies) that commonly occur in people who have connective tissue diseases. The test results will be negative for patients with the primary form of the disease, and may be positive for those with the secondary form.

The ESR test measures inflammation in the body and tests how fast red blood cells settle out of unclotted blood. Inflammation in the body will cause an elevated ESR. An abnormal reading is an indicator of the secondary form of the disease, whereas a normal reading indicates primary Raynaud's phenomenon.

How is Raynaud's phenomenon treated?

The aims of treatment are to reduce the number and severity of attacks and to prevent tissue damage and loss in the fingers and toes. Doctors may prescribe medications for some patients, usually those with secondary Raynaud's phenomenon; however, they most often prescribe non-drug treatments.

Non-Drug Treatments

Several non-drug treatments can help decrease the severity of a Raynaud's attack as well as promote overall well-being.

- *Be proactive during an attack*: A Raynaud's attack should not be ignored. By taking the proper steps both the length and the severity of the attack can be decreased. The first and most important action is to warm the hands or feet. In cold weather, people should go indoors. Running warm water over the fingers or toes or soaking them in a bowl of warm but not hot water will also warm them. Heat causes the vessels to dilate (good) but also increases the tissue's demand for oxygen (bad). Excessive heat can promote gangrene (very bad). Learning relaxation techniques as well as taking time to relax will further help to end an attack.

- *Keep warm*: Not only is it important to keep your hands and feet warm, but it is also helpful to avoid chilling any other part of the body. In cold weather, people with Raynaud's phenomenon should pay particular attention to the way they dress. Several layers of loose clothing, socks, hats, and gloves or mittens are recommended. Hats are particularly important because a great deal of body heat is lost through the scalp. The feet should be kept dry and warm. Chemical warmers, such as small heating pouches that can be placed in pockets, mittens, boots, or shoes, can give added protection during long periods outdoors. Patients with secondary Raynaud's should talk to their doctor before exercising outdoors in cold weather.

- *Quit smoking*: Nicotine causes the skin temperature to drop, which may lead to an attack.

- *Learn to control stress*: Because stress may trigger an attack, particularly for people who have primary Raynaud's phenomenon, learning to recognize and avoid stressful situations may help control the number of attacks. Many people have found that relaxation or biofeedback training can help decrease the number and the severity of attacks.

- *Exercise*: Many doctors encourage patients who have Raynaud's phenomenon to exercise regularly. Most people find that exercise promotes an overall well-being, increases energy level, helps control weight, and promotes restful sleep. Patients with Raynaud's phenomenon should talk to their doctors before starting an exercise program.

Medications

People with secondary Raynaud's phenomenon are more likely than those with the primary form to be treated with medications. Many health care professionals believe that the most effective and safest drugs are calcium-channel blockers, which relax smooth muscles and dilate the small blood vessels. These drugs decrease the frequency and severity of attacks in about two-thirds of patients who have primary or secondary Raynaud's phenomenon. These drugs also can help heal skin ulcers on the fingers or toes.

Other medications that have helped patients with Raynaud's include alpha blockers, which counteract norepinephrine, a hormone that constricts blood vessels, and vasodilators (drugs that relax the blood vessels), such as nitroglycerin paste, which is applied to the fingers, to help heal skin ulcers.

It is important to keep in mind that the treatment for Raynaud's phenomenon is not always successful. Often, patients with the secondary form will not respond as well to treatment as those with the primary form of the disorder. Patients may find that one drug works better than another and some people may experience side effects that require stopping the medication. For other people, a drug may become less effective over time. Regardless of the medication a patient is using, it is important to schedule follow-up appointments with the doctor to monitor effects of the medications.

Chapter 47

What You Need to Know about Vasculitis

What is vasculitis?

Vasculitis is a general term that refers to the inflammation of blood vessels. When blood vessels become inflamed, they can react in only limited ways. They may become weakened, stretch and increase in size, or become narrow—even to the point of closing off entirely.

What are the causes of vasculitis?

In many cases, the causes of vasculitis are not known. However, in a few cases, the cause may be traced to recent or ongoing infections, like those due to viruses such as hepatitis. Occasionally, an allergic reaction to a medicine may trigger vasculitis.

Vasculitis can sometimes develop after an infection has come and gone. Usually in these cases, the infection caused an abnormal response in the person's immune system, damaging the blood vessels.

Vasculitis may also be related to other diseases of the immune system that the patient had for months or years. For example, vasculitis could be a complication of rheumatoid arthritis, systemic lupus, or Sjögren's syndrome.

"What You Need to Know about Vasculitis" by Gary Hoffman, M.D., Chairman, Cleveland Clinic Department of Rheumatic and Immunologic Diseases. © 2004 The Cleveland Clinic Foundation. All rights reserved.

What are the consequences of vasculitis?

In an extreme situation, when a segment of a blood vessel becomes weakened, it may then stretch and bulge (called an "aneurysm"). The wall of the blood vessel can become so weak that it ruptures and bleeds. Fortunately, this is a very rare event.

If a blood vessel becomes inflamed and narrowed, blood supply to that area may be partially or completely eliminated. If collateral blood vessels (thought of as alternate routes of blood supply) are not available in sufficient quantity to carry the blood to such sites, the tissue supplied by the affected blood vessels will die. This is called infarction.

Because vasculitis can occur in any part of the body, any tissue or organ can be at risk.

Who is affected by vasculitis?

Vasculitis can affect people of all ages from childhood to adulthood. There are some types of vasculitis that occur in certain age groups more than others.

What are the types of vasculitis?

There are many types of vasculitis. Some forms may be restricted in their location to certain organs (these are called isolated forms of vasculitis).

Examples include vasculitis that occurs only in either the skin, eye, brain, or certain internal organs. There are also systemic (or generalized) types of vasculitis. Generalized vasculitis may affect many organ systems at the same time. However, the types of vasculitis that are generalized also differ a great deal from one another. Some of the generalized forms may be quite mild and may not require therapy. Other forms may be severe, affecting critical organs and, if left untreated, may lead to death within days or months.

What are the symptoms of vasculitis?

Because any organ system may be involved, an enormous number of symptoms are possible. If the skin is involved, there may be a rash. If nerves suffer loss of blood supply, there may initially be an abnormal sensation followed by a loss of sensation. Vasculitis in the brain may cause a stroke, or in the heart may result in a heart attack. Inflammation in the kidney may result in abnormalities noted on urinalysis and can lead to progressive kidney failure.

Sometimes the symptoms are nonspecific. When inflammation is present in the body, we tend to respond in ways that tell us that we are not well, but those responses may not be unique to vasculitis at all. For example, along with the symptoms mentioned previously, a person with vasculitis may also have a fever or experience loss of appetite, weight loss, and loss of energy.

How is vasculitis treated?

Treatment depends entirely upon diagnosis and the organs that are affected. When vasculitis represents an allergic reaction, it may be "self-limiting," or will go away on its own and not require treatment. In other instances, when critical organs such as the lungs, brain, or kidneys are involved, the outlook is less positive, and aggressive and timely treatment is necessary.

Treatment generally consists of corticosteroid medications (prednisone is the most commonly prescribed). Chemotherapeutic drugs (like those used to treat cancer) are also used, but in doses considerably lower than people with cancer may receive. The goal of this type of chemotherapy is to suppress the abnormal immune response that has led to blood vessel damage.

What is the outlook for people with severe vasculitis?

The outlook for a patient who has vasculitis will vary with the type of vasculitis that is present. Knowing the type of vasculitis (the diagnosis) allows the doctor to predict the likelihood of illness severity and outcome (called the prognosis).

In the past, people with severe vasculitis may have had anticipated survival of only weeks to months. However, today, with proper treatment, normal life spans are possible. The success of therapy is related to prompt diagnosis, aggressive treatment, and careful follow-up with patients to be sure that side effects that can be as bad as the disease do not develop.

Once vasculitis is "under control," medications may be cautiously withdrawn, with the hope that the patient will sustain a long remission or cure, independent of treatment. Because doctors cannot predict how long a patient may remain in remission, it is very important for patients with more severe forms of vasculitis to remain under the care of a knowledgeable physician for the rest of their lives.

Chapter 48

Diseases of the Veins

Three sets of vessels comprise the circulatory system: arteries, lymphatics, and veins. Arteries bring oxygen-carrying blood from the heart to the tissues. In the normal course of blood circulation, small amounts of fluid and protein leak from arteries and veins. Lymphatic vessels bring this protein-rich fluid back into the circulation. The third type of blood vessel is the vein.

Veins bring oxygen-depleted blood from the organs and tissues to the heart and lungs, where it is reoxygenated. Blood return to the heart tends to be passive and is enabled by muscle contraction in the arms and legs. Because the venous system is a low-pressure one, the telltale complaints and physical signs of venous disease on which your physician relies for diagnosis are often subtle and sometimes require further testing. Diseases of the veins fall into two broad categories: blockage from a blood clot (thrombosis) and inadequate venous drainage (insufficiency).

Thrombosis

The legs are the most common location for blood clot formation (thrombus) in the venous system. Today, the most commonly encountered causes for blood clots include cancer, prolonged immobility, an inherited tendency for blood clotting, pregnancy, and contraceptive use.

Reprinted from "Diseases of the Veins," by Joshua A. Beckman, M.D., M.S., *Circulation* 106, no. 17 (2002): 2170–72. © 2002 Lippincott Williams and Wilkins; reprinted with permission.

Superficial Thrombophlebitis

Blood clots may develop in the veins that lie either just under the skin or deep within the limb. In the skin-deep (superficial) veins, a blood clot commonly appears as a red streak along the course of an affected vein and is often accompanied by inflammation (phlebitis). The vein may feel warm and tender and may be swollen. This combination of clot and inflammation, known as superficial thrombophlebitis, commonly occurs in the setting of varicose veins. Cancer may be the cause for development of many episodes of superficial blood clots; this is known as Trousseau's syndrome.

Superficial thrombophlebitis is typically more annoying than dangerous because the likelihood that the clot(s) will break up and be transported in pieces to the lung is very low. Physicians commonly treat symptoms with leg elevation, moist heat, and nonsteroidal anti-inflammatory medications (such as ibuprofen). Rarely, blood clots with persistent symptoms will be treated with a short course of blood-thinning medication (anticoagulation).

Deep Vein Thrombosis

Blood clots in the veins deep within the legs (deep vein thromboses, or DVTs) are more difficult to diagnose because symptoms are present in only 50 percent of patients. When symptoms are present, patients may complain of pain with walking, typically in the ball of the foot; leg swelling; leg pressure; or leg fullness. DVTs are classified as primary or secondary. Primary DVTs occur in the absence of an obvious cause and are usually caused by an inherited tendency to clotting. Secondary DVTs occur as a result of a specific event, like immobilization after surgery or cancer.

When a clot forms, blood return to the heart is blocked. Smaller, alternate veins (collateral vessels) can return blood back to the heart, but not so efficiently as the central large vein. This backup increases both pressure within the vein and also fluid leakage from the vein, resulting in leg swelling. The clot itself can cause inflammation, producing warmth, redness, and tenderness. During examination, the doctor may note swelling, or fullness of the affected muscles, or feel the cord of clotted blood in the vessel.

Physicians focus treatment on the complication of blood clots. Without treatment, up to one-fourth of all leg DVTs will have a piece of clot detach, travel through the veins, and lodge within the lungs, where it can cause a pulmonary embolism (PE). Complications of a PE are significant shortness of breath, marked exercise limitation, and death.

The diagnosis of DVT is most commonly made with ultrasound. Ultrasound is very reliable for discovering blood clots at or above the knee, the location most likely to send off an embolism. In contrast, the veins below the knee are smaller, the anatomy of the veins commonly varies between people, and the ability of the test to diagnose a DVT is not as high. Only rarely is it necessary to perform more testing, such as magnetic resonance imaging (MRI) or a dye test (a venogram).

To decrease the symptoms of a DVT and prevent the embolization of a fragment to the lungs, physicians will prescribe blood-thinning medication (anticoagulants), first heparin (given intravenously or by injection) and then warfarin (administered by mouth). Anticoagulation dramatically reduces the rate of pulmonary embolism, should be continued for three to six months, and requires frequent measurement of the level of blood thinning. Appropriate therapy lowers the occurrence of pulmonary embolism from 25 percent to 5 percent over the first year but is associated with a small increase (about 2 percent to 3 percent) in the risk of significant bleeding.

Two areas of therapy are controversial: (1) use of a clot-dissolving (thrombolytic) agent and (2) use of blood thinners for clots in the calf. Thrombolytic agents carry a much higher risk of bleeding and are typically reserved for severe DVTs that seriously restrict blood flow in the leg arteries. Most physicians will prescribe a blood-thinning medication for calf blood clots, although the risk of embolization is lower. Anticoagulation should certainly be provided for patients with a calf DVT and an ongoing cause for clotting, such as cancer or orthopedic surgery. In some circumstances, physicians may opt for a repeat ultrasound five to seven days later, treating only those clots that have changed in appearance.

Insufficiency

Resulting from a blood clot or an inherited abnormality of the vein wall, inadequate venous drainage (venous insufficiency) can be classified similarly to thrombosis: superficial (varicose veins) and deep (chronic venous insufficiency).

Varicose Veins

Superficial venous insufficiency is also known as varicose veins. These are dilated, snake-like segments of veins that lie just below the skin. They are more common in women, and half of all patients being treated will have a family history. In the absence of a blood clot, there is most likely a structural abnormality of the vein wall or valve, allowing backflow of blood and increase in pressure within the vessel. Valves, which prevent backflow of blood, may become damaged, resulting in pooling of blood within the veins. Obesity, pregnancy, prolonged standing, and a sedentary lifestyle may exacerbate dilation of the veins.

Although most patients see a physician for the poor cosmetic appearance of varicose veins, they can also experience symptoms of burning, aching, or itchiness. Symptoms tend to be less severe in the morning after a night of leg elevation in bed and worsen through the day with standing. Occasionally, without proper care, varicose veins may progress and cause skin ulcers, skin infections, blood clots, and spontaneous bleeding.

Standard therapies for varicose veins are exercise, weight loss, blood pressure control, and compression stockings. Compression stockings are specially fit and apply pressure to prevent the veins from being engorged with blood and thus from worsening over time. The stockings should be applied in the morning when the veins are empty. Thus, after washing up in the morning, patients should get back into bed for a few minutes to elevate their legs and thereby drain the veins prior to putting on these stockings. Leg elevation is also helpful; in a reclining position, one should elevate the ankles to the level of the heart or higher. Sitting with legs elevated on a stool or ottoman is not sufficient to drain blood from the veins in the legs. Elevating the foot of the bed is also beneficial. The injection of a scarring agent and surgical removal are rarely needed, but may be used to remove specific varicose veins for cosmetic purposes. However, up to 50 percent of all patients will develop recurrent varicose veins after removal.

Chronic Venous Insufficiency

When drainage from the veins deep within the limbs is inadequate over a long period of time, patients develop chronic venous insufficiency. Inadequate venous drainage may occur as a result of obstructed blood flow between the limbs and the heart or because of reflux backward of blood into the veins caused by faulty valves. The most common cause of obstruction is a DVT; other causes are inherited abnormalities and compression of the vein, for example from a tumor or bandage. One-third of all patients with DVT will develop chronic venous insufficiency, usually within five years. Reflux, or excess flow back into the veins, may occur when the valves in the vein fail, most commonly as a result of clot-related scarring or an inherited valve abnormality.

Chronic venous insufficiency is characterized by leg swelling, pain, darkened skin color, and coarsening skin texture. Gravity is an important factor in the return of blood to the heart. Swelling is worsened when the leg is below the level of the heart (dependent) and improved after a night of leg elevation in bed. Leg pain, commonly described as heaviness or aching, is usually worse in the warmer weather and during menstruation. Changes in skin color and texture result from deposits of destroyed red blood cells that accumulate over time. Less commonly, patients may report burning, itching, pain, and the development of moist, irregular ulcers around the ankle.

Treatment for venous insufficiency is aimed at improving blood return to the heart and decreasing fluid escape from the veins. Compression stockings, leg elevation, specialized care of ulcers, and the occasional use of diuretics are the main options for therapy. Surgical options are limited and used rarely in this disorder.

Conclusion

Diseases of the veins are common, relatively easy to treat, and, with treatment, rarely life-threatening. Addressing the problems of thrombosis and insufficiency should improve physical functioning and quality of life. In the absence of appropriate medical care, patients risk marked disability and life-threatening complications, such as pulmonary embolism. Understanding the nature of these disorders will facilitate therapeutic communication between patient and physician, improving the proper use of appropriate therapies.

Additional Resources

American College of Cardiology. Peripheral vascular diseases and you. Available at: http://www.acc.org/media/patient/PVD/#vascular. Accessed July 30, 2002.

Goldhaber, SZ, Grasso-Correnti N. Treatment of blood clots. *Circulation* 106, no. 20 (2002): 138–40.

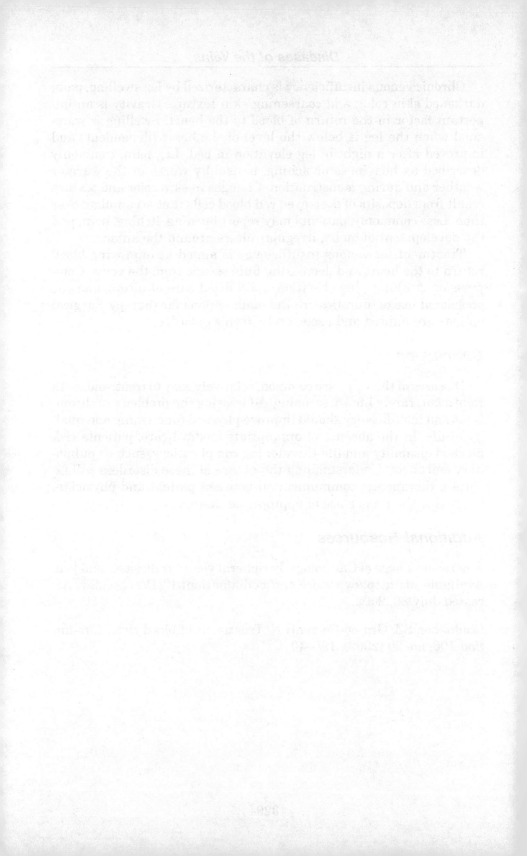

Chapter 49

Pulmonary Embolism and Deep Vein Thrombosis

The heart pumps oxygenated blood through the aorta to smaller arteries. After the blood supplies nutrients to vital organs, it returns through veins for reoxygenation in the lungs. Blood clots called deep vein thrombi (DVT) often develop in the deep leg veins. Pulmonary embolism (PE) occurs when clots break off from vein walls and travel through the heart to the pulmonary arteries. The broader term "venous thromboembolism" (VTE) refers to DVT, PE, or to a combination of both.

What is the epidemiology of venous thromboembolism?

VTE poses a public health threat with an estimated incidence in the United States of 250,000 to 2 million cases per year. Predisposition to VTE arises from acquired conditions, inherited disorders, or both. Many of the acquired risk factors can be modified, thus lessening the likelihood of PE or DVT.

What are the acquired risk factors?

Long-haul air travel is the most talked-about risk factor for PE. Other acquired risk factors include obesity, cigarette smoking, hypertension, immobilization, surgery, and trauma. Chronic medical illnesses such as congestive heart failure, chronic obstructive pulmonary

Reprinted from "Pulmonary Embolism and Deep Vein Thrombosis," by Samuel Z. Goldhaber and Ruth B. Morrison, *Circulation* 106, no. 12 (2002): 1436–38. © 2002 Lippincott Williams and Wilkins; reprinted with permission.

disease, and cancer also predispose to PE. PE is also a prominent women's health issue. Risk factors include oral contraceptives, pregnancy, and hormone replacement therapy.

What are the inherited disorders?

Heredity plays an important role in a patient's susceptibility to PE. We are just beginning to develop genetic tests (such as factor V Leiden and the prothrombin gene mutation) that can identify those who are predisposed. The presence of these risk factors is sometimes called a prothrombotic or thrombophilic state.

How is the diagnosis established?

DVT most often originates in the calf, with a persistent cramping or "charley horse" that intensifies over several days. Leg swelling and discoloration may accompany the increase in discomfort. Upper-extremity DVT may cause otherwise unexplained upper arm or neck swelling. The most frequently used diagnostic imaging test is the noninvasive venous ultrasound examination.

Many patients with PE have a vague sense that something is wrong but have difficulty defining or describing the problem. Consequently, they often delay seeking medical attention. At times, because symptoms are so vague and nonspecific, medical professionals will diagnose anxiety rather than PE. To establish the diagnosis of PE, the most frequently used noninvasive imaging test is the rapid-speed chest computed tomography (CT) scan.

What are the warning signals of PE?

- Unexplained shortness of breath (the most common symptom of PE)
- Chest discomfort, usually worse with a deep breath or coughing
- A general sense of anxiety or nervousness
- Lightheadedness or blacking out

What should I expect at the hospital?

Definitely expect:

- Questions about symptoms of chest or leg discomfort, breathing difficulties, or lightheadedness

- Questions about whether you or your family members have suffered prior VTE

- A check of your blood pressure, pulse rate, breathing rate, heart, lungs, and legs

- An ECG and chest x-ray

Possibly expect:

- A blood test (D-dimer) that screens for PE (If results are normal, PE is extremely unlikely.)

- A chest CT scan, which directly images blood clots causing blockages in the pulmonary arteries

- A lung scan, which indirectly identifies areas of decreased blood flow in the lung tissue as a consequence of PE

- Blood tests to detect a prothrombotic state, especially in relatively young and otherwise healthy patients with PE or DVT

What treatment will I receive?

PE can range from mild to severe. Mild PE is managed with blood thinners (anticoagulation). Severe PE requires additional measures, such as clot busters (thrombolytic therapy) or embolectomy, a procedure in which the clot is removed with either a catheter or surgery.

Anticoagulation begins with a combination of two blood thinners: (1) heparin, administered intravenously or by injection, and (2) warfarin, an oral blood thinner. Heparin comes in two principal forms. The traditional unfractionated form ordinarily requires intravenous administration. There is no fixed dose for this type of heparin. Instead, the dose is titrated to a blood test called the partial thromboplastin time. This blood test is usually performed several times daily for the first few days and then once daily thereafter. More recently, low-molecular-weight heparins have begun replacing unfractionated heparin. Low-molecular-weight heparins are ordinarily prescribed in proportion to the patient's weight, require no blood testing, and necessitate injection once or twice daily.

We overlap heparin treatment with warfarin until the oral blood thinner becomes effective, usually after five to ten days of combined therapy. We determine the proper dose of warfarin by a blood test reported as the International Normalized Ratio (INR). The target INR range is usually between 2.0 and 3.0. Interactions with food, alcohol, and other drugs can dramatically alter the INR. Sometimes, major fluctuations in the INR occur for no apparent reason. Too high an INR may result in bleeding as a side effect. Too low an INR may result in recurrent clotting. Patients may need their INR checked every few weeks or months, according to the stability of the readings. It is important for patients to keep a record of their values over time.

PE is usually treated in the hospital with intravenous unfractionated heparin as a bridge to warfarin. In contrast, DVT can often be managed successfully on an outpatient basis with low-molecular-weight heparin injections as a bridge to oral anticoagulation with warfarin. The most controversial area in VTE therapy is the optimal duration of warfarin anticoagulation. The current recommendation is usually at least six months of anticoagulation, but it can sometimes be longer, according to individual patient circumstances.

In patients who cannot tolerate anticoagulation or those for whom anticoagulation fails, a permanent metal filter is inserted into the inferior vena cava, the largest vein below the heart, to prevent large blood clots from reaching the pulmonary arteries and causing PE. Unfortunately, the filter devices do not halt the clotting process. Their presence predisposes to future venous clots on or below the filter.

What can be done to prevent venous thrombosis?

Maintaining ideal body weight with a healthy nutritional program and exercise regimen will generally reduce the likelihood of venous thrombosis. Specific other measures are as follows:

- To prevent immobility or inactivity: Walk, jog, bicycle, or swim.

- To prevent obesity: Limit caloric intake, exercise, and avoid saturated fats.

- To prevent VTE during air travel: Drink extra water, walk if feasible, wear vascular compression stockings, and avoid alcohol.

- To quit cigarette smoking: Use nicotine patch, gum, or spray, or consider the prescription drug bupropion.

- To control hypertension: Self-check blood pressure, and report elevated readings to primary care provider.

- To deal with a known genetic predisposition to VTE: Alert your healthcare provider about the family history and any abnormal blood tests related to a clotting tendency.

- To prevent VTE after trauma or surgery: Discuss with the treating physician the implementation of measures such as mechanical compression boots for the legs or blood thinners given either intravenously or as injections.

- To prevent VTE during a hospitalization precipitated by a medical condition: Discuss with the treating physician measures such as mechanical compression boots for the legs or blood thinners given either intravenously or as injections.

- To prevent VTE when planning birth control: Discuss VTE risks, and consider alternatives to oral contraceptives.

- To prevent VTE during pregnancy: Consider daily self-injected heparin if considered at high risk of VTE.

- To prevent VTE during hormone replacement therapy: Keep in mind that VTE risks with hormone replacement therapy are similar to those of oral contraceptives.

References

Goldhaber SZ. Pulmonary embolism. *N Engl J Med*. 1998; 339: 93–104.

Goldhaber SZ, Visani L, De Rosa M. Acute pulmonary embolism: clinical outcomes in the International Cooperative Pulmonary Embolism Registry (ICOPER). *Lancet*. 1999; 353: 1386–1389.

Goldhaber SZ, ed. Frequently asked questions of the Pulmonary Embolism Support Group, Brigham and Women's Hospital. Available at: http://icoper.cineca.com/faq_icoper.htm. Accessed August 23, 2002.

Geerts WH, Heit JA, Clagett GP, et al. Prevention of venous thromboembolism. *Chest*. 2001; 119: 132S–175S.

Goldhaber SZ, Ridker PM. *Thrombosis and Thromboembolism*. New York, NY: Marcel Dekker, Inc., 2002.

Chapter 50

Varicose Veins and Spider Veins

What are varicose veins and spider veins?

The heart pumps blood to supply oxygen and nutrients to all parts of the body. Arteries carry blood from the heart toward the body parts, while veins carry blood from the body parts back to the heart. As the blood is pumped back to the heart, veins act as one-way valves to prevent the blood from flowing backward. If the one-way valve becomes weak, some of the blood can leak back into the vein, collect there, and then become congested or clogged. This congestion will cause the vein to abnormally enlarge. These enlarged veins can be either varicose veins or spider veins.

Varicose veins are very swollen and raised above the surface of the skin. They are dark purple or blue in color, and can look like cords or very twisted and bulging. They are found most often on the backs of the calves or on the inside of the leg, anywhere from the groin to the ankle. During pregnancy, varicose veins called hemorrhoids can form in the vagina or around the anus.

Spider veins are similar to varicose veins, but they are smaller, are often red or blue in color, and are closer to the surface of the skin than varicose veins. They can look like a tree branch or spider web with their short jagged lines. Spider veins can be found on both the legs and the face. They can cover either a very small or a very large area of skin.

Reprinted from "Varicose Veins and Spider Veins," National Women's Health Information Center (www.4woman.gov), December 2000.

How common are abnormal leg veins?

As many as 60 percent of all American women and men suffer from some form of vein disorder, but women are more affected—up to 50 percent overall. It also is estimated that 41 percent of all women will suffer from abnormal leg veins by the time they are in their fifties.

What causes varicose and spider veins?

No one knows the exact cause of spider and varicose veins, but there are several factors that cause a person to be more likely to develop them. Heredity, or being born with weak vein valves, is the greatest factor. Hormones also play a role. The hormonal changes that occur during puberty, pregnancy, and menopause, as well as taking estrogen, progesterone, and birth control pills can cause a woman to develop varicose veins or spider veins. During pregnancy, besides the increases in hormone levels, there also is a great increase in the volume of blood in the body that can cause veins to enlarge. The enlarged uterus also puts more pressure on the veins. (Within three months after delivery, varicose veins usually improve. However, more abnormal veins are likely to develop and remain after additional pregnancies.)

Other factors that weaken vein valves and that may cause varicose or spider veins include aging, obesity, leg injury, and prolonged standing, such as for long hours on the job. Spider veins on the cheeks or nose of a fair-skinned person may occur from sun exposure.

Why do varicose and spider veins usually appear in the legs?

The veins in the legs have the toughest job of carrying blood back to the heart. They endure the most pressure—pressure that can overcome the strength of these one-way valves. The force of gravity, the pressure from body weight, and the task of carrying the blood from the bottom of the body up to the heart make the legs the primary location for varicose and spider veins.

Are varicose and spider veins painful or dangerous?

Medical treatment usually is not required for varicose or spider veins. However, varicose veins can become quite uncomfortable as well as look unattractive. Varicose veins usually enlarge and worsen over time. They can cause the legs and feet to swell. Although severe leg pain is not common, leg muscles may feel fatigued or heavy, or throb and cramp at night. The skin on the legs and around the ankles also can itch or burn.

In some cases, varicose veins and spider veins can cause more serious problems, and medical treatment will provide benefits. If the veins become severe, they can cause a condition called venous insufficiency, a severe clogging of the blood in the veins that prevents it from returning to the heart. This condition can cause problems like a deep-vein thrombosis (blood clot), or a severe bleeding infection. These usually are caused by injury to the varicose vein. A blood clot can be very dangerous because of the possibility of it traveling from the leg veins to the lungs, where it may block the heart and lungs from functioning. Lastly, because the skin tissue around the varicose vein may not receive enough nourishment, sores or skin ulcers may develop.

How can I prevent varicose and spider veins?

There are several easy things you can do to help prevent varicose and spider veins and to relieve discomfort from the ones you have:

- Protect your skin from the sun by wearing sunscreen to limit spider veins on the face.

- Exercise regularly to improve your leg strength, circulation, and vein strength. Focus on exercises that work your legs, such as walking or running.

- Control your weight to avoid placing too much pressure on your legs.

- Do not cross your legs when sitting. However, try to elevate your legs when resting.

- Do not stand for long periods of time. If you have to stand for long periods of time, shift your weight from one leg to the other every few minutes. If you have to sit for long periods of time, stand up and move around or take a short walk approximately every thirty minutes.

- Wear elastic support stockings, but avoid clothing that is too tight or that will constrict your waist, groin, or legs.

- Make sure to include high-fiber foods in your diet since constipation can contribute to varicose veins. High-fiber foods include fresh fruits and vegetables and whole grains, like bran. Control your salt intake. Salt, or sodium, can cause you to retain water or swell.

Should I see a doctor about varicose veins?

Remember these important questions when deciding whether to see your doctor:

- Has the varicose vein become swollen, red, or very tender or warm to the touch?
    - If yes, see your doctor.
    - If no, are there sores or a rash on the leg or near the ankle with the varicose vein, or are there circulation problems in your feet? If yes, see your doctor. If no, continue to follow the self-care tips listed here.

How are varicose and spider veins treated?

Besides a physical examination, your doctor can take x-rays or ultrasound pictures of the vein to assess the cause and severity of the problem. You may want to speak with a doctor who specializes in vein diseases (phlebology). You should discuss which treatment options are best for your condition and lifestyle. It is important to remember that not all cases of varicose veins are the same. Doctors may differ in the ways they treat you. Some available treatments or surgeries include:

Sclerotherapy

Of all available treatments, this one is most commonly used for both spider veins and varicose veins. It involves injecting a solution into the vein that causes the lining of the vein walls to swell, stick together, and eventually seal shut. The flow of blood is stopped and the vein turns into scar tissue. In a few weeks, the vein should fade. Although the same vein may need to be injected with the solution more than once, sclerotherapy is very effective if done correctly. The American Academy of Dermatology states that most patients can expect a 50 percent to 90 percent improvement. Also, a new and improved type of sclerotherapy called microsclerotherapy uses improved solutions and injection techniques that increase the success rate for removal of spider veins. Sclerotherapy does not require anesthesia, and can be done in the doctor's office.

Some side effects may occur at the site of the injection, such as stinging or painful cramps, red raised patches of skin, small skin ulcers, and bruises. Spots, brown lines, or groups of fine red blood vessels could appear around the vein being treated. These usually disappear. The treated vein could become inflamed or develop lumps of coagulated or congested blood. These are not dangerous. Applying heat and taking aspirin or antibiotics can relieve inflammation. Lumps of coagulated blood can be drained. Health insurance coverage varies. If the treatment is done for cosmetic reasons only, it may not be covered.

Electrodesiccation

This treatment is similar to sclerotherapy, except the veins are sealed off with an electrical current instead of the injection of solution. This treatment may leave scars.

Laser Surgery

Until recently, laser treatments mostly were used for treating spider veins on the face. Varicose veins in the legs did not respond consistently to this treatment, and some doctors doubted whether laser treatment actually worked. Furthermore, it was not covered by most health insurance plans. Now, however, new technology in laser treatments can effectively treat varicose veins in the legs.

Laser surgery works by sending very strong bursts of light onto the vein that make the vein slowly fade and disappear. Lasers are very direct and accurate, and damage only the area being treated. All skin types and colors can be safely treated with lasers. The American Academy of Dermatology believes that the new laser technology is more effective with fewer side effects. Laser surgery is more comfortable for patients because there are no needles or incisions. When the laser hits the skin, the patient feels only a small pinch, and the skin is soothed by cooling both before and after the laser is applied. There may be some redness or swelling of the skin right after the treatment, but this disappears within a few days. The skin also may be discolored, but this will disappear within one to two weeks. Treatments last fifteen to twenty minutes, and depending on the severity of the veins, two to five treatments are generally needed to remove varicose veins in the legs. Patients can return to normal activity right after treatment.

There are several types of lasers that can be used to treat varicose veins and spider veins on the legs and face. Although your doctor will decide which type is best to treat your condition, some of the lasers used to treat veins include yellow light lasers, green light lasers, and other intense pulsed light systems. Again, health insurance coverage varies. If the treatment is done for cosmetic reasons only, it may not be covered.

Closure Technique

The U.S. Food and Drug Administration (FDA) approved this new procedure in March 1999 for use in the United States. Although it is not as widely used as sclerotherapy, some doctors feel it may become the standard for treating varicose veins. It is not very invasive and can be done in a doctor's office. This method involves placing a special catheter or a very small tube into the vein. Once inside, the catheter sends radiofrequency energy to cause the vein wall to shrink and seal shut. Healthier veins surrounding the closed vein can then restore the normal flow of blood. As this happens, symptoms from the varicose vein decrease. The only side effect is slight bruising.

Surgery

Surgery is used mostly to treat very large varicose veins. Available surgical options include:

Surgical Ligation and Stripping. With this treatment, the veins are tied shut and completely removed from the leg. Removing the veins will not affect the circulation of blood in the leg because veins deeper in the leg take care of the larger volumes of blood. The varicose veins removed through surgery are superficial or surface veins, and collect blood only from the skin. This surgery requires either local or general anesthesia and must be done in an operating room on an outpatient basis.

Serious side effects or complications with this surgery are uncommon. However, with general anesthesia, there always is a risk of cardiac and respiratory complications. Similar to the risks of sclerotherapy, bleeding and congestion of blood can be a problem, but the collected blood usually settles on its own and does not require any further treatment. Wound infection, inflammation, swelling, and redness also can occur. This surgery also can leave permanent scars. A very common complication is the damage of nerve tissue around the treated vein. Small sensory nerve branches are difficult to avoid when veins are removed. This damage can cause numbness in small areas of skin, burning, or a change in sensation around the surgical scar. The most serious, but rare, complication of surgery is the creation of a deep vein blood clot that may travel to the lungs and heart. To be safe, many surgeons give injections of heparin, a drug that reduces blood coagulation, for one to two days before the surgery. However, heparin also can increase the normal amount of bleeding and bruising after the operation.

Ambulatory Phlebectomy. With this surgery, a special light source marks the location of the vein. Tiny incisions are made in the vein, and then with surgical hooks, the vein is pulled out of the leg. This surgery requires local or regional anesthesia. The vein usually is removed in one treatment. Side effects and complications are similar to those of ligation and stripping. The most common side effect is slight bruising. Compared to traditional surgery, ambulatory phlebectomy allows the removal of very large varicose veins while leaving only very small scars. Patients can return to normal activity the day after treatment.

Can varicose and spider veins return even after treatment?

Current treatments for varicose veins and spider veins have very high success rates. Although it is uncommon, these veins can return after treatment. One reason may be hidden areas in the body where there is a lot of pressure on the veins. This pressure may cause new spider veins. Doctors can diagnose this with ultrasound. Another cause may be new regrowth of vein branches. Doctors have found that tiny vein branches can grow through scar tissue to connect to both deep and superficial veins even after surgery.

Part Five

Diagnosing Cardiovascular Disorders

Chapter 51

Diagnosing Heart Disease

How can I find out if I have heart disease?

To diagnose heart disease, your doctor will first review your medical history, health behaviors, family history, and other risk factors for heart disease. Your doctor will ask you about having any chest pain, fatigue, shortness of breath, weakness, and swelling of the feet and ankles. These symptoms may mean that you could have heart disease.

Your doctor will then perform a physical exam and focus on your lungs, heart, and all of the blood vessels near and around the heart. He or she will place a stethoscope on your chest to listen to your heartbeat and to other areas to hear the heart valves. He or she will also listen to your lungs for sounds that indicate they could have fluid inside them (which can be the result of heart disease). Your doctor may order special heart tests to confirm or rule out heart disease, figure out the extent of disease, or help in planning a treatment that is best for you.

When a person develops heart disease, it is most often due to a number of risk factors (rather than a single factor). Some of the risk factors for heart disease are beyond your control, such as age, family history of heart disease, and prior heart disease. However, there are risk factors you can do something about. Risk factors you can control include smoking, high blood pressure, high blood cholesterol, overweight and obesity, physical inactivity, and diabetes. If you have one

Excerpted from "Diagnosing Heart Disease," National Women's Health Information Center (www.4woman.gov), November 2002.

or more of these risk factors, talk with your doctor to find out how to reduce your risk of getting heart disease.

What is an ECG or an electrocardiogram?

An electrocardiogram or ECG, also called an EKG, is a simple, painless test that records the electrical activity of your heart. It is done by placing patches with metal contacts (electrodes) on a person's arms, legs, and chest, which are hooked up to an ECG machine. These electrodes measure the electrical impulses in the heart and record them on a moving strip of paper. An ECG also gives information about the heart's rhythm and the size of the different heart chambers. A twelve-lead ECG means that there are twelve tracings that can give a view of the heart from twelve different angles. With this type of ECG, your doctor can tell which part of the heart is affected by a heart attack.

How can a chest x-ray help diagnose heart disease?

A chest x-ray shows the size and shape of the heart, which can be larger than normal (or enlarged) in conditions such as congestive heart failure. The lungs are also looked at for fluid buildup, which is most often caused by heart failure.

What is an echocardiogram (echo)?

An echo provides moving pictures of the heart using sound waves. It is an ultrasound test, very similar to the test done on pregnant women to look at the growing fetus. An echo takes pictures of the heart chambers, valves, and the major blood vessels running to and from the heart. It gives very detailed information about all areas of the heart and can detect abnormalities or problems with the heart's pumping action. Echocardiograms are not invasive (meaning there is nothing inserted into the body, such as needles, instruments, or fluids) and don't involve radiation.

How is an echocardiogram performed?

A standard echo procedure involves placing a small recording probe, called a transducer, on the chest. Before the echo is done, a technician or doctor will first place some clear jelly onto your chest to help the transducer, or wand, slide around easily to take pictures of different parts the heart. The image appears on a video screen and is recorded on videotape or paper.

What other tests might be performed with an echocardiogram?

A special exam, called the Doppler, can be done with an echo and gives information about the direction and speed of blood flow in the heart. From this, doctors can tell how heart valves are working, whether they are narrowed, and how much a valve is narrowed or leaking. Other types of echocardiograms include M-mode and 2-D echocardiograms. M-mode echocardiograms look at a one-dimensional view of a small section of the heart as it moves. 2-D echocardiograms produce a moving, two-dimensional slice of the heart.

In some cases, your doctor may do an echo in a slightly different way. This may include having you exercise while the echo is done (an exercise echo) or having medicine injected to increase your heart muscle's blood flow before the echo (a stress echo). These echocardiograms are a way to see whether or not your heart muscle gets enough blood flow and oxygen even when it is working its hardest.

I have heard many people talk about stress tests. What is a stress test?

Stress tests are done to diagnose many types of heart problems. They often look for blockages in the arteries that supply blood to the heart. A stress test most often involves monitoring your heart while you exercise. This is because the amount of exercise a person can endure, or handle, can tell a lot about heart disease and how severe it may be (when a person has heart disease). Your doctor may suggest this test if he or she feels that your arteries may be blocked. There are also stress tests for people who can't exercise.

What happens when a treadmill stress test is performed?

Before the treadmill stress test, an ECG will be performed and your blood pressure will be taken. A few plastic-coated wires will be taped to your arms and one leg, so that your heart's electrical pattern can be picked up while you exercise. Your heart rhythm and blood pressure are also watched the entire time the test is being done. You will be asked to walk on a treadmill for about ten minutes. The speed and steepness of the treadmill will be increased a few times during the test. Your doctor or a technician will be with you during the test, and you should let them know if you feel any chest pain, shortness of breath, leg pain, or other symptoms that do not usually happen when you exercise. Ask to stop the treadmill if you think you can't keep on exercising.

What are some different types of exercise stress tests?

The exercise stress test has a person walk on a treadmill or pedal an exercise bike. This test will tell if your heart muscle gets enough blood flow and oxygen even when it is working its hardest, such as during exercise.

The exercise stress test can sometimes be combined with other techniques to take pictures of your heart before and after exercise. A stress echo is one such test where an echo is done before and after exercise to see if the heart muscle responds the way it should to exercise. Sometimes your doctor may order a small amount of a liquid radioactive material called thallium or sestamibi be injected through a needle into your bloodstream before and after exercise. Pictures of the heart are then made after you lie down on an exam table that has a camera overhead. This test may also be called an exercise-thallium, thallium-stress, nuclear stress, or exercise-MIBI test. Your doctor will talk with you about the type of stress test that is best for you.

What about stress tests for people who can't exercise?

When you have a stress test without exercising, a medicine called dobutamine or dipyridamole/adenosine is injected through a needle into your bloodstream. This slowly makes the heart work harder, which simulates how your heart would function if you were exercising. Pictures of the heart are then taken, with either an echo or a thallium test, to look at the heart's pumping action and whether there are any problems with blood supply to one of the heart's walls.

My heart often skips beats and my doctor ordered a Holter Monitor test. What is this?

A Holter monitor is a test that lets your doctor see whether there are changes in the heart's rhythm or electrical appearance over a longer period of time than can be observed during one office visit. A few stickers with attached plastic-coated wires are placed onto the skin of your chest, and these connect to a small monitor that you wear. The monitor, a machine about the size of a purse that records your heart rhythm, is worn for twenty-four or forty-eight hours while you carry on with your normal daily activities. You will be given a small diary so you can write down any symptoms you may feel during the test, as well as the time they happened.

Another type of monitor, called an event monitor, is used for people who have heart-related symptoms only now and then. It is a small machine that you turn on only when you have a symptom that may be due to heart-rhythm changes. The event monitor may be kept for up to one month.

What is cardiac catheterization?

Cardiac catheterization is a common procedure that is done to detect problems with the heart and heart function. A small tube (catheter) is placed up into and around the heart through a blood vessel in the groin or arm. Moving x-rays (angiograms) are then taken to show any problems with the coronary (or heart) arteries, heart chambers, major blood vessels, heart valves, and congenital (at birth) heart defects. This test can also be used to treat blocked coronary arteries by blowing up a small balloon at the site of the blockage to create a larger opening, called an angioplasty. When a catheter is used to inject dye into the coronary arteries, the procedure is called coronary angiography or coronary arteriography.

How is a cardiac catheterization performed?

A doctor, called a cardiologist, usually does a cardiac catheterization, using equipment and cameras in a special lab. During the test, you lie on your back and your heart is hooked up to a monitor. After local anesthesia is given, a catheter (thin plastic tube) is placed inside your body through a blood vessel in your groin or arm. The catheter is gently guided up into your body to reach the arteries around the heart. The doctor will most likely measure pressures within the chambers of the heart, take blood samples, and carefully move the catheter into the arteries that deliver blood to your heart (or coronary arteries). While the catheter is pointed into each of the coronary arteries, the doctor will inject a special dye into the blood vessels. Pictures are taken with an x-ray machine. The pictures will show if there are any blockages in the arteries and how severe these blockages are. Other than the brief sting of the numbing medicine and soreness in your groin or arm afterward, you are not likely to feel any pain. If blockages are found, your doctor will discuss treatment options with you.

Are CT scans or MRI tests used to diagnose heart disease?

Yes, CT (computed tomography, or CAT) scans and MRI (magnetic resonance imaging) tests may be used to detect any problems with the structure or position of the heart, lungs, or blood vessels. The CT scan and the MRI provide a much clearer picture of your organs than an x-ray. These tests are sometimes used to avoid the potential risk of other invasive heart tests, such as angiography. Some of these tests are done by injecting through a needle a small amount of radioactive material into a vein.

CT scans use a unique x-ray machine that makes a circle around your body. Using measurements from every angle around this circle, the computer takes pictures, each showing a slightly different "slice" or "cross-section" of your body. MRI is often more costly and time-consuming, but it is preferred over other noninvasive heart tests. This is because MRI provides detailed pictures of the heart and blood vessels, shows the heart from many different views, clearly shows blood vessels, identifies structures (like clots) from moving blood, and helps to better understand findings from X-rays or CT scans. The main discomfort with CT scans and MRI is the closed in, or claustrophobic, feeling that some people have from being inside the scanner. An MRI may require you to lie still in the scanner for at least one hour. However, a technician watches you during the test and may enter the room to speak to you or may speak with you over an intercom in the MRI machine.

What is a MUGA scan and how is it performed?

The MUGA scan (multiple gated acquisition scan) is a tool that looks at how the heart functions. It takes a moving picture of the beating heart, and from this image, the health of the cardiac ventricles (the heart's major pumping chambers) can be determined. If a person has had a heart attack or any other disease that affects the heart muscle, the MUGA scan can identify the part of the heart muscle that was damaged. It can also figure out the degree of the damage.

When having a MUGA scan, a radioactive substance called Technetium 99 is attached to red blood cells, which are then injected into the person's bloodstream. The person is then placed under a special camera (called a gamma camera), which picks up the low-level radiation being given off by the Technetium-labeled red cells. (The level of radiation to which a person is exposed during a MUGA scan is felt by experts to be quite small—it is in the same range as the level of radiation you get with a chest x-ray.) An image is produced by the gamma camera that outlines the chambers of the heart. The final image is like a movie of the heart beating.

There are so many tests to diagnose heart disease. How do I know which one is right for me?

Today, there are many tests to look at the heart, and new tests are being developed. Your doctor will discuss the best test for you based on your symptoms, physical exam, health behavior, family history, and other risk factors. Remember also that new advances in the treatment of heart disease occur often, so it is important that you go to your doctor regularly for checkups and to get any new or changing symptoms evaluated.

Chapter 52

Blood Tests Used in the Diagnosis and Management of Heart Disease

A blood test is a test in which a medical professional takes a drop of the patient's blood from the finger, earlobe, or heel (in the case of a baby), or a more substantial amount of blood from a vein (venipuncture) or artery (arterial puncture). The blood is then tested for many different factors, depending on what tests the physician has ordered. For example, the physician may need to know the number of red or white blood cells that are present, or the amount of oxygen or carbon dioxide that is in the blood. Blood tests are essential to the diagnosis and management of most medical conditions, including heart disease. Obtaining a blood sample takes only about five minutes, and most patients find them to be virtually painless. For most blood tests, there is very little preparation beforehand, and people can generally go right back to their usual daily activities afterward.

What is a blood test?

A blood test uses a sample of blood from an artery or a vein to detect and measure various factors in the blood that could be signs of an abnormal condition. In some cases, it may be just as important to establish that a condition is "normal" as to establish that a condition is "abnormal." Blood tests serve a number of purposes when used with people who have cardiovascular conditions. These purposes include the following:

- To help diagnose heart disease
- To help establish that a heart attack has occurred
- To evaluate the extent of heart damage (e.g., after a heart attack)
- To monitor the patient's progress during treatment

Blood is part of the circulatory system that contains a variety of cells suspended in a light-colored fluid known as plasma. Plasma comprises over half of the blood volume. Dissolved in the plasma are many substances, such as electrolytes, nutrients, vitamins, clotting factors, hormones, enzymes, and antibodies. In addition, there are three types of blood cells that circulate in the plasma: red blood cells (that carry oxygen to the tissues), white blood cells (that fight invading organisms), and platelets (that control blood clotting). An analysis of various blood components can provide the physician with essential information about its microscopic contents, which include the following:

- Blood cells
- Nutrients, vitamins, and minerals
- Proteins, sugars, and fats
- Chemicals
- Hormones
- Antigens (foreign proteins that stimulate the formation of antibodies)
- Antibodies (factors that attack "foreign proteins" or, in the case of autoimmune diseases, mistakenly attack the patient's own cells)
- Blood gases (e.g., oxygen or carbon dioxide that is dissolved in the blood)
- Enzymes
- Clotting factors

Because blood carries all of these substances to where they are needed in the body, examining its contents can help to evaluate the health of major organs and organ systems, including the heart, lungs, and respiratory system. For example, blood tests can determine how well the liver, kidney, and lungs are functioning and whether there is any infection or inflammation.

What blood tests are used to check cardiovascular function?

The most common blood tests used in the diagnosis and management of cardiovascular disease include the following:

- **Antistreptolysin-O test.** Antistreptolysin-O (ASO) is an antibody that is present in the body in small amounts to "ward off" minor streptococcal ("strep") infections. High levels of ASO may indicate the presence of an infection from strep, such as endocarditis (an inflammation of the lining of the heart or valves).

- **Arterial blood gases.** This test takes a sample of blood from an artery in the side of a wrist (which carries oxygen-rich blood) instead of a vein in the crook of the arm (which carries oxygen-poor blood). The sample gives information about levels of oxygen (which should be high) and levels of carbon dioxide (which should be low).

- **Blood fat profile.** This test measures fats and fat-like substances in the blood that, if abnormally high, have been associated with heart disease. They include:
  - **Total cholesterol.** A high total cholesterol level is associated with heart disease.
  - **LDL cholesterol.** Low-density lipoprotein or "bad" cholesterol that is associated with atherosclerosis.
  - **HDL cholesterol.** High-density lipoprotein or "good" cholesterol" that protects against heart disease.
  - **Triglycerides.** High levels are associated with heart disease.
  - **VLDL (very low density lipoprotein).** Another carrier of fat in the blood.

- **Blood calcium test.** By measuring the calcium levels of blood, a physician may be able to support the diagnosis of a number of cardiovascular problems.

- **C-reactive protein test (CRP test).** CRP is an inflammatory marker—a substance that the body releases in response to inflammation. CRP levels can provide physicians with information about a patient's risk of having a heart attack or stroke.

- **Carbon dioxide content.** CO_2 levels are generally used as an investigative and diagnostic tool for patients with breathing problems. It may be helpful in the diagnosis of conditions such as chronic obstructive pulmonary disease.

- **Complete blood count (CBC).** This very common test can provide important information about the types of blood cells present, their condition, and number (percentage) in relation to other cells. High levels of white blood cells may occur at the time of a heart attack, infection, or an inflammatory disease such as rheumatoid arthritis. High levels of red blood cells, hematocrit (the term for the space taken up by red blood cells), or hemoglobin (the protein molecule in red blood cells that carry oxygen) may indicate a lack of oxygen in the body. This may be caused by smoking, congenital heart disease (cardiac abnormality, defect, or malformation that is present from birth), dehydration, or kidney disease.

- **Electrolyte panel.** Tests that measure the amount of potassium, sodium, chloride, and carbon dioxide in the blood in order to assess how well the major organ systems (e.g., the heart and cardiovascular system) are functioning.

- **Erythrocyte sedimentation rate (ESR).** A test that measures the rate at which red blood cells separate from plasma (the liquid part of blood) and fall to the bottom of a test tube to form a sediment. High levels may occur at the time of a heart attack, rheumatic fever, giant cell arthritis, severe anemia, cancer relapse, or other conditions. Low levels may be associated with heart failure, sickle cell anemia, or other conditions.

- **Cardiac enzyme tests.** Measuring a number of heart enzymes can be helpful in the diagnosis of various heart conditions. For example, creatine phosphokinase (CPK) is a valuable tool for determining whether a heart attack is the cause of chest pain, and cardiac troponin is helpful in detecting heart muscle damage and predicting risk of heart attack. AST/SGPT and ALT/SGPT are abbreviations for enzymes that become elevated after a recent heart attack.

- **Glucose test.** This is primarily used to screen for, diagnose, or monitor patients with diabetes, a metabolic condition in which blood glucose levels are too high because the body cannot produce enough insulin in the pancreas. Following a heart attack or other serious illness, fasting glucose levels may be temporarily high.

- **INR / prothrombin time test.** A type of coagulation test. Prothrombin is a protein substance that needs to be converted to thrombin in order for clotting to occur. The test is used to determine whether a patient's blood is clotting normally. People taking anticoagulants (such as warfarin) may have this test done regularly.

- **Serum myoglobin test.** A test sometimes used to measure the damage done to the heart muscle after a heart attack.

- **Total serum protein.** Blood contains large amounts of protein, and measuring these levels can give physicians valuable information about a patient's nutritional state and kidney and liver functions. Abnormal protein levels may indicate congestive heart failure, high blood pressure (hypertension), or kidney or liver disease.

- **Waste products test.** A group of blood tests that measure the levels of specific waste products in the blood. Abnormal results could be a sign of heart failure, heart attack, or kidney disease.

How does a patient prepare for a blood test?

Preparation for blood tests varies according to the requirements of each specific test. In most cases minimal preparation is necessary. The patient may need to reduce or stop certain medications at some point prior to the test. Additionally, food intake as well as exercise may be temporarily restricted or suspended. Alcohol and caffeine should be avoided prior to a blood test. On the day of the test, the procedure will be explained and patients will have the opportunity to ask questions. The medical professional will also ask questions about the patient's medical history before the test, to determine if the patient is taking any medications that will interfere with the test's accuracy or has any history of clotting problems.

How is a blood test done?

Drawing blood for a blood test is an easy and virtually painless process for most people. If the physician needs only a drop or two of blood, then a simple prick of the finger, earlobe, or heel can provide enough blood for testing. The technician will use a sterile, sharp lancet to prick the skin. The technician will then gently squeeze the puncture area to produce drops of blood that are collected in tiny glass tubes. Light pressure and sterile gauze is then applied to the puncture site to stop the bleeding. A bandage is not usually necessary.

If a substantial amount of blood is needed, it is usually drawn from a vein in a process called venipuncture. Blood samples may be more difficult to obtain from infants, overweight people whose veins are difficult to find, elderly people whose veins tend to roll away, or patients with scarred or collapsed veins due to multiple transfusions or drug use. During a venipuncture, a needle is inserted into a vein—usually at the inside of the elbow or on the back of the hand. The area around the puncture site is cleaned with rubbing alcohol and a wide elastic band or piece of latex tubing may be placed around the upper arm to slightly increase the pressure in the vein. One end of a sterile and disposable double-ended needle attached to an open-ended syringe (that contains an empty test tube) is inserted into the vein. Because the test tube contains a partial vacuum, blood flows directly from the vein through the double-ended needle, which has been inserted into the test tube.

The precise amount of blood to be drawn is determined by the type and number of tests to be done. It is usually around 7 milliliters. The technician may change test tubes once or twice during the venipuncture to either allow for more blood to be collected or to change the type of tube being used. Tubes are marked with different colored tops that indicate the way in which the collected blood will be preserved:

- Lavender tops indicate that the tube contains an anticoagulant, which prevents the collected blood from clotting.

- Red tops indicate that the tube contains no anticoagulants, allowing serum to separate and the blood to form a blood clot.

- Gray tops indicate that the tube contains a preservative, which keeps glucose (blood sugar) from breaking down in the tube.

After the necessary amount of blood is drawn, the needle is withdrawn and a small cotton ball or pad is applied with light pressure over the puncture site. After several minutes, the cotton will be discarded or replaced, and a small bandage will be placed on the puncture wound. The entire process takes less than ten minutes.

Despite the precautions taken to avoid bruising and soreness, it does sometimes occur. Typically, this is not a cause for great concern. To minimize soreness, patients may immediately apply a warm compress to the puncture site and repeat this application every three hours until the discoloration or pain subsides.

Blood tests can be made on different parts of the blood, such as:

- Whole blood (to which an anticoagulant has been added in the test tube to prevent clotting)

- Blood serum, the term for plasma (the liquid part of blood) that has had the clotting agents removed

- Blood plasma, the whitish yellow liquid that remains in unclotted blood once the blood cells have settled out to the bottom of the test tube

- Blood cells, the individual red, white, and platelet cells

If blood must be taken from an artery instead of a vein, (e.g., during an arterial blood gas study), it is usually drawn from a small artery located on the inside or the top side of the wrist.

What happens after the blood test?

Following the withdrawal of blood, patients may resume medications and food intake according to their physician's orders. Immediately after the blood sample is taken, the test tubes are labeled with the date and the patient's name, and they are sent to the laboratory for testing. Results are usually returned within twenty-four hours, depending on which tests need to be performed. Based on the test results, additional blood tests may be ordered.

Test results are always evaluated in relation to the "normal range" for that test. The range of values considered to be normal is the range of test results from the blood of normal, active healthy people. When someone has a disease or health problem, his or her blood test results may be higher or lower than normal (i.e. "outside of the normal range"). When a physician sees that a blood test is outside of the normal range, he or she may order a repeat test to verify the results or additional tests to determine the underlying causes behind the abnormality.

Normal ranges for some tests may vary slightly from lab to lab, especially between labs that use machines to perform blood tests and those that perform the tests by hand. Frequently, results of a patient's blood test are compared to another "known" blood sample taken from a healthy individual that is run at the same time and is designated as the "normal control." When the "normal control" sample falls within the normal range, or reaches a specific "known" measurement, the laboratory results confirm that the blood test has been carried out accurately.

What are the main types of blood tests?

Hundreds of blood tests are performed every day in today's modern labs. In general, there are four main types of blood tests:

- Hematology tests
- Biochemistry tests
- Microbiology tests
- Serology tests

Hematology tests examine the blood to identify:

- The types and numbers of blood cells that are present (e.g., red blood cells, white blood cells, and platelets)
- The appearance of the cells, especially their maturity
- The ability of the blood to form a blood clot and the speed at which clotting occurs

Biochemistry tests measure the amounts of normally occurring chemicals and biochemicals in the blood, both individually and in relation to other chemicals. These measurements are compared to normal ranges for that test and are used to determine whether blood biochemicals are in a proper and healthy balance. Biochemicals and other substances that may be studied include the following:

- Sodium
- Cholesterol and other fats
- Vitamins and minerals
- Hormones
- Blood gases
- Prescription drugs
- Recreational drugs
- Alcohol

Not only can biochemical tests precisely measure these substances, but they can also be used to indicate how well some organs and organ systems are functioning. For instance, the amount of blood sugar

362

(glucose) in the bloodstream can help to diagnose or monitor diabetes, and indirectly reflect how much insulin is being produced by the pancreas.

Microbiology tests examine blood for the presence of infectious microscopic organisms such as the following:

- Bacteria
- Fungi
- Viruses (in most clinical labs a serology test is used)
- Parasites

Microbiology tests include:

- Smears, in which a small amount of blood is placed on a glass slide for examination under a microscope. Sometimes the blood smear is stained with special dyes before examination.
- Blood cultures, in which a small amount of blood is placed in a nutrient broth, incubated for days or weeks, and then examined for growth of disease-causing bacteria.

Serology tests (tests done on blood serum) can detect the presence of antibodies that are produced by white blood cells to attack microscopic organisms. They are frequently used to detect viral diseases. Most hospital laboratories do not have the equipment or specially trained personnel necessary to isolate the viruses themselves, so serology tests are done instead to identify the infecting organism by studying the antibodies produced against it.

About HeartCenterOnline

HeartCenterOnline is a cardiovascular specialized health care website providing tools to help patients and their families better understand the complex nature of heart-related conditions, treatments, and preventive care. The website includes a library of physician-edited patient education information, interactive health-tracking tools, and an online cardiovascular community for patients, their families and other site visitors.

HeartCenterOnline
One South Ocean Boulevard, Suite 201
Boca Raton, FL 33432
http://www.heartcenteronline.com

Chapter 53

Exercise Stress Testing

What is a stress test?

Most people who have a heart problem have had a stress test somewhere along the way. It is a noninvasive test used to evaluate your heart. First, electrodes are placed on your chest, then you are asked to walk on a treadmill or ride a bike. You start exercising at a very low level, but the workload gradually increases every two to three minutes. Your blood pressure and EKG are measured throughout the test. This allows your doctor to detect and guide the treatment of your condition.

When will I have a stress test?

A stress test may be prescribed for the following reasons.

- If you are having chest discomfort, a stress test is often done to determine if your discomfort is heart related.

- If you have been in the hospital, it is also common to take a low-level stress test before discharge. This helps doctors determine the best treatment for you.

- Once you go home from the hospital, it is likely that you will be scheduled for a follow-up stress test in approximately three

"Exercise Stress Testing," a Heart Health Information Sheet from the Department of Cardiology at Johns Hopkins Bayview Medical Center, Baltimore, MD. © 2000. Reprinted with permission.

months, then once a year thereafter. This ensures that your medications are working and that any procedure you had (such as PTCA or bypass surgery) was successful.

- You also should take a stress test prior to entering a cardiac rehabilitation program. The test helps determine at what level you should be exercising.

How will I know if I passed or failed my stress test?

You don't necessarily "pass" or "fail" a stress test. Typically, you are asked to exercise for as long as you can. This may be two to three minutes for some people and ten to twelve minutes for others, depending on the condition of your cardiovascular system (heart and lungs). If your test is positive, it shows that your heart was not getting enough oxygen when you were exercising. This means you may have one or more blockages in your coronary arteries. Your doctor will then decide which form of treatment is best for you. If your test is negative, your heart responded well to the exercise, and you will probably not need further treatment.

What is a thallium stress test?

This test is similar to a regular stress test, except you will have an I.V. inserted in your arm before the test begins. As you exercise, you will be asked to let the technician know when you feel very tired. The thallium will then be injected into your I.V. You may feel a cool sensation as the thallium goes in, but most people feel nothing. You will walk for another minute and then sit down to rest for three to five minutes. At this time, you will be escorted to another room where you will lie under a large camera. The camera takes pictures of you heart for about thirty minutes. Then, in two hours, you will come back for a second set of pictures.

What does a thallium stress test show?

Thallium goes where blood goes, and the camera can detect the thallium. If there are any areas of your heart that are not getting enough oxygen during exercise, your doctor will be able to tell from these pictures. The pictures also indicate which area of your heart is not getting enough oxygen; an EKG alone cannot do this.

Chapter 54

Echocardiograms

What is an echocardiogram?

An echocardiogram is a safe, noninvasive procedure used to diagnose cardiovascular disease. It uses high-frequency sound waves to literally see all four chambers of the heart, the heart valves, the great blood vessels entering and leaving the heart, as well as the sack around the heart. Echocardiography allows doctors to visualize the anatomy, structure, and function of the heart. It can quickly diagnose the presence and severity of heart valve problems, as well as determine abnormal flow within the heart that occurs with congenital heart disease that you may have been born with. This window to the heart enables the doctors to diagnose a number of cardiovascular diseases, so that they can begin proper treatment.

How does it work?

It uses high-frequency sound waves to literally see all four chambers of the heart, the heart valves, blood vessels entering and leaving the heart, and the sack around the heart.

Who gets an echocardiogram?

The procedure can be performed on people of all ages, from fetuses to senior citizens.

"Frequently Asked Questions: Echocardiograms," copyright © 2004 American Society of Echocardiography (ASE). All rights reserved. Reprinted with permission. For additional information, visit http://www.seemyheart.org.

Why is an echocardiogram preformed?

Doctors use an echocardiogram to diagnose and evaluate conditions of the heart and surrounding veins and arteries. Echocardiography can be used to determine causes for chest pain, establish a baseline for reference in tracking chronic heart conditions, evaluate the effects of a heart attack, diagnose narrowed or leaking heart valves, or determine the need for intervention, or as a follow-up to evaluate the effectiveness of treatment. An echocardiogram also can determine if the heart or aorta has been damaged in an accident and can help evaluate a donor heart prior to a transplant. Young children or infants could have echocardiography performed if there is suspected congenital heart disease.

What types of echocardiograms are there?

The conventional echocardiogram usually performed is the **transthoracic echo**, which is performed by placing the probe on the outside of the chest wall with a gel-like substance to transmit sound waves into the body.

Doppler echocardiograms evaluate blood flow in the heart and blood vessels. This procedure measures the speed and direction of the blood flow within the heart. It screens the four valves for leaks or other abnormalities. With Doppler echocardiograms, as the transducer moves over your heart you will hear a "whooshing" sound much like that of a washing machine. This sound relates to the movement of blood within your heart chambers.

Stress echocardiograms combine the echo exam with a treadmill or bike exercise test, or medication that simulates the effect of exercise on the heart. Both forms of stress echocardiograms are used to diagnose the presence and severity of narrowing of the coronary arteries.

Contrast echocardiograms combine an echocardiogram with an administration, through a vein, of a sterile contrast solution, which allows visualization of the inside of the heart. This is a harmless agent that has no known side effects. You will need to have an IV started to receive a contrast echocardiogram.

Transesophageal echo is a form of echo where a miniature ultrasound camera is passed down the esophagus, or food pipe, behind the heart. This allows the physician to obtain very high quality images. Transesophageal echocardiograms are typically performed to evaluate strokes and transient ischemic attacks (TIA), previous valve replacements and bypass surgeries, and other serious heart conditions.

What type of information can echocardiography provide?

Echocardiography displays the size of the chambers of the heart, including the dimension or volume of the cavity and the thickness of the walls. The appearance of the walls may also help identify certain types of heart disease that predominantly involve the heart muscle.

Pumping function of the heart can also be assessed by echocardiography. One can tell if the pumping power of the heart is normal or reduced to a mild or severe degree. This measure is known as an ejection fraction. Echocardiography can also identify if the entire heart is pumping poorly due to a condition known as cardiomyopathy, or if one or more areas of the heart muscle have sustained prior damage (from heart attacks).

Echocardiography identifies the structure, thickness, and movement of each heart valve. It can help determine if the valve is normal, scarred from an infection or rheumatic fever, thickened, calcified (loaded with calcium), torn, and so on. It can also assess the function of prosthetic or artificial heart valves.

Echocardiography is used to diagnose mitral valve prolapse. The presence of mitral regurgitation frequently prompts the use of antibiotics prior to any dental or nonsterile surgical procedure. Such action helps reduce the rare complication of valve infection.

Echocardiography is useful in the diagnosis of fluid in the pericardium (the sac that surrounds the heart). It also determines when the problem is severe and potentially life-threatening. Other diagnoses made by Doppler or echocardiography include congenital heart diseases, blood clots or tumors within the heart, active infection of the heart valves, and abnormal elevation of pressure within the lungs.

How is each procedure performed?

The transthoracic echocardiogram is a painless procedure that involves the patient lying quietly while a small probe, called the transducer, is gently placed on various portions of the chest, from which to obtain the images or pictures of the heart in real-time. Because the sound waves do not readily pass through air, a clear, jelly-like substance is applied between the chest and the transducer to improve the contact of the transducer with the skin. Transesophageal echo involves the passage of a very small tube down the food pipe, or esophagus. Because the esophagus lies in close proximity (behind) the heart, outstanding images of the heart can be obtained. To minimize the amount of discomfort that a patient might have from swallowing the probe, patients are often given oral sprays of novocaine-like medicine, as well as intravenous medicine to relax them.

Where does the procedure take place?

An echocardiogram can be performed in any setting, that is, wherever the patient is. While it is usually performed in a hospital or doctor's office, it can be performed at bedside in the emergency room, in an intensive care unit, or in an operating room. A cardiac sonographer, a health care professional specially trained and certified in ultrasound imaging of the heart, usually performs the procedure, and the results are reviewed and interpreted by a cardiologist. In some cases, such as with transesophageal echocardiography or when the echo is performed in the operating room, the cardiologist both performs the exam and interprets the results.

How long does an echocardiogram take?

An echocardiogram takes approximately thirty to forty-five minutes.

Will I be exposed to radiation?

The sound waves are painless, and are not radioactive. This test is completely noninvasive in terms of needles and probes.

What happens if the doctor finds a problem?

The doctor will explain the findings of the echocardiogram to the referring physician. Then additional tests may be performed or treatment may be recommended. Treatment for heart problems includes medication, surgery, and lifestyle modification.

What is the difference between an echocardiogram and an EKG?

An echocardiogram shows an image of a beating heart on a television-like screen as the sonographer performs the test. An EKG, or electrocardiogram, measures the electrical currents in the heart. These are different diagnostic techniques used to obtain different information. The EKG tells us about the electrical health of the heart while the echocardiogram tells us about the structural health of the heart and its valves.

How long has echocardiography been around?

Echocardiography began to be used in a clinical setting in the late 1960s. Echocardiography is still being improved, and the development of new technologies has made the procedure more accurate.

Do health plans cover echocardiography?

Most health plans, HMOs, and Medicare cover echocardiography for established reasons.

How can I tell if my echocardiogram is being performed by qualified personnel?

The professionals involved in your echocardiogram should follow specific guidelines to provide high-quality service. Check with them to see if the sonographer has passed a nationally recognized certification exam such as the Registered Diagnostic Cardiac Sonographer (RDCS) exam, whether the physician has passed the ASCeXAM [adult special competency in echocardiography examination] for special competency in cardiac ultrasound, and whether the lab is accredited by the Intersocietal Commission of Accreditation of Echocardiographic Laboratories (ICAEL).

Chapter 55

Electrocardiograms (EKG; ECG)

Definition

An electrocardiogram (ECG) is a test that records the electrical activity of the heart.

ECG is used to measure the rate and regularity of heartbeats as well as the size and position of the chambers, the presence of any damage to the heart, and the effects of drugs or devices used to regulate the heart (such as a pacemaker).

How the Test Is Performed

You are asked to lie down, and electrodes are affixed to each arm and leg and to your chest. This requires cleaning the site and, if necessary, shaving or clipping hair. The standard number of leads attached is twelve to fifteen for a diagnostic ECG but may be as few as three to five for a monitoring procedure.

You are usually required to remain still, and you may be asked to hold your breath for short periods during the procedure. Sometimes this test is performed while you are exercising or under minimal stress to monitor changes in the heart. This type of ECG is often called a stress test.

The results are recorded on graph paper.

"ECG," © 2002 A.D.A.M., Inc. Reprinted with permission. Updated January 2004.

How to Prepare for the Test

Adults

Before the ECG, tell your health care provider if you are taking any medications.

There are no restrictions for food or fluids. However, ingestion of cold water immediately before an ECG may produce changes in one of the waveforms recorded (the T wave). Exercise (such as climbing stairs) immediately before an ECG may significantly increase your heart rate.

You may be asked to remove all jewelry and to wear a hospital gown.

Infants and Children

The physical and psychological preparation you can provide for this or any test or procedure depends on your child's age, interests, previous experience, and level of trust.

How the Test Will Feel

An ECG is painless. When first applied, the disks may be cold, and in rare circumstances you may develop a localized rash or irritation where the patches are placed.

Why the Test Is Performed

An ECG is very useful in determining whether a person has heart disease. If a person has chest pain or palpitations, an ECG is helpful in determining if the heart is beating normally. If a person is on medications that may affect the heart or if the patient is on a pacemaker, an ECG can readily determine the immediate effects of changes in activity or medication levels. An ECG may be included as part of a routine examination in patients over forty years old.

Normal Values

- Heart rate: fifty to one hundred beats per minute.
- Rhythm: consistent and even.

What Abnormal Results Mean

Abnormal ECG results may indicate the following:

- Myocardial (cardiac muscle) defect

- Enlargement of the heart
- Congenital defects
- Heart valve disease
- Arrhythmias (abnormal rhythms)
- Tachycardia (heart rate too fast) or bradycardia (too slow)
- Ectopic heartbeat
- Coronary artery disease
- Inflammation of the heart (myocarditis)
- Changes in the amount of electrolytes (chemicals in the blood)
- Past heart attack
- Present or impending heart attack

Additional conditions under which the test may be performed include the following:

- Alcoholic cardiomyopathy
- Anorexia nervosa
- Aortic dissection
- Aortic insufficiency
- Aortic stenosis
- Atrial fibrillation/flutter
- Atrial myxoma; left
- Atrial myxoma; right
- Atrial septal defect
- Cardiac tamponade
- Coarctation of the aorta
- Complicated alcohol abstinence (delirium tremens)
- Coronary artery spasm
- Digitalis toxicity
- Dilated cardiomyopathy
- Drug-induced lupus erythematosus
- Familial periodic paralysis
- Guillain-Barré
- Heart failure
- Hyperkalemia
- Hypertensive heart disease
- Hypertrophic cardiomyopathy
- Hypoparathyroidism
- Idiopathic cardiomyopathy
- Infective endocarditis
- Insomnia
- Ischemic cardiomyopathy
- Left-sided heart failure
- Lyme disease
- Mitral regurgitation; acute
- Mitral regurgitation; chronic
- Mitral stenosis
- Mitral valve prolapse
- Multifocal atrial tachycardia
- Narcolepsy
- Obstructive sleep apnea
- Paroxysmal supraventricular tachycardia
- Patent ductus arteriosus
- Pericarditis
  - Bacterial pericarditis
  - Constrictive pericarditis
  - Post-MI pericarditis
- Peripartum cardiomyopathy

- Primary amyloid
- Primary hyperaldoster-onism
- Primary hyperparathyroid-ism
- Primary pulmonary hyper-tension
- Pulmonary embolus
- Pulmonary valve stenosis
- Restrictive cardiomyopathy
- Right-sided heart failure
- Sick sinus syndrome
- Stable angina
- Stroke
- Systemic lupus erythemato-sus
- Tetralogy of Fallot
- Thyrotoxic periodic paralysis
- Transient ischemic attack (TIA)
- Transposition of the great vessels
- Tricuspid regurgitation
- Type 2 diabetes
- Unstable angina
- Ventricular septal defect
- Ventricular tachycardia
- Wolff-Parkinson-White syn-drome

What the Risks Are

There are generally no risks. Because this procedure merely monitors the electrical impulses and does not emit electricity, there is no risk of shock.

During an exercise electrocardiogram, some patients experience arrhythmias or heart distress. Equipment for dealing with these occurrences is located in the testing area.

Special Considerations

The accuracy of the ECG varies with the condition being tested. Some heart conditions are not detectable all the time, and others may never produce any specific ECG changes.

A person who suspects heart disease or has had a heart attack may need more than one ECG. There is no reason for healthy people to undergo annual testing unless they have inherited risks or a medical condition.

It is important to be relaxed and relatively warm during ECG recording. Any movement, including muscle tremors such as shivering, can alter the tracing.

Chapter 56

Computer Imaging and Tomography Used in the Diagnosis and Management of Cardiovascular Diseases

X-ray computed tomography, including conventional, helical, and electron-beam ("Ultrafast®") forms, provides cross-sectional images of the chest, including the heart and great vessels. In general, cardiac tomography (also called CT scan and coronary artery scanning) is useful to evaluate aortic disease (such as aortic dissection), cardiac masses and pericardial disease.

CT provides clinically relevant anatomic and functional information, is relatively noninvasive, and has very low short- and long-term risks (if the well-known potential hazards are avoided).

Computerized axial tomographic scan is also used to examine how the brain looks, functions, and gets its blood supply. This test can outline the affected part of the brain and help define the problem a stroke creates.

Electron-Beam Computed Tomography (EBCT or Ultrafast® CT)

EBCT is an especially fast form of x-ray imaging technology. It's particularly useful to:

- evaluate bypass graft patency, intra- and congenital cardiac lesions, and

---

"Computer Imaging/Tomography," reprinted with permission from www.americanheart.org © 2004, American Heart Association.

377

- quantify right and left ventricular muscle mass, chamber volumes, and systolic and diastolic function (such as cardiac output and ejection fraction).

Electron-beam CT can also measure calcium deposits in the coronary arteries. The amount of calcium detected by EBCT is related to the amount of underlying coronary atherosclerosis. The coronary calcium score, derived from EBCT scans of the coronary arteries, is known to predict the occurrence of cardiac events, such as fatal and nonfatal heart attacks or the need for coronary bypass surgery or coronary (balloon) angioplasty over the next one or two years. A negative calcium score implies a very low risk for obstructing coronary lesions and has a high negative predictive value for coronary events.

The increased predictive value of EBCT of the coronary arteries relative to traditional risk factor assessment isn't yet completely defined.

EBCT isn't a substitute for cardiac catheterization. EBCT measurement of coronary calcium is of no known value in patients who've already had a heart attack or undergone coronary bypass surgery or coronary angioplasty.

Cardiac Positron Emission Tomography (PET)

Positron emission tomography of the heart allows the study and quantification of various aspects of heart tissue function. Its use in research has provided novel observations in cardiac physiology and pathophysiology. PET combines

1. tomographic imaging with radionuclide tracers of blood flow metabolism and receptors and

2. tracer kinetic principles for noninvasively quantifying regional myocardial blood flow, substrate fluxes, biochemical reaction rates, and neural control.

Clinical studies suggest an important role for PET in diagnosing patients, describing disease, and developing treatment strategy. Two areas of clinical application have emerged:

- PET, which is noninvasive, is highly accurate for detecting, localizing, and describing coronary artery disease that impairs blood flow to the myocardium (heart muscle).

- PET accurately identifies injured but viable myocardium (heart muscle), such as reversible ventricular dysfunction.

Technological improvements have occurred in PET scanners, cyclotron production of tracer labels, and radiotracer synthesis. These have greatly enhanced the performance of cardiac PET studies, which now appear to be feasible. Cardiac PET studies can also be performed without an on-site cyclotron, using generator-produced isotopes such as rubidium-82 or tracers of metabolism produced off-site.

Digital Cardiac Angiography, Digital Subtraction Angiography (DCA or DSA)

This modified form of imaging records pictures by computer of the major blood vessels to the heart or brain. It lets a doctor know if there are any blockages, how severe they are, and what can be done about them. In this test, dye is injected into a vein in the arm, and an x-ray machine quickly takes a series of pictures of the chest or head and neck.

Magnetic Resonance Imaging (MRI)

Magnetic resonance imaging (MRI) is also called nuclear magnetic resonance (NMR) imaging. It uses powerful magnets to look inside the body. Computer-generated pictures can show the heart muscle, identify damage from a heart attack, diagnose certain congenital cardiovascular defects, and evaluate disease of larger blood vessels such as the aorta. It can outline the affected part of the brain and help define the problems created by stroke. Unlike radiographic imaging methods,

- It's non-ionizing and has no known biological hazards.

- It can produce high-resolution images of the heart's chambers and large vessels without the need for contrast agents.

- It's intrinsically three-dimensional.

- It produces images of cardiovascular structures without interference from adjacent bone or air.

- It has high tissue contrast.

MRI is an acceptable technique for evaluating diseases of the aorta such as dissection, aneurysm, and coarctation; diseases of the pericardium such as constrictive pericarditis or hematoma; congenital cardiac lesions before or after surgical repair; heart muscle diseases, including those affecting the right ventricle such as dysplasia; and cardiac masses such as intracardiac tumor or invasive lung malignancy.

Other proven but less common applications of MRI include evaluation of cardiac chamber morphology such as ventricular mass; global or regional ventricular function; and valve regurgitation.

Other potential applications are currently under active investigation, including evaluation of coronary artery anatomy and flow; evaluation of myocardial blood flow; assessment of myocardial viability with pharmacologic stress; and assessment of myocardial metabolism by spectroscopic techniques.

In summary, MRI provides clinically relevant anatomic and functional information noninvasively and with minimal risk, if the well-known contraindications (such as pacemakers) and potential hazards (such as attraction of metallic objects) are avoided.

Radionuclide Imaging or Radionuclide Angiography
(includes such tests as thallium test, MUGA scan, or acute infarct scintigraphy)

These tests involve injecting radioactive substances called radionuclides into the bloodstream. Computer-generated pictures can then find them in the heart. These tests show how well the heart muscle is supplied with blood, show how well the heart's chambers are working, or identify a part of the heart damaged by heart attack.

Radionuclide angiography can also be used as a nuclear brain scan. In it radioactive compounds are injected into a vein in the arm, and a machine similar to a Geiger counter creates a map showing their uptake into different parts of the head. The pictures show how the brain functions rather than its structure. This test can detect blocked blood vessels and areas where the brain is damaged.

Single Photon Emission Computed Tomography (SPECT)

SPECT of the heart is a well-established nuclear imaging technique. It involves taking a series of pictures around the chest after injecting a radioactive tracer into the blood. Then computer graphics are used to create images of slices through the heart. This technique has been applied to the heart for myocardial perfusion (blood flow) imaging with agents like thallium-201 and the technetium-based myocardial perfusion tracers. These agents are injected either at rest or with exercise or pharmacologic stress.

Cardiac SPECT was introduced for myocardial perfusion imaging to overcome some of the limitations of planar imaging and to improve the localization and quantification of perfusion defects. Cardiac SPECT has been shown to make it easier to detect and localize myocardial perfusion defects at rest and during stress. The ability of SPECT to localize coronary artery disease and assess the extent and severity of perfusion abnormalities is enhanced compared to planar imaging. As a result, SPECT imaging is now widely used in nuclear cardiology laboratories across the country.

Several large, published studies have demonstrated the quantitative methods of interpretation. When SPECT is used to image the technetium-based myocardial perfusion tracers, global and regional function of the ventricle can be obtained in addition to regional perfusion. SPECT imaging of the heart can also be used in conjunction with newer agents that evaluate metabolism, but these applications are at present investigational.

In summary, SPECT myocardial perfusion imaging is a well-established, clinically useful technique for diagnosing coronary artery disease and for managing patients with known coronary artery disease.

Chapter 57

What You Need to Know about Your Angiography Test

What Is Angiography?

Angiography is a way to produce x-ray pictures of the inside of blood vessels. When blood vessels are blocked, damaged, or abnormal in any way, chest pain, heart attack, stroke, or other problems may occur. Angiography helps your physician determine the source of the problem and the extent of damage to the blood vessel segments that are being examined.

Before the Test

Lab work may be needed before the angiogram to determine your blood's ability to clot.

Please follow these guidelines after midnight the night before your test:

Medications

Always consult with your primary physician or the physician requesting this test before discontinuing any medication. Here are some guidelines:

- Do NOT take any aspirin or any products containing aspirin.

- Do NOT take dipyridamole (Persantine) or warfarin (Coumadin) within seventy-two hours before the test, and twenty-four hours after the test. These medications are often referred to as blood-thinning pills.

- DO take your other medications on schedule as usual, especially any medications for high blood pressure.

If You Have Diabetes

- Take half of your usual dose of insulin and eat a light breakfast before 6 A.M. When you arrive for your test, please be sure to remind the physician that you have diabetes and have eaten breakfast.

- Do NOT take Glucophage (metformin hydrochloride) for forty-eight hours before the test or forty-eight hours after the test, to reduce the risk of kidney complications.

Eating and Drinking

- Drink only clear liquids for breakfast the day of your test. Clear liquids include clear broth, tea, strained fruit juices, strained vegetable soup, black coffee, plain gelatin, tomato juice, and ginger ale.

On the Day of the Test

Please make arrangements for transportation, as you should not drive until the day after the procedure.

Please do not bring valuables such as jewelry or credit cards.

You will meet with your physician and he or she will review further instructions and discuss any questions you may have. The physician will also review your medical history.

In almost all cases, laboratory tests ("blood work") will be needed, and your physician will need to study the results before beginning your angiography test. It may be several hours before the laboratory results are available.

Every effort will be made to perform your test at the scheduled time, but delays do occur. You may want to bring a book or magazine.

During the Test

You may be asked to change into a hospital gown.

The test itself will take approximately two to three hours. Mild sedation may be given.

During angiography, a long slender tube called a catheter is inserted into a large artery (generally, in the groin area).

The catheter is slowly and carefully threaded through the artery until its tip reaches the segment of vessel to be examined by angiography.

A small amount of contrast material is injected into the blood vessel segment through the catheter, and x-rays are taken. The contrast agent enables the blood vessels to appear on the x-ray pictures.

A physician specially trained in angiography studies the x-ray pictures to determine the source of the problem and the extent of damage to the blood vessel segments that are examined.

After the Test

You will be monitored for four to six hours. At that time, the radiology nurse will discuss post-angiogram instructions with you. You will be provided with a written form of these instructions—please follow these at home.

A radiologist will evaluate you before you are discharged. Then your physician will discuss the test results with you.

If you have diabetes, do NOT take Glucophage (metformin hydrochloride) for forty-eight hours after the test, to reduce the risk of kidney complications.

The Evening after the Test

We advise for your safety to spend a quiet, restful evening with a friend or relative in the immediate area. On rare occasions, it may be necessary for you to spend the night in the hospital.

Angiography allows your physician to view how blood circulates within vessels at specific locations in the body. This diagnostic test is used to locate the specific source of an abnormality in the neck, kidneys, legs, or other sites.

385

Chapter 58

Cardiac Catheterization

What is heart catheterization?

Heart (cardiac) catheterization is a procedure in which a narrow, flexible tube is inserted through a blood vessel into the veins, arteries, and chambers of your heart. The tube is called a catheter. It is usually inserted through a blood vessel in the arm, groin, or neck.

Heart catheterization can:

- Record the blood pressure in the blood vessels in the lungs and the heart and in the chambers of the heart.
- Measure blood flow and oxygen content of blood in different parts of the heart.
- Allow x-ray pictures (angiograms) outlining the heart chambers or coronary arteries to be taken with use of a special dye.
- Take a tissue sample (biopsy) of the heart muscle using an instrument passed through the catheter.

Usually you do not need to stay in the hospital overnight for this procedure.

When is it used?

Some of the reasons heart catheterization may be done are:

Reprinted from Clinical Reference Systems Cardiology Advisor, 2003.2 with permission from McKesson Health Solutions. © 2003 McKesson Health Solutions, LLC.

- **Coronary artery disease:** If your coronary arteries are partly or completely blocked, you have an increased risk of a heart attack, especially if your symptoms have gotten worse recently. Cardiac catheterization and the injection of dye into the arteries is the best way to study the coronary arteries. The dye study shows the location and the amount of the blockage. The procedure may be done to see if you need coronary bypass surgery or coronary angioplasty.

- **Open-heart surgery:** Sometimes catheterization is needed before open-heart surgery. The surgeon needs to check for any conditions that may increase the risk of problems during surgery.

- **Artificial heart valves:** If you have an artificial heart valve, you may need catheterization so the health care provider can see how the valve and the rest of the heart are working.

- **Biopsy:** The tissue sample of heart muscle can be checked for inflammation or other problems.

- **Angioplasty:** Catheters can be used to open a narrowed heart valve or artery. Balloon angioplasty, for example, uses pressure from a balloon to widen an artery.

- **Stenting:** Catheters may also be used to remove plaque buildup and to place stents that hold open arterial walls.

How do I prepare for the procedure?

You will be asked not to eat or drink anything for twelve hours before the procedure. Arrange for someone to drive you home afterward. Follow any other instructions your health care provider may give you.

What happens during the procedure?

You are given a sedative, which will make you feel relaxed, but you will stay awake. You are also given a shot (a local anesthetic) to numb the area where the catheter is inserted.

The doctor will insert the catheter through a small incision. The catheter is pushed through the blood vessels toward the heart. X-rays are used to follow the position of the catheter. You will not feel the catheter as it passes through your blood vessels.

The health care provider will direct the tip of the catheter to precise positions in the heart and its blood vessels. The catheter is attached to a device that measures blood flow and blood pressure in various places in the heart and blood vessels.

If pictures of the heart chambers, valves, or coronary arteries are needed, a special dye is injected through the catheter. During this injection, moving x-ray pictures are recorded. This procedure with dye is called angiography.

When the procedure is finished, the health care provider will remove the catheter and apply pressure over the area where the needle was inserted to control any bleeding.

What happens after the procedure?

The procedure may last thirty to sixty minutes. You will spend several hours in the recovery room. After that, you may go home. You should avoid strenuous activity for the rest of the day to prevent bleeding.

Ask your health care provider if you should take any precautions after the procedure, what symptoms to watch for, and when you should come back for a checkup.

A swollen bruise may appear near the puncture site and be uncomfortable for a few days.

What are the benefits?

Heart catheterization is considered the most accurate way to gather the information your health care provider needs to diagnose and treat heart problems most effectively. The health care provider will study the x-ray moving pictures to see if your heart valves are normal, to check how well the heart is pumping, and to look for possible blockages in the coronary arteries. He or she will take note of the direction and the amount of blood flow through the heart. With the knowledge gained from the procedure, heart valves may be repaired or replaced before heart failure occurs. Heart attacks may be prevented or delayed by treating coronary artery blockages.

What are the risks?

- You may feel some minor discomfort.
- In rare cases, you may have an allergic reaction to the drug used in the anesthesia.
- The procedure can cause irregular heart rhythms, which could require treatment.

- If the catheter is placed in an artery, a blood clot could form around the catheter. If this happens, your health care provider may give you a blood thinner and keep you in the hospital for a few days to dissolve the clot.

- You may have an allergic reaction to the dye and become nauseated or flushed. This reaction can be treated with medicine. The dye could also damage the kidneys.

- The catheter could puncture a blood vessel and cause internal bleeding.

- While not common, a heart attack or stroke might be triggered by the procedure.

Complications from this procedure are rare. The risk of death is very low. People with diabetes or kidney disease may be at higher risk for kidney damage from the dye. In general, the more skilled the health care provider, the less likely you are to have problems.

When should I call my health care provider?

Call your health care provider if you have:

- severe pain where the catheter was placed
- bleeding from the puncture site
- increased swelling and tenderness where the needle was inserted.

Chapter 59

Nuclear Ventriculography

Alternative Names

RNV; cardiac blood pooling imaging; nuclear heart scan; radionuclide ventriculography; MUGA [multigated acquisition]

Definition

Nuclear ventriculography (MUGA or RNV) is a test that uses radioactive tracers to make heart chambers and blood vessels visible. The procedure is noninvasive. The heart structures are not touched by instruments.

How the Test Is Performed

A radioactive isotope is injected into your vein. Commonly used isotopes include technetium and thallium. Radioactive isotopes attach to red blood cells and pass through the heart in the circulating blood. The radioactive isotope can be traced through the heart using special cameras or scanners. The images may be synchronized with an electrocardiogram.

You will be tested when you are resting, then tested again with exercise or after administering certain medications.

"Nuclear Ventriculography (MUGA or RNV)," © 2003 A.D.A.M., Inc. Reprinted with permission. Updated January 2004.

How to Prepare for the Test

Adults

You may be required to abstain from food or beverages containing caffeine or alcohol for several hours before the test.

Infants and Children

The physical and psychological preparation you can provide for this or any test or procedure depends on your child's age, interests, previous experiences, and level of trust.

How the Test Will Feel

Electrodes may be placed on your chest. An intravenous line will be placed in your arm to inject the radioactive isotope. A camera or scanner will be placed over the chest area to process the images. The scan may be repeated during exercise on a treadmill or stationary bicycle.

Why the Test Is Performed

The test is performed when it is important to very accurately measure the pumping function of the heart.

Normal Values

Normal results indicate normal heart function, or a normal cardiac response to exercise.

What Abnormal Results Mean

Abnormal results may indicate a myocardial infarction, coronary artery disease, heart valve disease, or other cardiac disorders.

Additional Conditions under Which the Test May Be Performed

- Atrial septal defect
- Dilated cardiomyopathy
- Heart failure

- Idiopathic cardiomyopathy
- Lyme disease, secondary
- Mitral stenosis
- Peripartum cardiomyopathy
- Senile cardiac amyloid
- SVC [superior vena cava] obstruction

What the Risks Are

Nuclear imaging tests carry a very low risk of complications. Exposure to radio tracers can be a concern for the nuclear lab staff, but not for patients undergoing an occasional nuclear imaging test.

Part Six

Medications and Procedures Used to Treat Cardiovascular Disorders

Chapter 60

Treating Heart Disease

Diagnosing a Heart Attack and Determining Treatment Options

Patients with heart disease or those with risk factors should seek emergency medical help immediately if they have any signs or symptoms of an attack. Early treatment is critical for recovery.

When a patient arrives at the hospital with a possible heart attack, the patient is given an electrocardiogram within ten minutes and put on constant monitoring. Blood and other tests are taken to determine the condition.

Depending on how severe the condition is, the patient is then given either medical treatments or more invasive approaches, such as angioplasty.

Immediate Treatments to Support the Patient

Oxygen. Oxygen is almost always administered right away, usually through a tube that enters through the nose. The patient is given aspirin if one was not taken at home.

Transfusions. A 2001 study suggested that giving transfusions to elderly heart attack patients with even mild anemia improved short-term survival rates.

Excerpted from "Heart Attack and Acute Coronary Syndrome," © 2003 A.D.A.M., Inc. Reprinted with permission.

Medications for Relieving Symptoms.

- *Nitroglycerin.* Most heart attack patients will receive nitroglycerin, usually under the tongue. Nitroglycerin decreases blood pressure and dilates the blood vessels around the heart, increasing blood flow. Nitroglycerin may be given intravenously in certain cases (e.g., those with recurrent angina, congestive heart failure, or high blood pressure). There is some evidence suggesting that intravenous administration may help reduce long-term heart muscle changes that can occur after a heart attack. (Patients with very low blood pressure or severely slow heart rate will not receive nitroglycerin.)

- *Morphine.* Morphine not only relieves pain and reduces anxiety but it also dilates blood vessels, thereby aiding the circulation of blood and oxygen to the heart. Morphine can decrease blood pressure and slow down the heart. In certain patients where such conditions can worsen their heart attacks, other drugs such as meperidine (Demerol) or nalbuphine (Nubain) may be used.

Anti-Clotting Medications. Appropriate anti-clotting medications are started immediately in all patients.

- Aspirin is given immediately unless the patient had taken aspirin before entering the hospital. It is continued afterward indefinitely.

- Clopidogrel (a more potent anti-platelet agent) is usually added and continued for one to nine months afterward. It is sometimes used in place of aspirin.

- Heparin is generally administered to moderate to high-risk patients. Low–molecular weight heparin (LMWH), such as enoxaparin, is now recommended over standard heparin.

- Glycoprotein IIb/IIIa inhibitors, most often tirofiban, are added for patients undergoing angioplasty.

Opening the Arteries: Thrombolytic Drugs or Emergency Angioplasty (PTCA)

After a heart attack, clots form in the injured artery within four to six hours in 90 percent of heart attack victims. Opening a clotted artery as quickly as possible is the best approach to improving survival.

The standard medical and surgical solutions for opening arteries are the following.

- Angioplasty, also called percutaneous transluminal coronary angioplasty (PTCA), is the major surgical procedure for opening the arteries.

- Thrombolytics are known as blood-clot-busting drugs and are the standard medications used to open the arteries. They are administered as soon as possible in centers where angioplasty is not available or in patients who are not good candidates for angioplasty.

Some studies suggest that a combination of early administration of a thrombolytic followed by angioplasty may have significant benefits for many patients, but such an approach is not routine.

Other Heart Supportive Agents

After a heart attack, the patient may need a number of different medications, depending on his or her risk factors for a future heart attack:

- Beta-blockers reduce the oxygen demand of the heart by slowing the heart rate and lowering arterial pressure. Intravenous administration of beta-blockers (metoprolol or esmolol) within the first few hours of a heart attack can reduce the destruction of heart tissue. Oral agents may be sufficient for some patients with unstable angina.

- Angiotensin converting enzyme (ACE) inhibitors should be given on the first day to all patients, unless there are medical reasons for not taking them.

- Calcium channel blockers may provide relief in patients with unstable angina whose symptoms do not respond to nitrates and beta blockers. They are also useful for patients with Prinzmetal's angina.

- Statins are important cholesterol-lowering agents that are beneficial for heart attack patients and may have heart-protective properties that go beyond lowering cholesterol. Of interest, however, was a 2003 study suggesting that cholesterol levels— whether high or low—had no effect on mortality rates among heart attack survivors over sixty-five. More research is needed.

- Atropine may be given for a very low heart rate (bradycardia) or signs of atrioventricular (AV) block, in which electric conduction of nerve impulses to specialized muscles in the heart is slowed or interrupted.

Treatment for Patients in Shock or with Congestive Heart Failure

Severely ill patients, particularly those in shock (a dangerous condition that includes a drop in blood pressure and other abnormalities) or with congestive heart failure, will be monitored closely and stabilized. Oxygen is administered, and fluids are given or replaced when it is appropriate to either increase or reduce blood pressure. Such patients may be given dopamine, dobutamine, or both. Other treatments depend on the specific condition.

Heart failure. Intravenous furosemide may be administered. Patients may also be given nitrates, and ACE inhibitors, unless they have a severe drop in blood pressure or other conditions that preclude them. Clot-busting drugs or angioplasty may be appropriate and life-saving in many of these patients, although they are less likely to be given these treatments. (A 2003 study suggested that drugs may be more beneficial in this group, but more research is needed to confirm this.)

Shock. A procedure called intra-aortic balloon counterpulsation (IABP) is proving to help these patients when used in combination with thrombolytic therapy. IABP involves inserting a catheter containing a balloon, which is inflated and deflated within the artery to boost blood pressure. Left ventricular assist devices and early angioplasty might be considered.

Treatment of Arrhythmias

An arrhythmia is a deviation from the heart's normal beating pattern caused when the heart muscle is deprived of oxygen and is a dangerous side effect of a heart attack. A very fast or slow rhythmic heart rate often occurs in heart attack patients and is not usually a dangerous sign.

Premature beats or very fast arrhythmias called tachycardia, however, may be predictors of ventricular fibrillation. This is a lethal rhythm abnormality, in which the ventricles of the heart beat so rapidly that they do not actually contract but quiver ineffectually. The pumping action necessary to keep blood circulating is lost.

Preventing Ventricular Fibrillation

People who develop ventricular fibrillation do not always experience warning arrhythmias, and to date, there are no effective agents for preventing arrhythmias during a heart attack.

- Potassium and magnesium levels should be monitored and maintained.

- Intravenous beta-blockers followed by oral administration of the drugs may help prevent arrhythmias in certain patients.

Treating Ventricular Fibrillation

Defibrillators. Patients who develop ventricular arrhythmias are given electrical shocks with defibrillators to restore normal rhythms. Some studies suggest that implantable cardioverter-defibrillators may prevent further arrhythmias in heart attack survivors of these events who are at risk for further arrhythmias. At this time, however, their use is investigative in these patients.

Antiarrhythmic agents. Antiarrhythmic drugs include lidocaine, procainamide, or amiodarone. Amiodarone or another antiarrhythmic drug may be used afterward to prevent future events.

Managing Other Arrhythmias.

People with an arrhythmia called atrial fibrillation have a higher risk for stroke after a heart attack and should be treated very aggressively. Other rhythm disturbances called bradyarrhythmias (very slow rhythm disturbances) frequently develop in association with a heart attack and may be treated with atropine or pacemakers.

Thrombolytic Drugs Used to Restore Blood Flow after a Heart Attack

Thrombolytic, or clot-busting, drugs are now mainstays in the early treatment of many patients with heart attacks. These drugs dissolve the clot, or thrombus, responsible for causing artery blockage and heart-muscle tissue death.

Specific Thrombolytics

The standard thrombolytic drugs used are recombinant tissue plasminogen activators or rt-PAs. They include alteplase (Activase and reteplase [Retavase]). They are similar in effectiveness, although reteplase is easier to administer. Tenecteplase (TNKase), a newer agent, can be delivered more rapidly than alteplase, and to date, survival rates are similar. Streptokinase (Kabikinase, Streptase) is sometimes used but is somewhat less effective that the others. Other agents include anistreplase (Eminase) and urokinase (Abbokinase), which is not available in the United States.

Thrombolytic Administration

The earlier thrombolytic drugs are administered, the better. The advantages of thrombolytics are highest in the first ninety minutes and are still considerable at three hours. Administering these drugs more than six hours after symptoms have started adds little or no benefit. Of interest, some of these agents can now be given by emergency medical technicians (EMTs) before the patient reaches the hospital. Whether this will improve survival compared to angioplasty or other blood-thinning approaches is not yet clear.

A thrombolytic agent, such as alteplase or tenecteplase, is typically administered with intravenous heparin, an anticoagulant agent. (Heparin, like aspirin, cannot destroy existing blood clots but can prevent clots from reforming after they are broken up.) Enoxaparin, a form of heparin called low–molecular weight heparin, may be more beneficial than standard heparin.

Other anti-clotting agents are being tested in combination with thrombolytic agents. For example, studies are reporting modest improvements with the addition of glycoprotein IIb/IIIa receptor antagonists to low-dose thrombolytics.

Complications

Hemorrhagic stroke, usually occurring during the first day, is the most serious complication of thrombolytic therapy, but fortunately it is rare. Streptokinase given without heparin poses the lowest risk (although it is also less effective than other regimens in restoring blood flow). In general, the mortality rate from bleeding is only three in every one thousand patients treated with thrombolytics, whereas thirty-nine patients out of one thousand would die without these clot-busting drugs. Recent evidence suggests that the survival benefits of thrombolytic therapy, particularly in combination with aspirin, last for years.

Surgical Procedures for Restoring Blood Flow after a Heart Attack

Revascularization Procedures for Opening Blocked Arteries

Percutaneous transluminal coronary angioplasty and coronary artery bypass graft surgery, known as revascularization procedures, are the standard operations for opening narrowed or blocked arteries.

Emergency angioplasty is the standard procedure for heart attack patients and more effective than the use of thrombolytic agents for most patients. Unfortunately, not all communities have the facilities for emergency angioplasty. (A 2002 study suggested that in spite of the delay, transporting patients to facilities where angioplasties are available may still be more beneficial than thrombolytics for many individuals.)

Coronary bypass surgery is typically used as elective surgery for patients with blocked arteries. It may be used after a heart attack if angioplasty or thrombolytics fail or are not appropriate. It is usually not performed for a few days to allow recovery of the heart muscles.

Angioplasty (PTCA) and Coronary Stents

Percutaneous transluminal coronary angioplasty (PTCA), usually simply called angioplasty, involves opening the blocked artery.

A typical angioplasty procedure follows the following steps:

- The surgeon threads a narrow catheter (a tube) containing a fiber optic camera directly to the blocked vessel.

- The physician opens the blocked vessel using balloon angioplasty, in which the surgeon passes a tiny deflated balloon through the catheter to the vessel.

- The balloon is inflated to compress the plaque against the walls of the artery, flattening it out so that blood can once again flow through the blood vessel freely.

- In order to keep the artery open afterward, surgeons now most often employ a device called a coronary stent, which is an expandable metal mesh tube that is implanted during angioplasty at the site of the blockage.

- Once in place, the stent pushes against the wall of the artery to keep it open. Stenting is improving outcome in patients with heart attack who have emergency angioplasty. A 2002 study reported that their safety and effectiveness was sustained for seven to eleven years.

Complications occur in about 10 percent of patients (about 80 percent within the first day). Serious ones include heart attack and the need for additional surgery. Outcomes are best in hospital settings with experienced teams and backup. According to a 2003 study, outcomes are also better if the procedure is done during routine working hours. It is not known if sleep deprivation in the medical professionals or increased clotting factors during the night are responsible for these differences.

Reclosure and blockage during or shortly after angioplasty. Reclosure of the artery during or shortly after angioplasty often occurs. A number of anti-clotting agents are used to help prevent this, although they are not wholly protective because reclosure in some cases is due to other, unknown causes.

Prevention of restenosis. Narrowing or reclosing of the artery (restenosis) occurs within a year of angioplasty in a large minority of angioplasty patients, often requiring a repeat operation. The narrowing of the artery in this case is not due to blood clots, so anti-clotting agents are not useful. Of great interest and promise are studies that show no restenosis in patients who have received stents that were coated with the drug sirolimus.

Coronary Artery Bypass Graft Surgery (CABG)

Coronary artery bypass graft surgery (CABG) is the alternative elective procedure to angioplasty for opening blocked arteries in patients with severe angina, particularly those who have two or more blocked arteries. It is a very invasive procedure, however:

- The chest is opened and the blood is rerouted through a lung-heart machine.

- The heart is stopped during the procedure.

- Segments of veins or arteries taken from elsewhere in the patient's body are fashioned into grafts, which are used to reroute the blood. The blood vessel grafts are placed in front of and beyond the blocked arteries, so the blood flows through the new vessels around the blockage.

Mortality rates with this procedure after a heart attack are much higher (6 percent) than when it is used electively (1 percent to 2 percent). How or when it should be used after a heart attack, then, is controversial. A 2002 study attempted to determine which patients are at highest risk for a poor outcome from CABG after a heart attack. They included women, patients over seventy-five, and those with heart failure or other severe heart problems.

Other Agents Used for Treatment of Heart Attack and Acute Coronary Syndrome

In addition to thrombolytics, a number of agents are now available for use during a heart attack and for treating acute coronary syndrome. Some of these and other medications are also important for preventing either a first or a second heart attack.

Aspirin and Other Anti-Clotting Agents

Anti-clotting agents that inhibit or break up blood clots are used at every stage of heart disease. They are generally either antiplatelet agents or anticoagulants. Investigators are also studying combinations of anti-clotting agents, which may be useful in patients with severe heart disease. All anti-clotting therapies carry the risk of bleeding, which can lead to dangerous situations, including stroke.

Anti-Platelet Drugs

These agents prevent formation of blood platelets. Platelets are very small disc-shaped blood cells that are important for blood clotting.

- *Aspirin.* Aspirin is an antiplatelet agent. It is the most common anti-clotting drug and nearly anyone with heart disease is advised to take it daily in low dose.

- *Glycoprotein IIb/IIIa Inhibitors.* These potent blood-thinning agents include abciximab (ReoPro, Centocor), eptifibatide (Integrilin), tirofiban (Aggrastat), and lamifiban. They are administered intravenously in the hospital and are being used with angioplasty and stent placement. They are proving to be

405

helpful for ACS patients with non-ST-segment elevation myocardial infarction.

- *Thienopyridines.* Clopidogrel (Plavix) and ticlopidine (Ticlid) are
  potent oral platelet inhibitors.

Anticoagulants

Anticoagulants help thin blood and include the following:

- *Heparin.* Standard, or unfractionated, heparin. Low–molecular
  weight heparin (LMWH), which include enoxaparin (Lovenox),
  dalteparin (Fragmin), tinzaparin (Innohep).

- *Warfarin (Coumadin).*

- *Direct thrombin inhibitors.* They include argatroban (Novastan),
  danaparoid (Orgaran), and lepirudin (Refludan)

How Anti-Clotting Agents Are Used in Heart Attack Patients.

Unlike the thrombolytic (clot-busting) agents, which are used to
break up blood clots during a heart attack, anti-clotting agents are
used to prevent blood clots from forming in the first place. Such agents
then may be used along with thrombolytics, immediately after a heart
attack, and also as ongoing maintenance to prevent a heart attack.
(See Table 60.1.)

- The physician usually gives the patient heparin or aspirin, either alone or in combination with thrombolytic therapy. Aspirin
  should be given immediately, and heparin is usually started
  during or at the end of the thrombolytic infusion.

- Other agents, such as glycoprotein IIb/IIIa receptor antagonists,
  are being tested in combination with thrombolytic agents.

All of these drugs pose a risk for bleeding.

Beta-Blockers

Beta-blockers reduce the oxygen demand of the heart by slowing
the heart rate and lowering pressure in the arteries. They are now
well known for reducing deaths from heart disease. They include propranolol (Inderal), carvedilol (Coreg), bisoprolol (Zebeta), acebutolol
(Sectral), atenolol (Tenormin), labetalol (Normodyne, Trandate), metoprolol (Lopressor, Toprol-XL), and esmolol (Brevibloc).

Administration during a Heart Attack

Intravenous administration of beta-blockers (metoprolol or esmolol) within the first few hours of a heart attack can reduce the destruction of heart tissue. Evidence strongly supports a lower incidence of complications and better survival rates after a heart attack in patients who had been treated with a beta-blocker. In spite of this evidence, beta blockers are greatly underutilized. In one major New York center, for example, 72 percent of patients who could have benefited from them were not given these important agents after a heart attack.

Prevention after a Heart Attack

Beta-blockers are also important after a heart attack in preventing another heart attack. In fact, among elderly heart attack patients, those who do not use these agents afterward have a much poorer outcome.

Side Effects

Side effects include the following: Some beta-blockers lower HDL cholesterol (the beneficial cholesterol) by about 10 percent. The effect is most marked in smokers. Fatigue and lethargy are the most common neurologic side effects. Some people experience vivid dreams and nightmares, depression, and memory loss. Exercise capacity may be reduced. Dizziness and lightheadedness, especially when getting up from a lying down position also can occur.

Other side effects may include cold extremities, asthma, decreased heart function, gastrointestinal problems (e.g., heartburn, gas, diarrhea, or constipation), and sexual dysfunction.

Because they can narrow bronchial airways and constrict blood vessels, patients with asthma, emphysema, and chronic bronchitis should avoid beta-blockers whenever possible. They should not be used by patients with severe heart failure or severe AV block.

If side effects occur, the patient should call a physician, but it is extremely important not to stop the drug abruptly. Angina, heart attack, and even sudden death have occurred in patients who discontinued treatment without gradual withdrawal.

Statins and Other Cholesterol and Lipid-Lowering Agents

In 2002, the National Cholesterol Education Program's Adult Treatment Panel issued its latest recommendations. The results of

Table 60.1. Anti-Clotting Agents and Their Use in Heart Disease and Heart Attack

Type of Agent	Time Administered	Reason for Use	Possible Negative Effects
Anti-Clotting Agents	During or immediately following a heart attack	For preventing heart attacks in high-risk patients with acute coronary syndrome or other high-risk patients	Side effects. All anti-clotting therapies carry the risk of bleeding, which can lead to dangerous situations, including stroke.
Anti-Platelet Agents			
Aspirin	*At the sign of a heart attack.* An aspirin tablet, chewed and swallowed is taken at the first signs of an attack. *With angioplasty.* Used with angioplasty in combination with other anti-clotting agents to prevent reclosure. *After a heart attack.* Used with warfarin [see below]. (Combination more effective than either agent alone.)	*Patients with heart disease or at risk for It.* Low-dose aspirin is the first choice for preventing heart attacks in patients who have had a heart attack, in people with stable angina, and in those with risk factors for a first heart attack.	Prolonged use may produce gastrointestinal ulcers and bleeding. Of concern is research suggesting that NSAIDs, which include aspirin, ibuprofen (Advil), and naproxen (Aleve), interfere with diuretics and ACE inhibitors. (A 2000 report has also suggested that taking ibuprofen (Advil) right before taking an aspirin may inhibit aspirin's benefits on the heart.) Recent use of NSAIDs, in fact, has been associated with a higher risk of hospitalization in heart failure patients. More research is needed.

Table 60.1. Anti-Clotting Agents and Their Use in Heart Disease and Heart Attack (continued)

Type of Agent	Time Administered	Reason for Use	Possible Negative Effects
Thienopyrindines: Clopidogrel (Plavix, Iscover), ticlopidine (Ticlid)	*With surgery.* Clopidogrel may be particularly useful in combination with aspirin for preventing blood clots after angioplasty. It also is more effective alone than aspirin in preventing a recurrent heart attack after surgery.	*Treatment of acute coronary syndromes.* Clopidogrel is now recommended along with aspirin for preventing a heart attack in all ACS patients and for patients undergoing angioplasty.	Severe risk of bleeding. Ticlopidine poses a high risk for thrombocytopenia (drastic reduction in blood platelets). Not as a high a risk with clopidogrel.
Glycoprotein IIb/IIIa receptor antagonists. Intravenous agents include abciximab (ReoPro, Centocor), eptifibatide (Integrilin), tirofiban (Aggrastat).	*With angioplasty.* These agents improve survival when used with angioplasty and coronary stent placement. *Combined with thrombolytics.* Studies are reporting benefits when these agents are combined with low-dose thrombolytics compared to the addition of standard heparin.	*For Treatment of Acute Coronary Syndromes.* They are beneficial for ACS patients who require angioplasty. In the absence of angioplasty, early use of these drugs in the emergency room may benefit selected patients with high-risk ACS.	Risk for bleeding and for thrombocytopenia, particularly in certain patients (e.g., thin, elderly, non-white, with more than one heart risk factor)

(continued on next page)

Table 60.1. Anti-Clotting Agents and Their Use in Heart Disease and Heart Attack (continued from previous page)

Type of Agent	Time Administered	Reason for Use	Possible Negative Effects
Anti-Coagulants			
Heparin. Administered intravenously or injected. Either standard (unfractionated) heparin or low–molecular weight heparin (LMWH). LMWHs including enoxaparin (Lovenox), dalteparin (Fragmin), tinzaparin (Innohep).	*With angioplasty.* Used with angioplasty. *With thrombolytic therapy.* May be used with alteplase. LMWH appears to be more beneficial in reducing heart events than unfractionated heparin, although poses a high risk for stroke, particularly in elderly patients, that may outweigh benefits.	*For treatment of acute coronary syndromes.* Low–molecular weight heparin (e.g., enoxaparin) is now preferred over standard heparin except in patients who are about to have bypass surgery.	High risk for bleeding. The major complication with standard heparin is thrombocytopenia (a severe drop in platelets). This is serious and can become life threatening, particularly if it produces bleeding in various body regions.
Warfarin (Coumadin). Oral anticoagulant. Prevents clots by inhibiting vitamin K.	*Immediately following a heart attack.* Combination with aspirin after a heart attack.	*For treatment of acute coronary syndromes.* May be more protective than aspirin in ACS patients. Some evidence that it might prevent disease progression itself in the arteries of the heart. *Other.* Very important for patients with atrial fibrillation.	Increases risk for bleeding. It must be monitored.

Table 60.1. Anti-Clotting Agents and Their Use in Heart Disease and Heart Attack (continued)

Type of Agent	Time Administered	Reason for Use	Possible Negative Effects
Direct Thrombin Inhibitors: Hirudin (derived from leech saliva), bivalirudin (a hirudin derivative) argatroban (Novastan) are standard agents. Others include inogatran, efegatran, danaparoid (Orgaran), lepirudin (Refludan), desirudin (Revasc). Ximelagatran (Exanta) new oral DTI.		*For treatment of acute coronary syndromes.* Proving to be useful along with warfarin for patients who develop heparin-induced thrombocytopenia. May be superior to heparin for preventing heart attack and death.	Risk for bleeding.

411

these guidelines would increase the number of Americans taking LDL-lowering agents from fifteen million to thirty-six million, with significant increases occurring in people under forty-five and over sixty-five years old and among men in all age groups. A number of agents are available for lowering cholesterol and other dangerous fat molecules (lipids). They include the following:

- Statins are now the standard agents for most people who require LDL-lowering therapy. Bile-acid binding resins or niacin may be considered. (Another LDL-lowering agent, probucol, is usually limited to people with genetic disorders that cause severely high cholesterol levels.) If LDL goals are not achieved, combinations of a statin with a bile-acid resin such as ezetimibe (Zetia) or niacin should be considered.

- Fibrates or niacin are beneficial for people who need to lower triglycerides and increase HDL.

Statins inhibit the liver enzyme HMG-CoA reductase, which is used in the manufacturing of cholesterol. They are the most effective drugs for the treatment of high cholesterol, and, according to a 2003 major analysis of over two hundred studies, they reduce risk for heart events by 60 percent and stroke by 17 percent.

Two studies in 2002 and 2003, however, muddied these positive findings. In one, lowering moderately high LDL cholesterol levels with a statin did not improve survival rates among high-risk patients. Some experts believe that statin treatment was not aggressive enough in this study. In the other 2003 study, however, cholesterol levels—whether high or low—had no effect on mortality rates among heart attack survivors over sixty-five. More research is needed on these findings.

Still, most experts estimate a 25 percent or more reduction in mortality rates when patients take statins after a heart attack. They may even become important agents for many people at risk for heart disease who have normal cholesterol levels. In fact, the benefits of statins may go beyond simply improving cholesterol levels.

Statins include lovastatin (Mevacor), simvastatin (Zocor), and pravastatin (Pravachol). These are the most studied statins and have proven effectiveness and good safety record. Newer synthetic statins including fluvastatin (Lescol), atorvastatin (Lipitor), and rosuvastatin (Crestor) are proving to be very beneficial.

In many studies the side effects reported by statin users were nearly the same as those taking placebos (inactive agents). Those reported include gastrointestinal discomfort, headaches, skin rashes, muscle aches, sexual dysfunction, drowsiness, dizziness, nausea, constipation, and peripheral neuropathy (numbness or tingling in the hands and feet).

The primary safety concern with statins has involved an uncommon condition called myopathy, which can cause muscle damage and in some cases, muscle and joint pain. Severe cases of myopathy warrant discontinuation. Patients should tell their physicians about any unusual muscle discomfort or weakness and if their urine becomes brown-colored.

Statins also can effect the liver, particularly at higher doses, so periodic liver function tests should be administered.

Angiotensin Converting Enzyme Inhibitors

Angiotensin converting enzyme (ACE) inhibitors are important agents after a heart attack, particularly in patients at risk for heart failure. Taking an ACE inhibitor at the onset of a heart attack may, in fact, reduce the damage. These agents are commonly used to treat hypertension and are recommended as first-line treatment for people with diabetes and kidney damage, for some heart attack survivors, and for patients with heart failure.

ACE inhibitors include captopril (Capoten), ramipril (Altace), enalapril (Vasotec), quinapril (Accupril), benazepril (Lotensin), perindopril (Aceon), and lisinopril (Prinivil, Zestril).

Side effects of ACE inhibitors are uncommon but may include an irritating cough, excessive drops in blood pressure, and allergic reactions. Of great concern is research suggesting that aspirin interferes with ACE inhibitors (and other so-called NSAIDs) and increases the risk for heart failure in patients taking ACE inhibitors. An encouraging 2003 analysis, however, reported that ACE inhibitors still significantly reduced risks for adverse heart events, including hospitalizations for heart failure, regardless of whether or not the patients were also taking aspirin.

Magnesium

Magnesium has blood-thinning properties and may help open blood vessels. It is important to correct any magnesium deficiencies in heart attack patients (such as in those who were on diuretics). For certain patients who cannot be given thrombolytic therapy, intravenous magnesium has been investigated. The most recent evidence suggests, however, that it offers no significant benefits for patients with heart attack.

Infection-Fighting Agents

Flu Shots. One study reported that influenza vaccinations might protect heart attack patients against another attack during flu season. A 2002 study reported that flu shots given to patients who had angioplasty were associated with a significantly lower risk for death from heart events.

Antibiotics. Researchers have been investigating antibiotics for treating patients with heart disease and past infection of *Chlamydia pneumoniae* or *H. pylori*. Results have been mixed. In one large 2002 study, patients with heart attack or ACS were treated with amoxicillin or azithromycin, two common antibiotics, for a week. A year later they had a 40 percent lower risk for adverse heart events than those not given antibiotics—regardless of whether they had evidence of infection. Other small studies have also been positive. Some experts believe the protection from antibiotics may be due to inflammatory effects, rather than anti-bacterial. Of note, some studies have found no protection for the heart from antibiotics.

Chapter 61

Cholesterol-Lowering Medicines

To reach an LDL-cholesterol goal of less than 100 mg/dL, you may need to take a cholesterol-lowering medicine in addition to making life habit changes. Heart disease patients and those at high risk for developing heart disease need to lower their LDL more than other people. As a result, medications are more often used by patients with heart disease and those at high risk than by those who do not have heart disease or who have a lower risk of developing it.

Cholesterol-Lowering Medications and You

If you have an LDL level of 130 mg/dL or greater, you will generally need to take an LDL-lowering medicine. If your LDL level is 100 to 129 mg/dL, your doctor will consider all the facts of your case in deciding whether to prescribe medication for further LDL lowering or for high triglycerides or low HDL if they are present. If you have been hospitalized for a heart attack, your doctor will likely start you on a medication at discharge if your LDL cholesterol is 130 mg/dL or greater. If your LDL cholesterol is between 100 and 129 mg/dL during your hospitalization, your doctor may choose to start you on an LDL-lowering medication before you are discharged. Also, if your LDL cholesterol is far above the goal level of less than 100 mg/dL when first measured, your doctor may choose to start a cholesterol-lowering

Reprinted from "Cholesterol-Lowering Medicines," National Cholesterol Education Program, National Heart, Lung, and Blood, Institute, National Institutes of Health, 2001.

medication together with diet and physical activity right from the beginning of treatment. If your doctor prescribes medicine, you also will need to:

- Follow your cholesterol-lowering diet.

- Be more physically active.

- Lose weight if overweight.

- Control all of your other heart disease risk factors, including smoking, high blood pressure, and diabetes.

Taking all these steps together may lessen the amount of medicine you need or make the medicine work better—and that reduces your risk for a heart attack. The following is a description of cholesterol-lowering medicines.

Statins

There are currently five statin drugs on the market in the United States: lovastatin, simvastatin, pravastatin, fluvastatin, and atorvastatin (cerivastatin was withdrawn from the market by the manufacturer in August 2001). The major effect of the statins is to lower LDL cholesterol levels, and they lower LDL cholesterol more than other types of drugs. Statins inhibit an enzyme, HMG-CoA reductase, that controls the rate of cholesterol production in the body. These drugs lower cholesterol by slowing down the production of cholesterol and by increasing the liver's ability to remove the LDL cholesterol already in the blood. Statins were used to lower cholesterol levels in the 4S, CARE, and LIPID studies. The large reductions in total and LDL cholesterol produced by these drugs resulted in large reductions in heart attacks and heart disease deaths. Thanks to their track record in these studies and their ability to lower LDL cholesterol, statins have become the drugs most often prescribed when a person with heart disease needs a cholesterol- lowering medicine.

Studies using statins have reported 20 to 60 percent lower LDL cholesterol levels in patients on these drugs. Statins also reduce elevated triglyceride levels and produce a modest increase in HDL cholesterol.

The statins are usually given in a single dose at the evening meal or at bedtime. It is important that these medications be given in the evening to take advantage of the fact that the body makes more cholesterol at night than during the day.

You should begin to see results from the statins after several weeks, with a maximum effect in four to six weeks. After about six to eight weeks, your doctor can do the first check of your LDL cholesterol while on the medication. A second measurement of your LDL cholesterol level will have to be averaged with the first for your doctor to decide whether your dose of medicine should be changed to help you meet your goal.

The statins are well tolerated by most patients, and serious side effects are rare. A few patients will experience an upset stomach, gas, constipation, and abdominal pain or cramps. These symptoms usually are mild to moderate in severity and generally go away as your body adjusts. Rarely a patient will develop abnormalities in blood tests of the liver. Also rare is the side effect of muscle problems. The symptoms are muscle soreness, pain, and weakness. If this happens, or you have brown urine, contact your doctor right away to get blood tests for possible muscle problems.

Bile Acid Sequestrants

Bile acid sequestrants bind with cholesterol-containing bile acids in the intestines and are then eliminated in the stool. The usual effect of bile acid sequestrants is to lower LDL cholesterol by about 10 to 20 percent. Small doses of sequestrants can produce useful reductions in LDL cholesterol. Bile acid sequestrants are sometimes prescribed with a statin for patients with heart disease to increase cholesterol reduction. When these two drugs are combined, their effects are added together to lower LDL cholesterol by over 40 percent. Cholestyramine, colestipol, and colesevelam are the three main bile acid sequestrants currently available. These drugs are available as powders or tablets. They are not absorbed from the gastrointestinal tract, and thirty years of experience with the sequestrants indicate that their long-term use is safe.

Bile acid sequestrant powders must be mixed with water or fruit juice and taken once or twice (rarely three times) daily with meals. Tablets must be taken with large amounts of fluids to avoid gastrointestinal symptoms. Sequestrant therapy may produce a variety of symptoms including constipation, bloating, nausea, and gas.

The bile acid sequestrants are not prescribed as the sole medicine to lower your cholesterol if you have high triglycerides or a history of severe constipation.

Although sequestrants are not absorbed, they may interfere with the absorption of other medicines if taken at the same time. Other medications therefore should be taken at least one hour before or four to six hours after the resin. Talk to your doctor about the best time to take this medicine, especially if you take other medications.

Nicotinic Acid

Nicotinic acid or niacin, the water-soluble B vitamin, improves all lipoproteins when given in doses well above the vitamin requirement. Nicotinic acid lowers total cholesterol, LDL cholesterol, and triglyceride levels, while raising HDL cholesterol levels. There are three types of nicotinic acid: immediate release, timed release, and extended release. Most experts recommend starting with the immediate-release form; discuss with your doctor which type is best for you. Nicotinic acid is inexpensive and widely accessible to patients without a prescription but must not be used for cholesterol lowering without the monitoring of a physician because of the potential side effects. (Nicotinamide, another form of the vitamin niacin, does not lower cholesterol levels and should not be used in the place of nicotinic acid.)

All patients taking nicotinic acid to lower serum cholesterol should be closely monitored by their doctor to avoid complications from this medication. Self-medication with nicotinic acid should definitely be avoided because of the possibility of missing a serious side effect if not under a doctor's care.

Patients on nicotinic acid are usually started on low daily doses and gradually increased to an average daily dose of 1.5 to 3 grams per day for the immediate release form, and 1.5 to 2 grams per day for the other forms.

Nicotinic acid reduces LDL cholesterol levels by 10 to 20 percent, reduces triglycerides by 20 to 50 percent, and raises HDL cholesterol by 15 to 35 percent.

A common and troublesome side effect of nicotinic acid is flushing or hot flashes, which are the result of blood vessels opening wide. Most patients develop a tolerance to flushing and, in some patients, it can be decreased by taking the drug during or after meals or by the use of aspirin or other similar medications prescribed by your doctor. The extended release form may cause less flushing than the other forms. The effect of high blood pressure medicines may also be increased while you are on niacin. If you are taking high blood pressure medication, it is important to set up a blood pressure monitoring system while you are getting used to your new niacin regimen. A variety of gastrointestinal symptoms including nausea, indigestion, gas, vomiting, diarrhea, and the activation of peptic ulcers have been seen with the use of nicotinic acid. Three other major adverse effects include liver problems, gout, and high blood sugar. Risk of the latter three increases as the dose of nicotinic acid is increased. Your doctor may possibly not prescribe this medicine for you if you have diabetes, because of the effect on your blood sugar.

Fibrates

The cholesterol-lowering drugs called fibrates are primarily effective in lowering triglycerides and, to a lesser extent, in increasing HDL cholesterol levels. Gemfibrozil, the fibrate most widely used in the United States, can be very effective for patients with high triglyceride levels. However, it is not very effective for lowering LDL cholesterol. It is used in some patients with heart disease for whom a goal of treatment is lowering triglycerides or raising HDL. One study found that patients with heart disease, somewhat elevated triglycerides, and low HDL who took fibrates had reduced risk for a heart attack. Fibrates are usually given in two daily doses thirty minutes before the morning and evening meals. The reductions in triglycerides generally are in the range of 20 to 50 percent with increases in HDL cholesterol of 10 to 15 percent.

Fibrates are generally well tolerated by most patients. Gastrointestinal complaints are the most common side effect, and fibrates appear to increase the likelihood of developing cholesterol gallstones. Fibrates can increase the effect of medications that thin the blood, and this should be monitored closely by your physician.

Hormone Replacement Therapy

The risk of heart disease is increased in postmenopausal women, whether the menopause is natural, surgical, or premature. This increasing risk may be related to the loss of estrogens after menopause. Hormone replacement therapy (HRT) is treatment with estrogen, either alone or with another hormone called progestin. HRT may be prescribed when women experience symptoms from menopause.

A recent study examined whether postmenopausal women with CHD who take HRT experience fewer CHD events than women who have CHD and do not take HRT. The Heart and Estrogen/Progestin Replacement Study (HERS) found that:

- In the first year of the study, women receiving HRT had more CHD events than those not taking it, despite a modest drop in their LDL cholesterol and a rise in their HDL cholesterol levels.

- By the fourth and fifth years of the study, women in the HRT group experienced fewer events than women not taking HRT.

- Women in the HRT group experienced more blood clots and gallbladder disease.

Overall, HERS found that women taking HRT did not benefit from a lower rate of CHD events. Although HERS looked at postmenopausal women with CHD, the results may also have implications for postmenopausal women who are trying to prevent heart disease. Postmenopausal women who are judged by their physician to need drug treatment to reduce their risk for a heart attack should consider cholesterol-lowering drugs instead of HRT, since cholesterol-lowering drugs have been shown to be safe and effective in lowering cholesterol and reducing CHD risk in such women. HRT is useful in reducing the risks for other conditions such as osteoporosis, and should not be discontinued if already started.

Combination Drug Therapy

If your goal LDL level is not reached after three months with a single drug, your doctor may consider starting a second medicine to go with it. Combination therapy can increase your cholesterol lowering, reverse or slow the advance of atherosclerosis, and further decrease the chance of a heart attack or death. The use of low doses of each medicine may help reduce the side effects of the drugs.

Chapter 62

Angiotensin Converting Enzyme (ACE) Inhibitors

Definition

Angiotensin converting enzyme inhibitors (also called ACE inhibitors) are medicines that block the conversion of the chemical angiotensin I to a substance that increases salt and water retention in the body.

Purpose

ACE inhibitors are used in the treatment of high blood pressure. They may be used alone or in combination with other medicines for high blood pressure. They work by preventing a chemical in the blood, angiotensin I, from being converted into a substance that increases salt and water retention in the body. Increased salt and water retention lead to high blood pressure. ACE inhibitors also make blood vessels relax, which helps lower blood pressure and allows more oxygen-rich blood to reach the heart.

Treating high blood pressure is important because the condition puts a burden on the heart and the arteries, which can lead to permanent damage over time. If untreated, high blood pressure increases the risk of heart attacks, heart failure, stroke, or kidney failure.

ACE inhibitors may also be prescribed for other conditions. For example, captopril (Capoten) is used to treat kidney problems in

From GALE ENCYCLOPEDIA OF MEDICINE 2nd EDITION, by Nancy Ross-Flanigan, Volume 1. © 2002 Gale Group. Reprinted by permission of The Gale Group.

people who take insulin to control diabetes. Captopril and lisinopril are also given to some patients after a heart attack. Heart attacks damage and weaken the heart muscle, and the damage continues even after a person recovers from the attack. This medicine helps slow down further damage to the heart. ACE inhibitors also may be used to treat congestive heart failure.

Description

ACE inhibitors are available only with a physician's prescription and come in tablet, capsule, and injectable forms. Some commonly used ACE inhibitors are benazepril (Lotensin), captopril (Capoten), enalapril (Vasotec), fosinopril (Monopril), lisinopril (Prinivil, Zestril), moexipril (Univasc), perindopril (Aceon), quinapril (Accupril), ramipril (Altace), and trandolapril (Mavik).

Recommended Dosage

The recommended dosage depends on the type of ACE inhibitor and the medical condition for which it is being taken. Check with the physician who prescribed the drug or the pharmacist who filled the prescription for the correct dosage.

This medicine may take weeks to noticeably lower blood pressure. Take it exactly as directed.

Do not stop taking this medicine without checking with the physician who prescribed it.

Precautions

A person taking an ACE inhibitor should see a physician regularly. The physician will check the blood pressure to make sure the medicine is working as it should and will note any unwanted side effects. People who have high blood pressure often feel perfectly fine. However, they should continue to see their physicians even when they feel well so that the physician can keep a close watch on their condition. It is also important for patients to keep taking their medicine even when they feel fine.

ACE inhibitors will not cure high blood pressure, but will help control the condition. To avoid the serious health problems that high blood pressure can cause, patients may have to take medicine for the rest of their lives. Furthermore, medicine alone may not be enough. Patients with high blood pressure may also need to avoid certain foods, such as salty snacks, and keep their weight under control. The health care professional who is treating the condition can offer advice on what measures may be necessary. Patients being treated for high blood pressure should not change their diets without consulting their physicians.

Anyone taking this medicine for high blood pressure should not take any other prescription or over-the-counter (OTC) medicine without first checking with his or her physician. Some medicines, such as certain cold remedies, may increase blood pressure.

Some people feel dizzy or lightheaded after taking the first dose of an ACE inhibitor, especially if they have been taking a water pill (diuretic). Anyone who takes these drugs should not drive, use machines, or do anything else that might be dangerous until they have found out how the drugs affect them. Such symptoms should be reported to the physician or pharmacist if they do not subside within a day or so. For the first one or two days of taking an ACE inhibitor, patients may become lightheaded when arising from bed in the morning. Patients should rise slowly to a sitting position before standing up.

While a goal of treatment with an ACE inhibitor is to lower the blood pressure, patients must be careful not to let their blood pressure get too low. Low blood pressure can lead to dizziness, lightheadedness, and fainting. To prevent the blood pressure from getting too low, observe these precautions:

- Do not drink alcohol without checking with the physician who prescribed this medicine.

- Captopril and moexipril should be taken one hour before meals. Other ACE inhibitors may be taken with or without meals.

- Avoid overheating when exercising or in hot weather. The loss of water from the body through heavy sweating can cause low blood pressure.

- Check with a physician right away if illness occurs while taking an ACE inhibitor. This is especially true if the illness involves severe nausea, vomiting, or diarrhea. Vomiting and diarrhea can cause the loss of too much water from the body, which can lead to low blood pressure.

Anyone who is taking ACE inhibitors should be sure to tell the health care professional in charge before having any surgical or dental procedures or receiving emergency treatment.

Some ACE inhibitors may change the results of certain medical tests, such as blood or urine tests. Before having medical tests, anyone taking this medicine should alert the health care professional in charge.

Do not use a potassium supplement or a salt substitute that contains potassium without first checking with the physician who prescribed the ACE inhibitor.

Patients who are being treated with bee or wasp venom to prevent allergic reactions to stings may have a severe allergic reaction to certain ACE inhibitors.

Special Conditions

People with certain medical conditions or who are taking certain other medicines can have problems if they take ACE inhibitors. Before taking these drugs, be sure to let the physician know about any of these conditions.

Allergies

Anyone who has had unusual reactions to an ACE inhibitor in the past should let his or her physician know before taking this type of medicine again. The physician should also be told about any allergies to foods, dyes, preservatives, or other substances.

Pregnancy

The use of ACE inhibitors in pregnancy can cause serious problems and even death in the fetus or newborn. Women who are pregnant or who may become pregnant should check with their physicians before using this medicine. Women who become pregnant while taking this medicine should check with their physicians immediately.

Breastfeeding

Some ACE inhibitors pass into breast milk. Women who are breastfeeding should check with their physicians before using ACE inhibitors.

Other Medical Conditions

Before using ACE inhibitors, people with any of these medical problems should make sure their physicians are aware of their conditions:

- diabetes
- heart or blood vessel disease
- recent heart attack or stroke
- liver disease
- kidney disease
- kidney transplant
- scleroderma
- systemic lupus erythematosus (SLE)

Use of Certain Medicines

Taking ACE inhibitors with certain other drugs may affect the way the drugs work or may increase the chance of side effects.

Side Effects

The most common side effect is a dry, continuing cough. This usually does not subside unless the medication is stopped. Ask the physician if the cough can be treated. Less common side effects, such as headache, loss of taste, unusual tiredness, and nausea or diarrhea also may occur and do not need medical attention unless they are severe or they interfere with normal activities.

More serious side effects are rare, but may occur. If any of the following side effects occur, check with a physician immediately:

- swelling of the face, lips, tongue, throat, arms, legs, hands, or feet
- itchy skin
- sudden breathing or swallowing problems
- chest pain
- hoarseness
- sore throat
- fever and chills
- stomach pain
- yellow eyes or skin

In addition, anyone who has any of the following symptoms while taking an ACE inhibitor should check with his or her physician as soon as possible:

- dizziness, lightheadedness, fainting
- confusion
- nervousness
- fever
- joint pain
- numbness or tingling in hands, feet, or lips
- weak or heavy feeling in the legs
- skin rash
- irregular heartbeat
- shortness of breath or other breathing problems

Other side effects may occur. Anyone who has unusual symptoms after taking an ACE inhibitor should get in touch with his or her physician.

Interactions

ACE inhibitors may interact with certain foods and other medicines. For example, captopril (Capoten) interacts with food and should be taken one hour before meals. Anyone who takes ACE inhibitors should let the physician know all other medicines he or she is taking and should ask about foods that should be avoided. Among the foods and drugs that may interact with ACE inhibitors are:

- water pills (diuretics)
- lithium, used to treat bipolar disorder
- tetracycline, an antibiotic
- medicines or supplements that contain potassium
- salt substitutes that contain potassium

The preceding list may not include everything that interacts with ACE inhibitors. Be sure to check with a physician or pharmacist before combining ACE inhibitors with any other prescription or nonprescription (over-the-counter) medicine.

Chapter 63

Angiotensin Receptor Blockers (ARBs)

Angiotensin receptor blockers (also known as ARBs) are a class of medications that are widely used by patients with high blood pressure, kidney disease, and heart failure. This chapter provides information for patients who receive this type of medication. Table 63.1 lists the brand and chemical names for the angiotensin receptor blockers that are available in the United States.

How do angiotensin receptor blockers work?

Angiotensin receptor blockers work by inhibiting the effects of a hormone called angiotensin 2, which produces a number of effects in the body: Constriction of blood vessels, increased salt and water retention, activation of the sympathetic nervous system, stimulation of blood vessel and heart fibrosis (stiffening), and promotion of heart cell growth. Together, these effects can increase blood pressure and in some situations be harmful to the heart and kidneys. For angiotensin 2 to produce its effects in the body, it must bind to a receptor in much the same way that a key must fit into a lock to open a door. Angiotensin receptor blockers prevent angiotensin 2 from binding to its receptor and thus reduce the effects of angiotensin 2.

Most of the angiotensin receptor blockers, except for Benicar (Sankyo Pharma, Inc.), are also available in combination with an additional

Reprinted from "Angiotensin Receptor Blockers," by Steven G. Terra, *Circulation* 107, no. 24 (2003): 215–16. © 2003 Lippincott Williams and Wilkins; reprinted with permission.

medication called hydrochlorothiazide (HCTZ), a diuretic that is very effective in lowering blood pressure. The blood pressure–lowering effects of angiotensin receptor blockers are made more effective by the addition of HCTZ. Therefore, your doctor may prescribe a combination product containing an angiotensin receptor blocker plus HCTZ if you require additional blood pressure lowering.

What conditions are treated with an angiotensin receptor blocker?

All angiotensin receptor blockers can be used to treat high blood pressure. In addition, both Cozaar (Merck) and Avapro (Bristol-Myers Squibb) are also used to prevent kidney damage in patients who have high blood pressure, and one angiotensin receptor blocker is used to treat patients who have heart failure but who cannot tolerate a related class of medications called angiotensin-converting enzyme (ACE) inhibitors. However, angiotensin receptor blockers can be used to treat

Table 63.1. List of Angiotensin Receptor Blockers Available in the United States

Trade Name (Manufacturer)	Chemical Name
Cozaar (Merck)	losartan
Hyzaar (Merck)	losartan/hydrochlorothiazide
Avapro (Bristol-Myers Squibb)	irbesartan
Avalide (Bristol-Myers Squibb)	irbesartan/hydrochlorothiazide
Diovan (Novartis)	valsartan
Diovan HCT (Novartis)	valsartan/hydrochlorothiazide
Atacand (AstraZeneca)	candesartan cilexetil
Atacand HCT (AstraZeneca)	candesartan cilexetil/hydrochlorothiazide
Teveten (Solvay Pharma Inc.)	eprosartan
Teveten HCT (Solvay Pharma Inc.)	eprosartan/hydrochlorothiazide
Micardis (Boehringer Ingelheim)	telmisartan
Micardis HCT (Boehringer Ingelheim)	telmisartan/hydrochlorothiazide
Benicar (Sankyo Pharma, Inc.)	olmesartan

other heart conditions, so speak with your doctor if you are not clear about the reason that you are receiving this class of medication.

What are the common side effects of angiotensin receptor blockers?

Any medication that lowers blood pressure can cause dizziness. Frequent dizziness or lightheadedness may be an indication that your blood pressure is too low. If this occurs, you should speak with your doctor. You may find that changing positions slowly (such as going from lying down to standing up) may minimize dizziness. In very rare cases, patients receiving this class of medication have developed swelling of the lips, tongue, or face. You should contact your physician immediately if you experience any facial swelling or trouble breathing. You should also notify your physician if you have experienced facial swelling or difficulty breathing with any other medications in the past.

In some susceptible individuals, angiotensin receptor blockers can cause increases in potassium and changes in kidney function. To monitor for these side effects, your doctor may do routine blood work. Many patients with high blood pressure are told to minimize their use of sodium. Some of these patients use salt substitutes instead. However, some of these salt substitutes contain potassium (instead of sodium), which when taken with an angiotensin receptor blocker may increase the amount of potassium in your blood. It is a good idea to talk with your doctor before using any of these salt substitutes, especially if you have kidney disease or heart failure.

You should not take angiotensin receptor blockers if you are pregnant or plan on becoming pregnant because this class of medication can cause harm to the unborn fetus.

Are there any medications that I should not combine with my angiotensin receptor blocker?

You should always inform your doctor and pharmacist of all the medications you are taking. This includes prescription and over-the-counter medications, along with any vitamins and herbal products. If you are taking an angiotensin receptor blocker for either high blood pressure or heart failure, you should speak with your doctor before taking any decongestants. Decongestants, which are available in many over-the-counter cough and cold products, can increase blood pressure. The most widely used decongestant is pseudoephedrine. In addition, in some individuals, nonsteroidal anti-inflammatory drugs such as ibuprofen, naproxen, and indomethacin may elevate blood pressure, thus blunting the blood pressure–lowering effect of angiotensin receptor blockers. Speak with your doctor before taking these medications. One angiotensin receptor blocker, Micardis (Boehringer Ingelheim) may interact with the medication Lanoxin (GlaxoSmithKline; digoxin). Therefore, the level of digoxin in your blood should be monitored when you begin taking Micardis or have the dose increased or decreased. Because of this interaction, another angiotensin receptor blocker may be more appropriate if you are also receiving Lanoxin (digoxin).

Does it matter if I take my angiotensin receptor blocker with or without food?

Angiotensin receptor blockers can be taken with or without food. It is, however, important that you take your medication at approximately the same time each day to maintain a consistent concentration of the medication in your body.

Chapter 64

Are ARBs Better than ACE Inhibitors?

Introduction

It was in the early 1970s that Brunner, Laragh, and Gavras first outlined the role of angiotensin II in the pathogenesis of hypertensive vascular damage. They showed that excess angiotensin caused damage to the myocardium and renal parenchyma, independent of its elevation of blood pressure; and that subjects with high blood pressure but low renin levels were less likely to have heart attacks or strokes than those with high renin levels. Thirty years later we are defining the clinical role of the first angiotensin receptor blockers (ARBs); Brunner and Gavras have recently summarized the progression of our knowledge in this area, up to this point.

Effective medical treatment of hypertension has been available for the last fifty years, and with each new class of drugs introduced there has been a reduction in the frequency and severity of adverse effects. This is extremely important, as antihypertensive therapy is, for the most part, a lifelong effort without motivation provided by obvious symptoms of the disease. In comparative studies, attention has mainly been directed at the side-effect profiles of the candidates. With the arrival of the angiotensin-converting enzyme (ACE) inhibitors and the selective angiotensin-type-1-receptor blockers (ARBs) the safety profiles are almost as good as can be expected for effective medications. However, there is still a lot to be learned about their full cardiovascular profile.

Some recent studies led to the view that there were no advantages of ACE inhibitors over thiazides or beta-blockers with regard to mortality and morbidity in hypertensive patients. However, when patients with higher absolute cardiovascular risk are examined, differences emerge. ACE inhibitors, in placebo-controlled studies, have been shown to be more effective than older antihypertensives in patients with coronary heart disease, congestive cardiac failure, diabetic nephropathy, and stroke; head-to-head comparisons were not reported, however. ARBs have provided similar results for diabetic nephropathy and congestive cardiac failure.

The LIFE Study Results

The concept that blockade of the renin-angiotensin system can provide benefits beyond merely lowering blood pressure gets further support from the LIFE [Losartan Intervention For Endpoint reduction in hypertension] study.[1] In this trial, over nine thousand hypertensive patients with left ventricular hypertrophy were given an ARB (losartan) or a beta-blocker (atenolol) for at least four years. Not only did the ARB prevent more cardiovascular morbidity and mortality—chiefly with respect to stroke—than the beta-blocker for a similar reduction in blood pressure, but also it was associated with a significantly decreased frequency of new-onset diabetes.

About 13 percent of the LIFE study population had diabetes at entry into the study.[2] Analysis of the results from this subset showed that all-cause mortality was reduced by 39 percent, cardiovascular mortality by 37 percent, and congestive heart failure by 40 percent in the losartan group, compared with the results for atenolol. Findings for stroke and myocardial infarction were less impressive.

Measurements of left ventricular hypertrophy (Cornell voltage-duration product and Sokolow-Lyon measured on ECG) showed that losartan treatment was associated with a greater regression of hypertrophy, compared with atenolol treatment. This was seen in both the total study population (in those who had these parameters measured) and in the diabetic subset. The finding is not totally surprising, as angiotensin II is a myocardial growth factor, and an independent risk factor for cardiovascular disease.

Stroke was an endpoint that was particularly lessened with the ARB. It was not related to thiazide use—patients in both treatment arms took hydrochlorothiazide equally—nor was it apparently associated with the presence of atrial fibrillation. The finding fits with the observed greater reduction in ventricular hypertrophy, which is itself an independent risk factor for cerebrovascular events.

The decrease in the numbers of new-onset diabetes in the losartan group may represent, in fact, a relative increase in the atenolol group; beta-blockers are known to decrease insulin sensitivity, and therefore increase the likelihood of the development of the metabolic syndrome (Syndrome X).

Other Recent Studies

Brunner and Gavras reference previous studies of ACE inhibitors in hypertensive patients showing their benefits with respect to cardiovascular events. Similar results to those in the LIFE study have been reported for the HOPE [Heart Outcomes Prevention Evaluation] study, which employed the ACE inhibitor ramipril, and the CAPPP [Captopril Prevention Project] study, which used captopril. There is little doubt that both ACE inhibitors and ARBs have similar effects on raised blood pressure, as well as other angiotensin II-related conditions, like left ventricular hypertrophy. Although they haven't been compared head-to-head, both ACE inhibitors and ARBs have the ability to provide a degree of renal protection in patients with type 2 diabetes and diabetic nephropathy. And one ARB, valsartan, has proved to be valuable in congestive heart failure, providing additional benefit when added to an ACE inhibitor.

Conclusions

To quote Brunner and Gavras, "To date, all evidence suggests that the beneficial effects of ACE inhibitors can be duplicated with ARBs without the nuisance of side effects". The chief ACE-inhibitor side effect that falls under the rubric "nuisance" is a dry, persistent cough. Different studies have shown that candesartan, eprosartan, losartan, and valsartan have virtually no potential to cause cough in subjects who developed cough with an ACE inhibitor. On the other hand, in these studies in hypertensive patients, the beneficial effects of the ACE inhibitors and the ARBs on blood pressure were virtually identical.

Other possible differences between ACE inhibitors and ARBs remain to be teased out in future studies. In the meantime, it seems safe to conclude that the benefits of both drug classes are extremely similar, their actions beyond lowering blood pressure are also similar, but they differ in that the ACE inhibitors have the propensity to cause an irritating dry cough.

Source

Angiotensin blockade for hypertension: a promise fulfilled. HR. Brunner, H. Gavras, Editorial. Lancet, 2002, vol. 359, pp. 990–91.

Notes

1. Cardiovascular morbidity and mortality in the Losartan Intervention For Endpoint reduction in hypertension study (LIFE): a randomized trial against atenolol. B. Dahlof, RB. Devereux, SE. Kjeldsen, et al., *Lancet*, 2002, vol. 359, pp. 995–1003.

2. Cardiovascular morbidity and mortality in patients with diabetes in the Losartan Intervention For Endpoint reduction in hypertension study (LIFE): a randomized trial against atenolol. LH. Lindholm, H. Ibsen, B. Dahlof, et al., *Lancet*, 2002, vol. 359, pp. 1004–10.

Chapter 65

Anticoagulation Medications

Some people with congenital heart defects, especially those who are cyanotic (blue), have had heart valve replacements, or have had complicated surgeries such as the Fontan operation, may need to take anticoagulants (blood-thinners). These medicines slow blood clotting. They're used to prevent major complications, such as vessel or valve obstruction, or strokes. Anticoagulants may be given by mouth. In some cases they're given intravenously or by injecting them just under the skin. Bleeding may be a complication of taking these medications, so tell your cardiologist if you begin to have easy bruising, bleeding gums, or nosebleeds.

Oral Medications

These mainly include aspirin (and other antiplatelet medications) and warfarin (Coumadin). Each of these medicines works on a different part of the blood-clotting cycle. Your cardiologist will decide which of these medications is right for you.

Aspirin tends to cause fewer bleeding complications. However, it may upset your stomach and be ineffective for treating your specific heart problem.

Warfarin increases your risk of serious bleeding problems. If you take warfarin, you may need to limit your activity to reduce the chance of injury, particularly a head injury. Warfarin also can cause malformations in an unborn child, so don't take it during pregnancy. Some

"Anticoagulation," reprinted with permission from www.americanheart.org © 2004, American Heart Association.

form of anticoagulant medication as prescribed by your cardiologist and obstetrician is recommended throughout pregnancy, however. (See the section below on Subcutaneous Medications.)

Intravenous Medications

Heparin is the main intravenous blood thinner. It's used mostly in hospitals after heart operations while the dosage of the oral medication, warfarin or aspirin, is being adjusted. Oral anticoagulants are longer acting, so if you need elective surgery (including dental surgery), these medications may need to be stopped and intravenous or subcutaneous, shorter-acting heparin begun in the hospital before surgery. Your doctor will decide if this is necessary.

Subcutaneous Medications

Heparin also can be given by an injection just underneath the skin. This is sometimes done if it's required for a longer time (e.g., during pregnancy). This usually eliminates a long-term need for an intravenous line. Both heparin and low-molecular-weight heparin are available for subcutaneous injection. Your cardiologist will determine which is best for you.

Medication Monitoring

If you're taking warfarin, to be sure your dosage is correct, your doctor will regularly monitor blood-clotting indicators. A value called the INR (international normalized ratio) tests how quickly your blood clots. Your warfarin dosage will be carefully adjusted to maintain an INR level appropriate for your heart condition. You must take your medicine exactly as prescribed. You also must have your blood tested regularly according to your doctor's orders.

Medication and Diet Interactions with Warfarin

Many over-the-counter or prescription medicines can interact with warfarin and change your INR, which can be hazardous. These include erythromycin, cimetidine, and several pain medicines (e.g., ibuprofen and other nonsteroidal anti-inflammatory drugs). There are others, too. You also shouldn't take aspirin when you're being treated with warfarin.

Certain foods also interfere with how your body processes warfarin. Your cardiologist will discuss foods to avoid or eat regularly while taking Coumadin. If you're on warfarin, always ask your doctor about your diet and before taking any other medicines, including vitamins and herbal preparations.

Chapter 66

Beta-Adrenergic Blockers

What is a beta blocker?

A beta blocker is a medicine used to treat high blood pressure and heart problems. Some beta blockers are atenolol (brand name: Tenormin), metoprolol (brand names: Lopressor, Toprol XL) and propranolol (brand name: Inderal). A beta blocker blocks the harmful effects of stress hormones on your heart. This medicine also slows your heart rate. Beta blockers can also be used to prevent migraine headaches in people who get them frequently.

What kinds of heart problems are treated with a beta blocker?

A beta blocker is often used to treat high blood pressure or an irregular heartbeat. This medicine can also be used to treat congestive heart failure, but people with severe heart failure may not be able to take a beta blocker. A beta blocker reduces the risk of another heart attack for people who have already had one.

What are some of the possible side effects of beta blockers?

Most people who take beta blockers do well and have no side effects. But because beta blockers slow your heart, they may make you feel tired. You also may notice that you can't exercise as hard as you used to. For example, you may get out of breath when you take a walk or climb stairs. Some men can have trouble with erections when they take beta blockers. Talk to your doctor if you have these problems after you start taking a beta blocker.

The beta blocker may make you feel a little dizzy or lightheaded. Because this might happen to you, you shouldn't drive a car or operate dangerous machines until you know if your beta blocker is going to make you feel dizzy. The dizziness usually goes away after you have been taking the medicine for a few days. If you keep feeling dizzy or lightheaded after a few days, tell your doctor.

Call your doctor right away if you have trouble breathing when you're taking a beta blocker. You should also call your doctor if you gain weight for an unknown reason. Tell your doctor if you have fluid retention (if your hands, feet, or legs start swelling). Call your doctor right away if you have chest pain or a very slow heartbeat (less than fifty heartbeats per minute).

Can I take a beta blocker if I have diabetes?

Yes, you can take a beta blocker if you have diabetes. However, a beta blocker may hide some of the warning signs of low blood sugar. For example, when you take a beta blocker, your heart rate may not increase in response to a low blood sugar level. You will need to check your blood sugar levels carefully after you start taking a beta blocker. If you have low blood sugar often, your doctor may want to change the dosages of your diabetes medicine.

Can I take a beta blocker if I have asthma or chronic lung disease?

Beta blockers are generally not used in people with asthma. A beta blocker can cause asthma attacks.

Sometimes people with a chronic lung disease such as emphysema or bronchitis can take beta blockers. If you have lung disease and are taking a beta blocker, call your doctor right away if you start having breathing problems.

What about other medicines?

Taking other medicines—even medicines that don't require a prescription—while you're taking a beta blocker can cause serious problems.

Tell your doctor about any other medicines that you take, and check with him or her before starting any new medications.

What is the best way to take beta blockers?

You should take your beta blocker exactly as your doctor tells you. Beta blockers are usually taken once or twice a day. Try to take the medicine at the same time every day. Do not stop taking your beta blocker without talking to your doctor first.

If you forget to take a dose and it has been a few hours or less since you missed the dose, take your beta blocker as soon as you remember. However, if it has been four to six hours or longer since you missed the dose, don't take the dose you missed. Instead, wait and take the next regular dose. Never take a double dose to catch up.

Chapter 67

Calcium Channel Blockers

Definition

Calcium channel blockers are medicines that slow the movement of calcium into the cells of the heart and blood vessels. This, in turn, relaxes blood vessels, increases the supply of oxygen-rich blood to the heart, and reduces the heart's workload.

Purpose

Calcium channel blockers are used to treat high blood pressure, to correct abnormal heart rhythms, and to relieve the type of chest pain called angina pectoris. Physicians also prescribe calcium channel blockers to treat panic attacks and bipolar disorder (manic depressive illness) and to prevent migraine headache.

Precautions

Seeing a physician regularly while taking calcium channel blockers is important. The physician will check to make certain the medicine is working as it should and will watch for unwanted side effects. People who have high blood pressure often feel perfectly fine. However, they should continue to see their prescribing physician even when they feel well so that he or she can keep a close watch on their condition. They should also continue to take their medicine even when they feel fine.

Calcium channel blockers will not cure high blood pressure, but will help to control the condition. To avoid the serious health problems associated with high blood pressure, patients may have to take this type of medication for the rest of their lives. Furthermore, the blockers alone may not be enough. People with high blood pressure may also need to avoid certain foods and keep their weight under control. The health care professional who is treating the condition can offer advice as to what measures may be necessary. Patients being treated for high blood pressure should not change their diets without consulting their physicians.

Anyone taking calcium channel blockers for high blood pressure should not take any other prescription or over-the-counter medication without first checking with the prescribing physician, as some of these drugs may increase blood pressure.

Some people feel drowsy or less alert than usual when taking calcium channel blockers. Anyone who takes these drugs should not drive, use machines, or do anything else that might be dangerous until they have found out how the drugs affect them.

People who normally have chest pain when they exercise or exert themselves may not have the pain when they are taking calcium channel blockers. This could lead them to be more active than they should be. Anyone taking calcium channel blockers should therefore consult with the prescribing physician concerning how much exercise and activity may be considered safe.

Some people get headaches that last for a short time after taking a dose of this medication. This problem usually goes away during the course of treatment. If it does not, or if the headaches are severe, the prescribing physician should be informed.

Patients taking certain calcium channel blockers may need to check their pulse regularly, as the drugs may slow the pulse too much. If the pulse is too slow, circulation problems may result. The prescribing physician can show patients the correct way to check their pulse.

This type of medication may cause the gums to swell, bleed, or become tender. If this problem occurs, a medical physician or dentist should be consulted. To help prevent the problem, care should be taken when brushing and flossing the teeth. Regular dental checkups and cleanings are also recommended.

Older people may be unusually sensitive to the effects of calcium channel blockers. This may increase the chance of side effects.

Special Conditions

People with certain medical conditions or who are taking certain other medicines may develop problems if they also take calcium channel blockers. Before taking these drugs, the prescribing physician should be informed about any of these conditions:

Allergies

Anyone who has had a previous unusual reaction to any calcium channel blocker should let his or her physician know before taking the drugs again. The physician should also be notified about any allergies to foods, dyes, preservatives, or other substances.

Pregnancy

The effects of taking calcium channel blockers during pregnancy have not been studied in humans. However, in studies of laboratory animals, large doses of these drugs have been reported to cause birth defects, stillbirth, poor bone growth, and other problems when taken during pregnancy. Women who are pregnant or who may become pregnant should check with their physicians before using these drugs.

Breastfeeding

Some calcium channel blockers pass into breast milk, but there have been no reports of problems in nursing babies whose mothers were taking this type of medication. However, women who need to take this medicine and want to breastfeed their babies should check with their physicians.

Other Medical Conditions

Calcium channel blockers may worsen heart or blood vessel disorders.

The effects of calcium channel blockers may be greater in people with kidney or liver disease, as their bodies are slower to clear the drug from their systems.

Certain calcium channel blockers may also cause problems in people with a history of heart rhythm problems or with depression, Parkinson's disease, or other types of parkinsonism.

Use of Certain Other Medicines

Taking calcium channel blockers with certain other drugs may affect the way the drugs work or may increase the chance of side effects.

As with most medications, certain side effects are possible and some interactions with other substances may occur.

Side Effects

Side effects are not common with this medicine, but some may occur. Minor discomforts, such as dizziness, lightheadedness, flushing, headache, and nausea, usually go away as the body adjusts to the drug and do not require medical treatment unless they persist or they are bothersome.

If any of the following side effects occur, the prescribing physician should be notified as soon as possible:

- breathing problems, coughing, or wheezing
- irregular, fast, or pounding heartbeat
- slow heartbeat (less than fifty beats per minute)
- skin rash
- swollen ankles, feet, or lower legs

Other side effects may occur. Anyone who has unusual symptoms after taking calcium blockers should contact the prescribing physician.

Interactions

Calcium channel blockers may interact with a number of other medications. When this happens, the effects of one or both of the drugs may change or the risk of side effects may increase. Anyone who takes calcium channel blockers should not take any other prescription or nonprescription (over-the-counter) medicines without first checking with the prescribing physician. Substances that may interact with calcium channel blockers include:

- Diuretics (water pills). This type of medicine may cause low levels of potassium in the body, which may increase the chance of unwanted effects from some calcium channel blockers.

- Beta-blockers, such as atenolol (Tenormin), propranolol (Inderal), and metoprolol (Lopressor), used to treat high blood pressure, angina, and other conditions. Also, eye drop forms of beta blockers, such as timolol (Timoptic), used to treat glaucoma. Taking any of these drugs with calcium channel blockers may increase the effects of both types of medicine and may cause problems if either drug is stopped suddenly.

- Digitalis heart medicines. Taking these medicines with calcium channel blockers may increase the action of the heart medication.

- Medicines used to correct irregular heart rhythms, such as quinidine (Quinidex), disopyramide (Norpace), and procainamide (Procan, Pronestyl). The effects of these drugs may increase if used with calcium channel blockers.

- Anti-seizure medications such as carbamazepine (Tegretol). Calcium channel drugs may increase the effects of these medicines.

- Cyclosporine (Sandimmune), a medicine that suppresses the immune system. Effects may increase if this drug is taken with calcium channel blockers.

- Grapefruit juice may increase the effects of some calcium channel blockers.

The preceding list does not include every drug that may interact with calcium channel blockers. The prescribing physician or pharmacist will advise as to whether combining calcium channel blockers with any other prescription or nonprescription (over-the-counter) medication is appropriate or not.

Description

Calcium channel blockers are available only with a physician's prescription and are sold in tablet, capsule, and injectable forms. Some commonly used calcium channel blockers include amlodipine (Norvasc), diltiazem (Cardizem), isradipine (DynaCirc), nifedipine (Adalat, Procardia), nicardipine (Cardene), and verapamil (Calan, Isoptin, Verelan).

The recommended dosage depends on the type, strength, and form of calcium channel blocker and the condition for which it is prescribed. Correct dosage is determined by the prescribing physician and further information can be obtained from the pharmacist.

Calcium channel blockers should be taken as directed. Larger or more frequent doses should not be taken, nor should doses be missed. This medicine may take several weeks to noticeably lower blood pressure. The patient taking calcium channel blockers should keep taking the medicine, to give it time to work. Once it begins to work and symptoms improve, it should continue to be taken as prescribed.

This medicine should not be discontinued without checking with the prescribing physician. Some conditions may worsen when patients stop taking calcium channel blockers abruptly. The prescribing physician will advise as to how to gradually taper down before stopping the medication completely.

Risks

A report from the European Cardiology Society in 2000 found that patients taking certain calcium channel blockers had a 27 percent greater risk of heart attack, and a 26 percent greater risk of heart failure than patients taking other high blood pressure medicines. However, there are many patients affected by conditions that still make calcium channel blockers the best choice for them. The patient should discuss this issue with the prescribing physician.

Normal Results

The expected result of taking a calcium channel blocker is to either correct abnormal heart rhythms, return blood pressure to normal, or relieve chest pain.

Chapter 68

Digoxin

Why is digoxin prescribed?

Digoxin (say "dih-jock-sin") is a drug used to treat some heart problems. One of these problems, heart failure, results when the heart can't pump blood well enough to supply the body's needs. If you have heart failure, digoxin can improve your heart's ability to pump blood. Better pumping of the heart will often improve symptoms such as shortness of breath. Digoxin can also help a rapid or irregular heartbeat, such as atrial fibrillation (sometimes called "a-fib"). Digoxin helps by slowing down and controlling the heart rate.

It may take several weeks to several months for digoxin to start working. Don't be surprised if you don't feel better right away. Keep taking your digoxin. Digoxin is used to treat heart conditions that last for a long time, so you may take digoxin the rest of your life. Call your doctor if you have any problems taking the drug.

How should I take my digoxin?

Digoxin is usually taken once a day. You should try to take the drug at the same time every day. It's very important to take your digoxin exactly as your doctor tells you. If you miss a dose, you may go ahead and take it if no more than twelve hours have passed from the time you should have taken it. If more than twelve hours have passed, skip that dose.

Don't double up on digoxin doses. Don't suddenly stop taking your digoxin, either, because this could make your heart problems worse.

Some medicines and foods can decrease the amount of digoxin your body absorbs. These include the following:

- Liquid antacids (such as Maalox or Mylanta)
- Some cholesterol-lowering drugs (cholestyramine and colestipol)
- Some antidiarrheal medicines (such as Kaopectate)
- Bulk laxatives (such as psyllium, Metamucil, or Citrucel)
- High-fiber foods (such as bran muffins) or nutritional supplements (such as Ensure)

Taking these medicines or eating high-fiber foods too close to the time you take your digoxin may result in too little digoxin in your bloodstream to help your heart. For this reason, it is better to take digoxin on an empty stomach. Check with your doctor before taking any of the medicines listed here. If your doctor says it's okay to take these medicines, keep two hours between a dose of digoxin and a dose of these medicines.

Digoxin interacts with many other drugs. You should always tell your doctor and your pharmacist about all the medicines you are taking, including any over-the-counter drugs, natural remedies, and herbal medicines. Always talk to your doctor or pharmacist before you take any new medicines.

How will my doctor know if I am getting enough digoxin?

The digoxin dose needed to treat heart conditions is different for different people. Your doctor may do a blood test to make sure you have the right amount of digoxin in your body. This blood test has to be done at least six hours after your last dose of digoxin. For this reason, you should tell your doctor when you normally take your digoxin. Ask your doctor if there is any special way to take your digoxin on the days your blood is drawn. Your doctor may want you to wait to take your dose. Or he or she may want to schedule your appointment so that you will have your blood drawn at the right time.

When should I call the doctor?

If you have heart failure, the following symptoms may mean that you are not getting enough digoxin. Call your doctor immediately if you have any of these symptoms:

- More shortness of breath than usual
- A decrease in your ability to climb stairs or walk
- Waking up short of breath at night
- Shortness of breath when you lie flat or sleep on more pillows than usual
- More frequent trips to the bathroom during the night
- Increased ankle swelling or tightness of your shoes

If you have atrial fibrillation, the following symptoms may mean that you are not getting enough digoxin. If you develop any of these symptoms, call your doctor immediately:

- A rapid pulse (more than one hundred beats per minute)
- Palpitations, or a feeling that your heart is racing
- A change in your heart rate
- Dizziness
- Fainting or blackouts

What are the side effects of digoxin?

Most people can take digoxin without many side effects. However, you could have side effects, especially if you get too much digoxin. These side effects include nausea, vomiting, diarrhea, stomach pain, loss of appetite, unusual tiredness or weakness, slow heartbeat, palpitations, irregular heartbeat, drowsiness, confusion, fainting, or changes in your vision (seeing a yellow, green, or white halo around objects). It is important to pay attention to these side effects, because too much digoxin is dangerous. You should call your doctor right away if you experience any of these side effects.

Chapter 69

Nitroglycerin

Brand name(s): Nitro-Bid; Nitrocine; Nitroglyn; Nitrolingual; Nitrong; Nitrostat.

Why is this medication prescribed?

Nitroglycerin is used to prevent chest pain (angina). It works by relaxing the blood vessels to the heart, so the blood flow and oxygen supply to the heart is increased.

This medication is sometimes prescribed for other uses; ask your doctor or pharmacist for more information.

How should this medicine be used?

Nitroglycerin comes as a sublingual tablet, buccal tablet, extended-release (long-acting) capsule, or spray to be used orally. The buccal extended-release tablets and the extended-release tablets and capsules are usually taken three to six times a day. Do not crush, chew, or divide the extended-release tablets or capsules. The sublingual tablet and spray are used as needed to relieve chest pain that has already started or to prevent pain before activities known to provoke attacks (e.g., climbing stairs, sexual activity, heavy exercise, or cold weather). The buccal extended-release tablets also may be used during an attack and just before situations known to provoke attacks. Follow the directions on your prescription label carefully, and ask your doctor or pharmacist to explain any part you do not understand. Take nitroglycerin exactly as directed. Do not take more or less of it or take it more often than prescribed by your doctor.

Nitroglycerin controls chest pain but does not cure it. Continue to use nitroglycerin even if you feel well. Do not stop taking nitroglycerin without talking to your doctor. Stopping the drug abruptly may cause chest pain.

Nitroglycerin can lose its effectiveness when used for a long time. This effect is called tolerance. If your angina attacks happen more often, last longer, or are more severe, call your doctor.

If you are using the buccal extended-release tablet, place the tablet between your cheek and gum and allow it to dissolve. Do not chew or swallow it. If you feel dizzy, sit down after placing the tablet in your mouth. Try not to swallow saliva until the tablet dissolves. Buccal extended-release tablets start to work within two to three minutes. To make the tablet dissolve faster, touch it with your tongue before placing it in your mouth or drink a hot liquid. If an attack occurs while you have a buccal extended-release tablet in place, place a second tablet on the opposite side of your mouth. If chest pain persists, use sublingual tablets, call for emergency assistance, or go to a hospital emergency department immediately.

If you are taking nitroglycerin sublingual tablets or spray for acute chest pain, you should carry the tablets and spray with you at all times. Sit down when an acute attack occurs. The drug starts to work within two minutes and goes on working for up to thirty minutes. If you are taking nitroglycerin tablets and your chest pain is not relieved within five minutes, take another dose. If you are using nitroglycerin spray and your chest pain is not relieved in three to five minutes, repeat the process. Call for emergency assistance or go to a hospital emergency department if pain persists after you have taken three tablets (at five-minute intervals) or have used three sprays (at three- to five-minute intervals) and fifteen minutes have passed.

To use the tablets, place a tablet under your tongue or between your cheek and gum and allow it to dissolve. Do not swallow the tablet. Try not to swallow saliva too often until the tablet dissolves.

To use the spray, follow these steps:

- Do not shake the drug container. Hold it upright with the opening of the spray mechanism as close as possible to your opened mouth.

- Press the spray mechanism with your forefinger to release the spray. Spray the drug onto or under your tongue and close your mouth immediately. Do not inhale or swallow the spray.

Are there other uses for this medicine?

Nitroglycerin tablets also are used with other drugs to treat congestive heart failure and heart attacks. Talk to your doctor about the possible risks of using this drug for your condition.

What special precautions should I follow?

Before taking nitroglycerin,

- tell your doctor and pharmacist if you are allergic to nitroglycerin, isosorbide (Imdur, Isordil, Sorbitrate), or any other drugs.
- tell your doctor and pharmacist what prescription and nonprescription medications you are taking, especially aspirin; beta blockers such as atenolol (Tenormin), carteolol (Cartrol), labetalol (Normodyne, Trandate), metoprolol (Lopressor), nadolol (Corgard), propranolol (Inderal), sotalol (Betapace), and timolol (Blocadren); calcium channel blockers such as amlodipine (Norvasc), diltiazem (Cardizem), felodipine (Plendil), isradipine (DynaCirc), nifedipine (Procardia), and verapamil (Calan, Isoptin); dihydroergotamine (D.H.E. 45); sildenafil (Viagra); and vitamins.
- tell your doctor if you have low red blood cell counts (anemia), glaucoma, or recent head trauma.
- tell your doctor if you are pregnant, plan to become pregnant, or are breastfeeding. If you become pregnant while taking nitroglycerin, call your doctor.
- if you are having surgery, including dental surgery, tell the doctor or dentist that you are taking nitroglycerin.
- you should know that this drug may make you drowsy or dizzy. Do not drive a car or operate machinery until you know how it affects you.
- ask your doctor about the safe use of alcoholic beverages while you are taking nitroglycerin. Alcohol can make the side effects from nitroglycerin worse.

What special dietary instructions should I follow?

Take nitroglycerin extended-release tablets and capsules on an empty stomach with a full glass of water.

What should I do if I forget a dose?

Take the missed dose as soon as you remember it. However, if it is almost time for the next dose, skip the missed dose and continue your regular dosing schedule. Do not take a double dose to make up for a missed one.

What side effects can this medication cause?

Side effects from nitroglycerin are common. Tell your doctor if any of these symptoms are severe or do not go away:

- headache
- rash
- dizziness
- upset stomach
- flushing (feeling of warmth)

If you experience any of the following symptoms, call your doctor immediately:

- blurred vision
- dry mouth
- chest pain
- fainting

What storage conditions are needed for this medicine?

Keep this medication in the container it came in, tightly closed, and out of reach of children. Store it at room temperature and away from excess heat and moisture (not in the bathroom). Avoid puncturing the spray container and keep it away from excess heat. Do not open a container of sublingual nitroglycerin until you need a dose. Do not use tablets that are more than twelve months old. Throw away any medication that is outdated or no longer needed. Talk to your pharmacist about the proper disposal of your medication.

What to do in case of emergency or overdose

In case of overdose, call your local poison control center at 1-800-222-1222. If the victim has collapsed or is not breathing, call local emergency services at 911.

What other information should I know?

Keep all appointments with your doctor and the laboratory. Nitroglycerin extended-release capsules should not be used for acute angina attacks. Continue to use nitroglycerin tablets or spray to relieve chest pain that has already started.

If headache continues, ask your doctor if you may take acetaminophen. Your nitroglycerin dose may need to be adjusted. Do not take aspirin or any other medication for headache while taking nitroglycerin unless your doctor tells you to.

The tablets may cause a sweet, tingling sensation when placed under your tongue. This sensation is not an accurate indicator of drug strength; the absence of a tingling sensation does not mean that the drug is not working.

Do not let anyone else take your medication. Ask your pharmacist any questions you have about refilling your prescription.

Chapter 70

Questions and Answers about Carotid Endarterectomy

What is a carotid endarterectomy?

A carotid endarterectomy is a surgical procedure in which a doctor removes fatty deposits blocking one of the two carotid arteries, the main supply of blood for the brain. Carotid artery problems become more common as people age. The disease process that causes the buildup of fat and other material inside the artery walls is called atherosclerosis, popularly known as "hardening of the arteries." The fatty deposit is called plaque; the narrowing of the artery is called stenosis. The degree of stenosis is usually expressed as a percentage of the normal diameter of the opening.

Why is surgery performed?

Carotid endarterectomy is performed to prevent stroke. Two large clinical trials supported by the National Institute of Neurological Disorders and Stroke (NINDS) have identified specific individuals for whom the surgery is beneficial when performed by surgeons and in institutions that can match the standards set in those studies. The surgery has been found highly beneficial for persons who have already had a stroke or experienced the symptoms of a stroke and have a severe stenosis of 70 to 99 percent. In this group, surgery reduces the

Reprinted from "Questions and Answers about Carotid Endarterectomy," National Institute of Neurological Disorders and Stroke, National Institutes of Health, reviewed July 2001.

estimated two-year risk of stroke or death by more than 80 percent, from greater than one in four to less than one in ten.

For patients who have already had transient or mild stroke symptoms due to moderate carotid stenosis (50 to 69 percent), surgery reduces the five-year risk of stroke or death by 6.5 percent. The failure rate for ipsilateral stroke or death for the medical group is 22.2 percent, and for the surgery group is 15.7 percent from greater than one in four to less than one in seven. Individuals who have already had stroke symptoms, and who have carotid stenosis greater than 50 percent, may wish to consider surgery to prevent future stroke. With the completion of the North American Symptomatic Carotid Endarterectomy Trial, patients with moderate (50 to 69 percent) stenosis will be better able to make more informed decisions.

In another trial, the procedure has also been found highly beneficial for persons who are symptom-free but have a carotid stenosis of 60 to 99 percent. In this group, the surgery reduces the estimated five-year risk of stroke by more than one-half, from about one in ten to less than one in twenty.

What is a stroke?

A stroke occurs when blood flow is cut off from part of the brain. In the same way that a person suffering a loss of blood to the heart can be said to be having a "heart attack," a person with a loss of blood to the brain can be said to be having a "brain attack." There are two kinds of stroke, hemorrhagic and ischemic. Hemorrhagic strokes are caused by bleeding within the brain. Ischemic strokes, which are far more common, are caused by a blockage of blood flow in an artery in the head or neck leading to the brain. Some ischemic strokes are due to stenosis, or narrowing of arteries due to the build up of plaque, fatty deposits, and blood clots along the artery wall. A vascular disease that can cause stenosis is atherosclerosis, in which deposits of plaque build up along the inner wall of large and medium-sized arteries, decreasing blood flow. Atherosclerosis in the carotid arteries, two large arteries in the neck that carry blood to the brain, is a major risk factor for ischemic stroke.

What are the symptoms of a stroke?

Symptoms of stroke include:

- Sudden numbness, weakness, or paralysis of face, arm, or leg, especially on one side of the body.

- Sudden confusion, trouble talking or understanding speech.
- Sudden trouble seeing in one or both eyes.
- Sudden trouble walking, loss of balance, or coordination.
- Sudden severe headache with no known cause (often described as the worst headache in a person's life).

Symptoms may last a few moments and then disappear. When they disappear within twenty-four hours, it is called a transient ischemic attack (TIA).

How important is a blockage as a cause of stroke?

A blockage of a blood vessel is the most frequent cause of stroke and is responsible for about 80 percent of the approximately 700,000 strokes in the United States each year. With nearly 150,000 stroke deaths each year, stroke ranks as the third leading killer in the United States after heart disease and cancer. Stroke is the leading cause of adult disability in the United States with two million of the three million Americans who have survived a stroke sustaining some permanent disability. The overall cost of stroke to the nation is $40 billion a year.

How many carotid endarterectomies are performed each year?

In 1995, the most recent year for which statistics are available from the National Hospital Discharge Survey, there were about 132,000 carotid endarterectomies performed in the United States. The procedure was first described in the mid-1950s. It began to be used increasingly as a stroke prevention measure in the 1960s and 1970s. Its use peaked in the mid-1980s when more than 100,000 operations were performed each year. At that time, several authorities began to question the trend and the risk-benefit ratio for some groups, and the use of the procedure dropped precipitously. The NINDS-supported North American Symptomatic Carotid Endarterectomy Trial (NASCET) and the NINDS-supported Asymptomatic Carotid Atherosclerosis Study (ACAS) were launched in the mid-1980s to identify the specific groups of people with carotid artery disease who would clearly benefit from the procedure.

What are the risk factors and how risky is the surgery?

Important risk factors, in addition to the degree of stenosis, include gender, diabetes, the type of stroke symptoms, and blockage

of the carotid artery on the opposite side. Without other compli-
cating illnesses, age alone is not a worrisome risk factor. Risk factors can affect patients in two ways. They can, particularly in
combination, greatly increase a person's risk of having a stroke. In
addition, these risk factors can increase the likelihood of surgical
complications.

How is carotid artery disease diagnosed?

In some cases, the disease can be detected during a normal checkup
by a physician. In other cases further testing is needed. Some of the
tests a physician can use or order include ultrasound imaging, arteriography, and magnetic resonance angiography (MRA). Frequently
these procedures are carried out in a stepwise fashion: from a doctor's
evaluation of signs and symptoms to ultrasound, MRA, and arteriography for increasingly difficult cases.

- **History and physical exam.** A doctor will ask about symptoms of a stroke such as numbness or muscle weakness, speech
  or vision difficulties, or lightheadedness. Using a stethoscope, a
  doctor may hear a rushing sound, called a bruit (pronounced
  "broo-ee"), in the carotid artery. Unfortunately, dangerous levels
  of disease sometimes fail to make a sound, and some blockages
  with a low risk can make the same sound.

- **Ultrasound imaging.** This is a painless, noninvasive test in
  which sound waves above the range of human hearing are sent
  into the neck. Echoes bounce off the moving blood and the tissue
  in the artery and can be formed into an image. Ultrasound is
  fast, risk-free, relatively inexpensive, and painless compared to
  MRA and arteriography.

- **Arteriography.** This can be used to confirm the findings of ultrasound imaging which can be uncertain in some cases. Arteriography is an x-ray of the carotid artery taken when a special
  dye is injected into the artery. A burning sensation may be felt
  when the dye is injected. An arteriogram is more expensive and
  carries its own small risk of causing a stroke.

- **Magnetic Resonance Angiography (MRA).** This is a new
  imaging technique that avoids most of the risks associated
  with arteriography. An MRA is a type of image that uses mag-
  netism instead of x-rays to create an image of the carotid arteries.

What is the "best medical therapy" for stroke prevention?

The mainstay of stroke prevention is risk factor management: smoking cessation, treatment of high blood pressure, and control of blood sugar levels among persons with diabetes. Additionally, physicians may prescribe aspirin, warfarin, or ticlopidine for some individuals.

What is the "best medical therapy" for stroke prevention?

The patients at risk for stroke are the same as those for transient ischemic attack and include treatment of high blood pressure and control of blood sugar levels in persons with diabetes. Additionally, persons who smoke should be urged to quit, or to decrease the amount they smoke.

Chapter 71

Angioplasty and Stenting Procedures

Coronary Angioplasty

What is coronary angioplasty?

Coronary angioplasty (AN-jee-oh-plas-tee) is a medical procedure used to open narrowed or clogged blood vessels of the heart. A thin balloon or other device is threaded through a blood vessel in the groin or arm into a heart (coronary) artery. The balloon is inflated to compress the blockage and stretch the artery open. It is used in patients with coronary artery disease (CAD) to:

- Relieve chest pain caused by reduced blood flow to the heart
- Minimize damage to the heart muscle during a heart attack, which occurs when blood flow is totally cut off to an area of the heart

CAD develops over time as fatty deposits, called plaque, build up on the inside walls of the coronary arteries. The buildup of plaque narrows the arteries, reducing the flow of blood to the heart. This is called atherosclerosis.

Angioplasty was first used in 1977. A tiny balloon was used to open or widen narrowed arteries. Since then, new devices and medications

"Coronary Angioplasty" is reprinted from "Angioplasty," National Heart, Lung, and Blood Institute Diseases and Conditions Index, 2004. "Stenting" is reprinted from "Stent," U.S. Food and Drug Administration, updated February 2004.

have improved the procedure and made it appropriate for more people. The improvements include:

- **Stents:** A stent is a tiny mesh tube that looks like a small spring. It is inserted in the area where the artery is narrowed to keep it open. Some stents are "coated" with medication to help prevent the artery from closing again. Most people will have a stent placed unless the artery is too small.
  - When a stent is placed, only two out of every ten people have the artery close again in the first six months.
  - When a stent is not used, four out of ten people have the artery close again in the first six months.
- **Plaque removers:** These devices are used to cut away plaque that narrows the inside of the arteries. There are many kinds.
- **Laser:** A laser is used to dissolve or vaporize plaque. The first laser device was approved in 1992. It is used in many major U.S. medical centers.

Today, over one million people in the U.S. receive angioplasty each year. They are best done:

- By doctors who do at least seventy-five angioplasties a year
- In hospitals that do at least four hundred angioplasties a year.

Research on angioplasty continues to:

- Make it even safer
- Prevent the artery from closing again
- Make it an option for more people.

Are there other names for coronary angioplasty?

- Percutaneous coronary intervention (or PCI)
- Percutaneous transluminal angioplasty (or PCTA)
- Balloon angioplasty
- Coronary artery angioplasty

When is coronary angioplasty done?

Your doctor may consider angioplasty if lifestyle changes and medications do not improve your symptoms of coronary artery disease

(CAD). It is an alternative to coronary bypass surgery, which is a major operation.

Your doctor will recommend angioplasty or bypass surgery based on:

- The number of blocked arteries you have
- Severity of the blockages
- Location of the blockages
- Whether you have other medical conditions
- Your surgical risk for bypass
- Your preference.

Angioplasty is often selected if:

- The blockage is small
- The blockage can be reached by angioplasty
- The artery affected is not the main artery that supplies blood to the left side of the heart
- You do not have heart failure.

The advantages of angioplasty are that it:

- Is not surgery
- Is done with local anesthesia and mild sedation
- Has a shorter recovery period than bypass surgery
- Provides similar survival outcomes as bypass surgery in some patients.

The disadvantage of angioplasty is that the artery may close again. If this happens, you will need a second angioplasty or bypass surgery. Also, bypass surgery tends to do a more complete job of restoring the heart's blood supply.

Your doctor will discuss treatment options with you and recommend the best procedure for you.

Coronary angioplasty is also used as an emergency procedure during a heart attack to quickly open a blocked coronary artery. This minimizes the damage during a heart attack and restores blood flow to the heart muscle. There are also drugs that can be used to dissolve clots in a coronary artery. These drugs are most effective when given soon after the heart attack begins (within three hours). Early angioplasty, without drugs that dissolve clots, also minimizes damage to the heart muscle.

What are the risks of coronary angioplasty?

Angioplasty is a common medical procedure and major complications are rare. However, there are risks with any medical procedure. The risks of angioplasty include:

- Bleeding from the blood vessel where the catheter (small flexible tube) was inserted
- Damage to the blood vessel from the catheter
- Infection
- Allergic reaction to dye given during the angioplasty.

Other less common complications include:

- Heart attack
- Need for emergency open-heart surgery during the procedure
- Stroke
- Death.

The risk of complications is higher in:

- Older persons (ages seventy-five and older)
- Women
- Persons with diabetes.

What happens before coronary angioplasty?

Meeting with Your Doctor

A heart specialist (cardiologist) performs the angioplasty. If your angioplasty is not done as an emergency, you will meet with your cardiologist before the procedure to have a physical exam and discuss the procedure. Your doctor will order:

- Blood tests
- An electrocardiogram (EKG)
- A chest x-ray

Your angioplasty will be scheduled at a hospital. You will also be told:

- When to begin fasting (not eating or drinking) before coming to the hospital

- What medications you should and should not take on the day of the angioplasty

- The time to come to the hospital and where to go.

What to Expect

- Angioplasty usually takes one to two hours, depending on the treatment options your doctor uses.

- During the procedure, you will be awake, but sleepy.

- You will be given medications to help you relax. These medications may make you feel sleepy. You may feel like you are floating or numb.

- A catheter or tube may be left in the blood vessel in the leg after the procedure. It is removed four to six hours later. Some doctors use a special device to seal the opening in the blood vessel.

- You will need to lie still for several hours until the blood vessel in your leg seals.

- Most people return home within a day or two.

What happens during coronary angioplasty?

Angioplasty is performed in a special part of the hospital called the cardiac catheterization lab. This lab is equipped with special video screens and x-ray machines. Your doctor will use this equipment to see enlarged pictures of the blocked areas in your coronary arteries.

Preparation or Prep

You will be taken into the cardiac catheterization lab, where you will lie on a table. The doctor will use an intravenous (IV) line to give you fluids and medications. The medications are given to relax you and prevent blood clots. The rest of your prep includes:

- Shaving the area where the catheter or tube will be inserted (usually the groin or arm)

- Cleaning the shaved area to make it germ free

- Numbing the area (the numbing medicine may sting as it is going in).

Steps in Angioplasty

Once you are comfortable, the doctor will begin the procedure:

- A small cut in your groin or arm is made. The doctor threads a very thin catheter or tube through a blood vessel to the area of the coronary artery that is blocked.

- A small amount of dye is injected into the tube. An x-ray is taken so that your doctor will be able to see the coronary arteries, valves, and chambers of your heart. This is called an angiogram.

- Once the blockage is reached, your doctor expands or inflates the balloon attached to the tube. The balloon will widen the artery to increase the flow of blood to the heart muscle.

- A special device may be used to remove some of the plaque from the wall of the artery.

- A stent is usually placed at the site to keep the artery open. The stent remains in place forever.

- When the doctor finishes, the inner catheter and other tools are removed from the blood vessels. A special outer catheter may remain in place, or if a closure device is used, all tubes will be removed.

During the procedure, potent antiplatelet medicines are given through the IV to prevent clots from forming in the artery or on the stent. These medicines are usually started just before the angioplasty to help thin your blood. You may receive them for twelve to twenty-four hours after your angioplasty.

Recovering

After the procedure, you will be moved to a special care unit where:

- You will lie flat without bending your legs. You will need to lie flat longer if no closure device is used. If the angioplasty was performed in your arm, you will not need to lie flat.

- If the catheter is removed later, pressure will be applied to the site.

- You will lie still for several hours to allow the blood vessels in your leg to seal completely.

- Afterward, you may walk with assistance.

As you recover, the nurses will check:

- Your heart rate and blood pressure
- Your groin or arm for bleeding.

The place where the tube was inserted may feel sore or tender. This may last for about one week.

In most cases, you should be able to go home in a day or two after the procedure.

What happens after coronary angioplasty?

Angioplasty is not a cure for CAD. You need to discuss with your doctor what led to CAD and the need for angioplasty.

Going Home

When you are ready to leave the hospital, you will be given instructions to follow at home. These instructions may include:

- How much activity or exercise you will be allowed
- When you should follow up with your doctor
- What medications you should be taking
- Checking the area where the tube was inserted every day for signs of infection
  - Redness
  - Swelling
  - Drainage
- Calling your doctor if you have a fever or signs of infection
- Calling your doctor for pain or bleeding where the tube was inserted
- For any chest pain call 9-1-1.

Your doctor will prescribe medication to prevent blood clots from forming. It is very important that you take them as directed. They can prevent the stent from becoming blocked. The medications may include:

- Anticoagulants (an-tee-ko-AG-u-lants)
- Antiplatelet drugs such as aspirin and clopidogrel (Plavix)

Most people return to work and other normal activities in about one week.

Cardiac Rehab

Your doctor may recommend that you participate in a cardiac rehabilitation (rehab) program. Cardiac rehab offers medical guidance and support to help you return to work or daily activities.

Stenting

What is a stent?

A stent is a small, lattice-shaped, metal tube that is inserted permanently into an artery. The stent helps hold open an artery so that blood can flow through it.

Drug-eluting stents are stents that contain drugs that potentially reduce the chance the arteries will become blocked again.

When is it used?

A stent is used to hold open an artery that has become too narrow due to atherosclerosis. In atherosclerosis, plaque builds up on the inner walls of arteries, the blood vessels that carry oxygen-rich blood throughout the body.

As the artery walls thicken, the pathway for blood narrows. This can slow or block blood flow.

How does it work?

The stent acts as a scaffold, remaining in place permanently to help keep the artery open.

A stent is inserted through a main artery in the groin (femoral artery) or arm (brachial artery) and threaded up to the narrowed section of the artery with a tiny catheter (balloon catheter.)

When it reaches the right location, the balloon is slightly inflated to push the plaque out of the way and expand the artery (balloon angioplasty). Some stents are stretched open (expanded) by the balloon at the same time as the artery. Other stents are inserted into the artery immediately after the angioplasty procedure.

Once in place, the stent helps holds the artery open so that the heart muscle gets enough blood.

Drug-eluting stents contain a drug that is released locally over time.

What will it accomplish?

The stent opens the narrowed artery so that an adequate supply of blood can be restored.

What are the risks?

The stent placement procedure can cause infection, blood clots, or bleeding. Other rare complications of coronary stents include chest pain, heart attack, or tearing of the blood vessel. The stent can move out of place (stent migration). In some cases, plaque can reappear in the stented artery (in-stent restenosis).

Drug-eluting stents have additional risks other than those listed here.

Your doctor can tell you more about the risks associated with stents and drug-eluting stents.

When should a stent not be used?

Stents should not be used in patients who cannot tolerate angioplasty, or who are sensitive (allergic) to the stent materials. They cannot be used in patients who cannot be placed on blood-thinning (anti-platelet) medication.

Drug-eluting stents have additional restrictions. Your doctor can tell you more about whether or not you are an appropriate candidate for this technology.

Chapter 72

Cardiac Ablation

Normally, electricity flows throughout the heart in a regular, measured pattern. This normally operating electrical system is the basis for heart muscle contractions.

Sometimes, the electrical flow gets blocked or travels the same pathways repeatedly, creating something of a "short circuit" that disturbs normal heart rhythms. Medicine often helps. In some cases, however, the most effective treatment is to destroy the tissue housing the short circuit. This procedure is called cardiac ablation.

Cardiac ablation is just one of a number of terms used to describe the nonsurgical procedure. Other common terms are: cardiac catheter ablation, radiofrequency ablation, cardiac ablation, or simply ablation.

The Ablation Process

Like many cardiac procedures, ablation no longer requires a full frontal chest opening. Rather, ablation is a relatively noninvasive procedure that involves inserting catheters—narrow, flexible wires—into a blood vessel, often through a site in the groin or neck, and winding the wire up into the heart. The journey from entry point to heart muscle is navigated by images created by a fluoroscope, an x-ray-like machine that provides continuous, "live" images of the catheter and tissue.

Once the catheter reaches the heart, electrodes at the tip of the catheter gather data and a variety of electrical measurements are made. The data pinpoints the location of the faulty electrical site. During this "electrical mapping," the cardiac arrhythmia specialist, an electrophysiologist, may sedate the patient and instigate some of the very arrhythmias that are the crux of the problem. The events are safe, given the range of experts and resources close at hand, and are necessary to ensure the precise location of the problematic tissue.

Once the damaged site is confirmed, energy is used to destroy a small amount of tissue, ending the disturbance of electrical flow through the heart and restoring a healthy heart rhythm. This energy may take the form of radiofrequency energy, which cauterizes the tissue, or intense cold, which freezes, or cryoablates, the tissue. Other energy sources are being investigated.

Patients rarely report pain, more often describing what they feel as discomfort. Some watch much of the procedure on monitors and occasionally ask questions. After the procedure, a patient remains still for four to six hours to ensure the entry point incision begins to heal properly. Once mobile again, patients may feel stiff and achy from lying still for hours.

When Is Ablation Appropriate?

Many people have abnormal heart rhythms (arrhythmias) that cannot be controlled with lifestyle changes or medications. Some patients cannot or do not wish to take life-long antiarrhythmic medications and other drugs because of side effects that interfere with their quality of life.

Most often, cardiac ablation is used to treat rapid heartbeats that begin in the upper chambers, or atria, of the heart. As a group, these are known as supraventricular tachycardias, or SVTs. Types of SVTs are:

- Atrial Fibrillation
- Atrial Flutter
- AV (atrioventricular) Nodal Reentrant Tachycardia
- AV Reentrant Tachycardia
- Atrial Tachycardia

Less frequently, ablation can treat heart rhythm disorders that begin in the heart's lower chambers, known as the ventricles. The most common, ventricular tachycardia, may also be the most dangerous type of arrhythmia because it can cause sudden cardiac death.

For patients at risk for sudden cardiac death, ablation often is used along with an implantable cardioverter device (ICD). The ablation decreases the frequency of abnormal heart rhythms in the ventricles and therefore reduces the number of ICD shocks a patient may experience.

For many types of arrhythmias, catheter ablation is successful in 90–98 percent of cases—thus eliminating the need for open-heart surgeries or long-term drug therapies.

Chapter 73

Electrical Cardioversion

What is electrical cardioversion?

Electrical cardioversion is used to make your heart beat normally by passing an electric shock across and through the chest. The electric shock is used most often to revive a person when the heart stops. It restores normal heart rhythm and has saved many lives. It is a very safe way to change an abnormal heart rhythm to normal.

The single, rapid, high-voltage electric shock to the heart causes all the heart muscle cells to stop beating for a moment. This allows your heart to restart itself with a normal heart rhythm. The heart then beats normally again. To be successful, the shock must be delivered at just the right time during a heartbeat.

When is it used?

Abnormal heart rhythms (arrhythmias), such as atrial tachycardia and ventricular tachycardia, may cause very rapid heart rates. The heart rate may be so fast that the blood does not circulate well. For some people with coronary artery or heart valve disease, this fast heartbeat may be life threatening. Cardioversion can quickly restore normal circulation.

Some other rhythm problems, such as atrial flutter or atrial fibrillation, are not very fast but are abnormal and inefficient. Having such

Reprinted from Clinical Reference Systems Cardiology Advisor, 2003.2 with permission from McKesson Health Solutions. © 2003 McKesson Health Solutions, LLC.

rhythms for days or weeks can lead to serious problems, such as heart failure and strokes.

Medicine is sometimes used to try to return the heart to a normal rhythm. In many cases electric cardioversion is safer and more effective than drug treatment.

How do I prepare for electrical cardioversion?

If the arrhythmia is life threatening, cardioversion is done without delay or special preparation.

For a planned cardioversion, follow any instructions your health care provider may give you. You may eat a light meal, such as soup or salad, the night before the procedure. Do not eat or drink anything after midnight and the morning before the procedure.

Plan for your care and recovery after the procedure.

What happens during the procedure?

You will be given a tranquilizer and a sedative (a light general anesthetic). These drugs will relax your muscles and put you to sleep. You will not feel pain during the procedure. The health care provider will put electrodes on your chest and back and deliver an electric shock through your chest for a fraction of a second. The electrical charge passes through two large, hand-held electrode paddles or two large adhesive patches placed on your chest. Abnormal heart rhythms usually return to normal with the first shock, but more shocks may be needed. Your health care provider will check your heart rhythm with an electrocardiogram (ECG, or EKG).

You will probably be unconscious from the anesthesia for less than five minutes and will not remember the shock.

What happens after the procedure?

You will be monitored in the recovery room or coronary care unit for a short time. Your chest might be a little sore. You may have ring-like marks on your chest where the electrode paddles were placed. These marks will fade after several days.

When you are fully recovered from the anesthesia, you will probably be allowed to go home. Sometimes you may need to stay in the hospital overnight. The health care provider may prescribe drugs to help your heart keep its new rhythm.

Ask your health care provider what you should do to take care of yourself and when you should come back for a checkup.

What are the benefits of this procedure?

- Your heart usually returns to a normal beat, reducing any discomfort and abnormal work for your heart.

- The procedure has fewer complications than treatment with most drugs.

What are the risks associated with this procedure?

- There are risks from the light general anesthesia, but harmful reactions rarely occur. Discuss these risks with your health care provider.

- You may have more problems with your heart rhythm. The health care provider may need to treat these problems after or even during the procedure.

- The procedure may not be successful and your heart rhythm may not change.

- Your heart could develop a more dangerous rhythm or possibly even stop.

- You may develop a small area of burn on your skin where the paddles were placed.

- A blood clot may become dislodged from the heart and cause a stroke.

Ask your health care provider how these risks apply to you.

When should I call my health care provider?

Call your health care provider right away if your heart rhythm becomes irregular or very rapid. Symptoms of a change in your heart rhythm are shortness of breath, chest pain or pressure, pounding in your chest, or dizziness.

Chapter 74

Cardiac Pacemakers,
Ventricular Assist Devices,
and
Cardiac Resynchronization

Cardiac Pacemakers

What Is a Cardiac Pacemaker?

A pacemaker is a small, battery-powered device that is implanted permanently into the body. The pacemaker monitors the electrical impulses in the heart and, when needed, delivers electrical stimuli to make the heart beat (contract) in a more normal rhythm.

When Is a Pacemaker Used

A pacemaker is used when the heart beats too slowly (bradycardia) or has other abnormal rhythms (arrhythmias). In some cases, pacemakers are also used to treat the symptoms of heart failure.

How Does a Pacemaker Work?

A pacemaker consists of a battery and electrical circuitry (pulse generator). The battery powers the pacemaker. The circuitry checks

"Cardiac Pacemakers" is reprinted from "Cardiac Pacemaker (Implanted)," U.S. Food and Drug Administration, updated February 2004. "Ventricular Assist Devices" is reprinted from "Ventricular Assist Device (VAD)," U.S. Food and Drug Administration, updated February 2004. "Cardiac Resynchronization" is reprinted from "Cardiac Resynchronization Therapy," Heart Rhythm Society, updated October 2003, © Heart Rhythm Society. The material is reprinted with the permission of the Heart Rhythm Society. No reproduction allowed without written permission from the Heart Rhythm Society.

the heart rate and produces tiny electrical pulses that keep the heart beating at the correct pace.

The pacemaker is connected to the heart through one to three insulated wires (leads) that are attached directly to the heart's chambers. Some pacemakers can be customized to meet specific needs.

- **Rate-Responsive Pacemakers.** These pacemakers may be programmed to increase or decrease heart rate to match your activities (i.e., resting or walking).

- **Single-Chambered Pacemakers.** These pacemakers use only one lead placed into the right upper chamber of the heart (right atrium) or the right lower chamber (right ventricle).

- **Dual-Chambered Pacemakers.** These pacemakers have two leads. One is placed in the right atrium, the other in the right ventricle.

- **Cardiac Resynchronization Therapy Pacemakers.** These pacemakers have three leads. One is in the right atrium, one is in the right ventricle, and one is placed through the heart's veins to the left ventricle.

What Will a Pacemaker Accomplish?

A pacemaker can restore a normal heart rate so that the heart can pump more effectively. This can reduce or stop the symptoms of abnormal heartbeats (arrhythmias), such as dizziness, confusion, fainting, or fatigue.

What Are the Risks?

Risks Due to Surgical Procedure

Risks from the surgery to implant the pacemaker include:

- Bleeding
- Swelling or bruising under the skin
- Blood clot formation
- Infection
- Blood vessel damage

Your doctor will tell you about additional risks from the surgical procedure.

Need for Additional Surgeries to Replace or Repair Pacemaker

Additional surgeries may become necessary to replace the pacemaker, or to repair it should it become damaged.

Electromagnetic Interference

Some devices in your surroundings may interfere with your cardiac pacemaker. Currently available pacemakers are more resistant to this problem than earlier models. Always carry your wallet I.D. card with you.

- Household devices and appliances may cause the pacemaker to enter a mode to prevent inappropriate behavior or cause it to stop delivering therapy until the interference source is removed.

- Some medical equipment can damage your pacemaker. If you are visiting your doctor or dentist, tell him or her that you have a pacemaker *before* they do any testing or treatment.

- Some security devices may temporarily stop your pacemaker from working properly or give you cardiac symptoms. A general rule of thumb is "Don't lean, don't linger" when moving through these devices.

- Welders and electric generators may stop your pacemaker from working properly.

When Should a Pacemaker Not Be Used?

A pacemaker should not be implanted in people who cannot tolerate the device or the surgical procedure, or who are sensitive (allergic) to the exposed parts of the pacing system.

Some pacemakers are designed to treat only specific conditions and should not be used to treat other conditions.

Ventricular Assist Devices

What Is a Ventricular Assist Device?

A ventricular assist device (VAD) is a mechanical pump that helps a heart that is too weak to pump blood through the body. It is sometimes referred to as "a bridge to transplant," since it can help a patient survive until a heart transplant can be performed.

When Is a VAD Used?

A VAD is used to aid the pumping action of a weakened heart ventricle (a major pumping chamber of the heart).

VADs were originally intended for short-term use to support failing hearts until donor hearts became available.

Some VADs are now used for long-term (destination) therapy in severe heart failure patients who are not candidates for heart transplants.

How Does a VAD Work?

A VAD does not replace the heart. Instead, it works with the patient's own heart to pump sufficient blood throughout the body.

The VAD consists of a pump, a control system, and an energy supply. Some VADs rely on a battery for their energy supply; others use compressed air (pneumatic). The energy supply and the control system are located outside the body; the pump can be either inside or outside the body.

In a VAD, blood flows from the ventricles into a pump. A left ventricular assist device (LVAD) receives blood from the left ventricle and delivers it to the aorta—the large artery that carries the blood from the heart to the rest of the body. A right ventricular assist device (RVAD) receives blood from the right ventricle and delivers it to the pulmonary artery—the artery that carries blood from the heart to the lungs.

What Will a VAD Accomplish?

A VAD will partially relieve the symptoms of severe heart failure, such as breathlessness and fatigue.

The VAD will "buy time" for a patient needing a heart transplant or nearing the end of life. Since many VADs are portable, patients can live at home and resume some activities while waiting for a heart transplant.

What Are the Risks?

VAD implant surgery carries risks of severe complications. Potential complications include bleeding, development of blood clots, respiratory failure, kidney failure, infection, stroke, and device failure.

Your doctor will tell you more about the risks associated with ventricular assist devices.

When Should a VAD Not Be Used?

A VAD should be used only in patients who are eligible for heart transplants or who have severe end-stage congestive heart failure and are not candidates for heart transplants.

Some VADs cannot be used with very short or very thin patients who have low body surface areas.

Poor candidates for VADs include people with:

- Irreversible kidney failure
- Severe liver disease
- Blood clotting disorders
- Severe lung disease
- Infections that do not respond to antibiotics

Cardiac Resynchronization

More than twenty-two million people worldwide suffer from congestive heart failure (CHF), a potentially debilitating disease. Until recently, lifestyle changes, medication, and, sometimes, heart surgery were the only treatment options. Patients with severe symptoms, however, received little, if any, relief from such approaches. To make matters worse, up to 40 percent of patients with CHF also have an arrhythmia that further reduces the heart's ability to beat properly.

Cardiac resynchronization therapy (CRT) is an innovative new therapy that can relieve CHF symptoms by improving the coordination of the heart's contractions. CRT builds on the technology used in pacemakers and implantable cardioverter devices. CRT devices also can protect the patient from slow and fast heart rhythms.

About Congestive Heart Failure

Damaged heart muscle can become so weak that it can no longer pump effectively, leading to cardiomyopathy and CHF.

Coronary artery disease and heart attacks are the most frequent causes of CHF, but inherited disorders, viral infections, and toxins, such as alcohol, also can cause heart muscle damage. Symptoms of CHF typically include shortness of breath, swelling of the feet and legs, abdominal swelling, fatigue, exercise intolerance, diminished appetite, and depression.

Most often, medications aim to control CHF symptoms, such as the buildup of excess fluid that causes leg swelling and makes it difficult to breathe. Medications can reduce fluid retention, strengthen the heart's squeezing ability, and relax blood vessels, thereby reducing the resistance to blood flow and easing the heart's workload.

In addition, lifestyle changes, such as low-salt diets and exercise, can help control symptoms.

Overview of a Heartbeat

The heart is comprised of four chambers: two upper atria, and two lower ventricles. An electrical system controls the synchronized pumping action of these chambers.

The normal heartbeat originates in a section of the right atrium known as the sinoatrial, or SA, node. The electrical signal from the sinoatrial node spreads through both atria, causing them to contract and squeeze blood into the ventricles. The electrical signal then passes through an electrical bridge known as the atrioventricular, or AV, node. After a split second delay, the signal continues to the ventricles by way of a specialized network known as the left and right bundle branches.

The bundle branches separate to the left and right ventricles, which enables the electrical signal to stimulate both ventricles simultaneously. This coordinated contraction, or squeezing, of the ventricles is necessary for optimal pumping of blood to the body and lungs.

Uncoordinated Contractions

When there is a delay in electrical signal transmission through the left bundle branch, this causes left bundle branch block (LBBB). Because the electrical signal to the left ventricle is delayed, the right ventricle begins to contract a fraction of a second before the left ventricle, instead of simultaneously. The result is an asynchronous, or uncoordinated contraction of the ventricles and a mis-timing in the contraction pattern of the left atrium and ventricle. Other conduction abnormalities, such as right bundle branch block (RBBB), also may contribute to less efficient contraction of the heart. This further reduces the pumping ability of the already weakened heart muscle.

Cardiac Resynchronization Therapy

The concept behind CRT is quite simple. Resynchronization restores the normal coordinated pumping action of the ventricles by overcoming the delay in electrical conduction caused by bundle branch block. This is accomplished by means of a special type of cardiac device.

These powerful, "built-in" devices have enormous potential to improve the quality of life and probably survival for patients with heart failure.

The CRT Device

Pacemakers are typically used to prevent symptoms due to an excessively slow heartbeat. The pacemaker continuously monitors the heartbeat and, when necessary, delivers tiny, imperceptible electrical signals to stimulate the heartbeat. Most pacemakers have two electrode wires, or leads, one in the right atrium and one in the right ventricle. This ensures the pacemaker will maintain the normal coordinated pumping relationship between the upper and lower chambers of the heart.

The wires that carry the electrical signals connect to an electrical pulse generator placed under the skin in the upper chest. In addition to the two leads (right atrium and right ventricle) used by a common pacemaker, the CRT device has a third lead that is positioned in a vein on the surface of the left ventricle.

This allows the CRT device to simultaneously stimulate the left and right ventricles and restore a coordinated, or "synchronous," squeezing pattern. This is sometimes referred to as "bi-ventricular pacing" because both ventricles are electrically stimulated (paced) at the same time. This reduces the electrical delay and results in a more coordinated and effective heartbeat.

CRT Results

The response to CRT can vary greatly among patients. Clinical studies involving more than two thousand patients worldwide demonstrate modest improvements in exercise tolerance, CHF severity, and quality of life in most patients. Improvement may happen quickly, but sometimes it can take several months.

When Is CRT the Right Choice?

The ideal candidate for a CRT device is someone with:

- Moderate to severe CHF symptoms, despite lifestyle changes and medication
- A weakened and enlarged heart muscle
- A significant electrical delay in the lower pumping chambers (bundle branch block)

Some CRT candidates also have a high risk of sudden cardiac death. For these patients, a special CRT device can stop potentially life-threatening rapid heartbeats by delivering an electrical shock known as defibrillation. This device incorporates a standard implantable cardioverter defibrillator (ICD) with a CRT pacemaker creating a "CRTD" device. (The "D" refers to defibrillation.)

Chapter 75

Implantable Cardioverter Defibrillators (ICDs)

Information about Implantable Cardioverter Defibrillators

What is an implantable cardioverter defibrillator?

An implantable cardioverter defibrillator (ICD) is a device that monitors heart rhythms, and delivers shocks if dangerous rhythms are detected.

Many ICDs record the heart's electrical patterns whenever an abnormal heart beat occurs. Doctors can review this record during regular checkups to help plan future treatment options.

When is an ICD used?

ICDs are used to treat patients whose lower heart chambers (ventricles) beat too quickly (tachycardia) or quiver ineffectively (fibrillation). They are also used in patients who are at risk of these conditions due to previous cardiac arrest, heart failure, or ineffective drug therapy for abnormal heart rhythms.

"Information about Implantable Cardioverter Defibrillators" is reprinted from "Implantable Cardioverter Defibrillator (ICD)," U.S. Food and Drug Administration, updated February 2004. "Common Questions about ICDs," updated February 2003, © Heart Rhythm Society, is reprinted with permission of the Heart Rhythm Society. No reproduction allowed without written permission from the Heart Rhythm Society.

How does an ICD work?

Like a pacemaker, an ICD consists of a battery and electrical circuitry (pulse generator) connected to one or more insulated wires. The pulse generator and batteries are sealed together and implanted under the skin, usually near the shoulder. The wires are threaded through blood vessels from the ICD to the heart muscle.

The ICD continuously checks the heart rate. When it detects a too-rapid or irregular heartbeat, it delivers a shock that resets the heart to a more normal rate and electrical pattern (cardioversion).

Stopping the potentially fatal fibrillation is called defibrillation.

What will an ICD accomplish?

ICDs protect against sudden cardiac death (SCD) from ventricular tachycardia and ventricular fibrillation.

What are the risks?

Potential risks from the surgical procedure include infection, bleeding, and bruising. Other rare complications include stroke, heart attack, blood clots, or perforation of a major vessel, a lung, or the heart muscle.

Your doctor will tell you about additional risks from ICDs.

Electromagnetic Interference: Some devices in your surroundings may interfere with your ICD. You may need to avoid certain types of security devices. Always carry your wallet ID card with you.

- Household devices and appliances may affect your ICD. Ask your doctor which devices to avoid.

- Some medical equipment can damage your ICD. If you are visiting your doctor or dentist, tell him or her that you have an ICD *before* he or she does any testing or treatment.

- Some security devices may affect your ICD. A general rule of thumb is "Don't lean, don't linger" when moving through these devices.

- Welders and electric generators may affect your ICD.

When should an ICD not be used?

ICDs should not be used in patients whose heart conditions are reversible or temporary. They should not be used in patients who will not benefit from the devices, or who are sensitive (allergic) to the exposed components.

Common Questions about ICDs

What is an ICD?

ICDs are pacemaker-like devices that continuously monitor the heart rhythm, and deliver life-saving shocks if a dangerous heart rhythm is detected. They can significantly improve survival in certain groups of patients with heart failure who are at high risk of ventricular fibrillation (VF).

Modern ICD devices have an electronic memory that records the electrical patterns of the heart whenever an abnormal heartbeat, or arrhythmia, occurs. This record is available for review during regular checkups by the physician, who can monitor the frequency and severity of problems in the heart's electrical conduction system that may lead to cardiac arrest or other serious heart disorders.

Can an ICD prevent a heart attack?

No! An ICD cannot prevent a heart attack, which is different from sudden cardiac arrest. A heart attack, or myocardial infarction (MI), is a "plumbing problem" caused by clogged or blocked blood vessels that reduce or block the normal supply of oxygen-rich blood to the heart. Without oxygen, heart muscle dies. An area of dead muscle is called an "infarct." Although a heart attack and SCD are separate conditions, they are related. Often, the damage done by a prior heart attack is an underlying cause of SCD.

SCD is the result of an "electrical problem" in the conduction system that regulates the normal, rhythmic contractions of the heart muscle that pumps blood throughout the body. In SCD, the electrical signals that regulate the pumping action of the lower chambers of the heart (ventricles) suddenly and without warning become rapid and chaotic. When the rhythmic contractions of the ventricles stop, the heart can't pump blood. The brain is starved of oxygen, and the individual loses consciousness in seconds. The heart cannot recover on its own from ventricular fibrillation. Unless immediate emergency help is available, death follows in minutes.

How does an ICD differ from a pacemaker?

Both an ICD and a pacemaker are devices that are implanted under the skin and connected to wires, or leads, that are placed in the heart. Both continuously monitor the heart to detect changes in its natural rhythm. A pacemaker, however, is used to detect a too-slow heart rate (bradycardia). When it senses that the rhythm is too slow, it sends an electrical signal to stimulate (pace) the heart so it continues its normal electrical beat. The electrical signal that is sent from the pacemaker is strong enough to stimulate the heart to beat, but not strong enough for the patient to feel. An ICD, on the other hand, detects a too-rapid or chaotic heartbeat and delivers a stronger electrical shock to restore the heart to its natural beat. Some ICDs also act as pacemakers.

How can an ICD help a patient who has suffered a heart attack?

The damage done by a heart attack, or MI, can affect the heart's electrical system and its ability to pump blood effectively. The damaged heart muscle that results from a heart attack may give rise to abnormal electrical signals that sometimes cause deadly heart rhythms, which the ICD detects and corrects.

The most common underlying problem seen in victims of SCD is coronary artery disease. This is a condition in which the arteries that supply blood to the heart are narrowed or blocked, usually due to arteriosclerosis (sometimes called "hardening of the arteries"). In this disease, a fatty substance called "plaque" builds up in the blood vessels, and can affect the normal flow of blood to the heart and other parts of the body.

Can I use a microwave oven or other appliances if I have an ICD?

Yes, normal household appliances and woodworking tools will not cause interference. You should avoid strong magnetic fields and large magnets, antennas, arc welders, and industrial equipment. If you work near industrial equipment, discuss your specific situation with your physician or nurse.

Can I use a cellular phone?

Yes, with these general guidelines:

- Hold the phone to the ear on the side of the body opposite to the implanted device.

- Do not carry the phone in the ON position in a breast pocket over or within six inches of the ICD.

- Maintain a minimum of six inches between the ICD and the phone.

Are security systems and airports a problem?

Walk normally through theft detector systems. Carry your ID card with you at all times. Show the airport security people the card, and ask to be hand searched.

Can an ICD patient drive a car?

Many physicians recommend no driving for six months after implantation of an ICD, or after a shock. Discuss this issue with your physician to maintain your safety as well as that of others.

What do I do when I receive a shock?

If one shock occurs and recovery is immediate, a call to the device clinic may be reassuring for the patient as well as the family. However, if one or more than one shock occur without rapid recovery, 911 emergency services should be called. If CPR and other lifesaving activities are needed, they should be started immediately.

How does it feel?

Fast pacing therapy may feel like a flutter or palpitation in the chest, or nothing at all. The shocks may feel like a sudden painful kick in the chest. It occurs in an instant and then is gone. If a blackout occurs, the shock may not be felt. Someone touching the patient may feel a small muscle jerk. It will not harm them.

How and when is the battery replaced?

The battery check at each visit will determine when the ICD should be replaced. The electronic circuitry as well as the battery are sealed inside the ICD. When replacement time arrives the lead(s) will be tested and then a new ICD will be attached to the lead(s). Usually the original lead(s) will be reused.

How effective are ICDs?

Studies of ICDs show they are 99 percent effective in detecting and stopping deadly heart rhythm disorders. In clinical trials, ICDs have been shown to be the most successful therapy to prevent sudden cardiac death in certain groups of high-risk patients.

Who is a candidate for an ICD?

The American College of Cardiology and the American Heart Association, along with representatives of the Heart Rhythm Society, have developed guidelines to help physicians and patients decide whether an ICD is the best treatment for an individual at risk for SCD. For example, it is agreed that ICD therapy is of benefit for:

Secondary Prevention. This includes individuals who have suffered a prior cardiac arrest or who experience spontaneous, sustained episodes of ventricular tachycardia (VT) that is not self-correcting, especially if they also have episodes of unexplained fainting. VT is a too-rapid heartbeat that can lead to VF.

Primary Prevention. This is treatment for patients who have never experienced the deadly heart rhythm disorders that lead to SCD, but have significant risk factors for the conditions. This includes certain patients with an ejection fraction of less than 35–40 percent and documented episodes of VT that are self-correcting and cause no adverse symptoms, but in whom sustained VT can be induced during the electrophysiology study. Ejection fraction is a measure of the amount of blood pumped out of the heart with each beat. An ejection fraction below 55 is considered abnormal. Vice President Cheney's ICD is for primary prevention.

How can people find out if they are at risk for SCD?

There are a number of tests that will help determine if heart attack survivors and people with other conditions that may put them at risk for SCD will benefit from ICD therapy. These include:

- **Echocardiogram.** The first test performed is usually an echocardiogram, which will determine whether the heart's pumping function is impaired. In this painless, noninvasive test, a device called a transducer is placed on the chest and sound waves are bounced off the heart. This provides a moving picture of the heart.

- **Holter monitor.** A Holter monitor is an external device worn by an individual who may be at risk for heart rhythm disorders. The monitor automatically records a continuous electrocardiogram (ECG) of the heart's electrical activity; it usually is worn for twenty-four to forty-eight hours.

- **Event recorder.** An event recorder is a small, pager-sized device that also records the electrical activity of the heart. Unlike a Holter monitor, it does not operate continuously, but instead is activated by the individual whenever he or she feels the heart begin to beat too fast or chaotically. After the device is activated to record the heart rhythm, the patient can report the event and transmit the recording by phone to a doctor or other health care provider.

- **Electrophysiology study.** An electrophysiology study (EPS) is a test that can predict if an individual is at high risk for SCD. In this study, electrical signals are administered to the heart muscle through a thin tube called a pacing catheter to see if they will stimulate ventricular tachycardia, the too-rapid heart rate that often leads to VF and SCD. The test is performed in a safe and controlled electrophysiology laboratory at a hospital or clinic and the patient is in no danger. In an EP study, local anesthetics are used to numb areas in the groin or near the neck, and small tubes called catheters are passed into the heart to record its electrical signals. During the test, the physician studies the speed and flow of electrical signals through the heart, identifies rhythm problems, and pinpoints areas in the heart's muscle that give rise to abnormal electrical signals. An electrophysiology study can:

  - Identify which patients who have had a prior heart attack, or MI, are at risk for serious heart rhythm disturbances and, perhaps, SCD.

  - Help determine which patients may require aggressive treatment to prevent SCD.

  - Identify individuals whose hearts cannot be induced into dangerous arrhythmias. They appear at lower risk for developing rhythm disorders that can lead to SCD.

How common is SCD?

SCD is a leading cause of death in adults in the United States and affects approximately three hundred thousand adults each year. Controlling the abnormal heart rhythm that leads to most cases of SCD might significantly reduce death from heart diseases. About half of all deaths from heart disease are sudden and unexpected, regardless of the underlying cause. This includes 50 percent of all deaths due to arteriosclerosis (clogged blood vessels—a condition sometimes called "hardening of the arteries") as well as 50 percent of deaths due to degeneration of the heart muscle, or to enlargement of the heart in patients with congestive heart failure.

SCD is particularly devastating because of its unexpectedness. Although studies have shown that most victims have underlying disease, many victims of SCD are outwardly healthy, active individuals who do not know they are at risk. Although economic studies have not yet been done and the direct medical costs are less than for lingering illnesses, the economic and social impacts of SCD are huge. Sudden cardiac death claims many people during their most productive years and devastates unprepared families.

Can patients without an ICD survive the cardiac arrest that causes SCD?

Cardiac arrest is reversible in most victims if it's treated within a few minutes with a defibrillator, an electrical device that shocks the heart back into normal rhythm. In as many as 95 percent of cases, however, patients die before emergency help can reach them. This number can be reduced by the recent development of small automated external defibrillators (AEDs) that are easy to use, portable, and relatively inexpensive. The Heart Rhythm Society, the American Heart Association, and other organizations advocate the widespread availability of these devices on airplanes and in public buildings. Studies in which police cars are equipped with AEDs have shown a reduction in the number of deaths from SCD in certain communities.

Is ICD therapy the only treatment for SCD?

A number of treatments have been investigated to help people at risk for SCD. These include:

- *Medications.* ACE inhibitors, beta blockers, channel blockers, and other medications are prescribed to control abnormal heart rhythms or treat other conditions that may contribute to heart disease or SCD. There have been many clinical trials and other studies of medications currently available to prevent cardiac arrest. Medications often are helpful in treating other symptoms of cardiovascular disease. Sometimes, more than one medication is prescribed at the same time. These medications also often are prescribed for patients who have an ICD. The results of drug therapy alone have been disappointing. In some cases, certain medications have actually increased patients' risk of SCD. ICD implantation remains the most effective way to prevent SCD in high-risk patients.

- *Radiofrequency Catheter Ablation (RFA).* In this technique, radiofrequency energy is used to destroy small areas of heart muscle that give rise to the abnormal electrical signals that cause rapid or irregular heart rhythms. RFA often is used in conjunction with ICD therapy to decrease the frequency of abnormal heart rhythms in the ventricles. It is not a substitute for an ICD.

Chapter 76

Coronary Artery Bypass Grafting (CABG)

Coronary artery disease (also known as CAD) is the most common cardiovascular disorder in adults. It is caused by the buildup of cholesterol deposits in the wall of the coronary arteries that convey the blood to the heart muscle (myocardium). These deposits limit the flow of blood through the coronary arteries. Coronary artery disease often results in heart attack (myocardial infarction) or chest pain (angina pectoris), even in the absence of prior symptoms. Warning signs of a heart attack have been well outlined in a previous publication.[1] Treatment for coronary artery disease can include changes in lifestyle, diet modification, weight reduction, and cholesterol reduction,[2] as well as control of diabetes and high blood pressure (if either or both are present). Smoking cessation is essential.[3] Many patients can be adequately treated with medications. Some individuals, however, will require invasive treatments such as stretching (dilatation) of the coronary arteries with a balloon (percutaneous transluminal coronary angiography or PTCA) or coronary artery bypass surgery.

What is coronary artery bypass surgery?

Coronary artery bypass surgery (CABG) involves creating new arteries to provide blood to the heart by use of other blood vessels as conduits to bypass the obstructions in the patient's coronary arteries.

Reprinted from "Coronary Artery Bypass Surgery," by Charles J. Mullany, *Circulation* 107, no. 3 (2003): 21–22. © 2003 Lippincott Williams and Wilkins; reprinted with permission.

In most cases, the surgeon constructs at least one of the bypasses by using an artery called the internal mammary artery that is located behind the breastbone or sternum. Other bypasses may be constructed by using a vein from the leg (saphenous vein) or an artery from the forearm (radial artery). In almost all cases, the operation requires an incision in the midline of the chest (sternotomy). During most bypass operations, the heart is stopped and is connected to a heart-lung machine that does the work of both the heart and the lungs (cardiopulmonary bypass). If the surgeon's assessment is that the operation could be done without the heart-lung machine, the surgery may be performed while the heart continues to beat (off-pump CABG). Not all patients are suitable for off-pump surgery, however, and off-pump surgery still requires a sternotomy.

Which patients need coronary artery bypass surgery?

Many patients with coronary artery disease will require more aggressive therapy other than medications and lifestyle modification. For patients who have severe chest pain (angina) or severe obstruction of the coronary arteries, further treatment may involve either enlargement of the coronary arteries by balloon dilatation (PTCA) or bypass surgery. Your cardiologist and cardiac surgeon will decide what is the most appropriate treatment for you. The location, the extent, and the number of obstructions in the arteries often dictate what is the most appropriate treatment for any particular individual. Patients who have undergone PTCA in the past may need bypass surgery in the future if their coronary disease progresses. Patients who have no symptoms but who have evidence of impaired blood supply to the heart muscle (ischemia) or poor function of the pumping chamber of the heart (left ventricle) may require surgery to improve heart function and prolong survival. This applies particularly to diabetic patients. CABG is also often performed at the same time as a heart valve operation or before other major surgery, such as abdominal aneurysm surgery.

What should I expect in the hospital?

In non-urgent cases, patients are usually admitted to hospital on the same morning as the surgery. General anesthesia is always used, and surgery may take three to five hours, depending on the complexity of the case. Under anesthesia in the operating room, a breathing tube (endotracheal tube) is inserted through the mouth. This tube helps patients breathe both during and after the surgery and allows the medical staff to clear secretions from the lungs. After surgery, patients are usually admitted to an intensive care unit for one or two days. While in the intensive care unit, breathing is assisted for several hours with a ventilator. The breathing tube is usually removed within two to four hours after surgery. Medications are given to relieve pain, and intravenous fluids are used to maintain hydration. One or more temporary drainage tubes exit from the chest cavity to drain any excess blood or fluid that may build up after the surgery. Many patients will require blood transfusions during or after the operation.

Within twenty-four hours of surgery, most patients are out of bed, and they are able to walk within one or two days. Over the next few days, patients usually regain sufficient strength so that they can be discharged within five to seven days after surgery. The most common complication after bypass surgery is an irregular rapid heart rate (atrial fibrillation). In most cases this can be adequately treated with medications. More serious but less common complications are stroke (in 1 percent to 2 percent of patients) and infection of the sternum (in 1 percent to 2 percent of patients).

What should I expect after leaving the hospital?

In most instances recovery is rapid. Most patients are able to drive in about three weeks. Sexual activity can be resumed in three to four weeks. The main limitation to activity is healing of the sternum. Like any bone that is divided, the sternum may take up to twelve weeks to fully heal. Therefore, strenuous upper limb activities that would put extra stress on the sternum should be avoided during this time.

When can I return to work?

Return to work will depend on rate of recovery, as well as the physical and emotional demands of your job. If you have a relatively sedentary job, then you may be able to return to work as early as four to six weeks after the operation. However, if your occupation involves heavy manual activity (for example, construction work or lifting heavy weights), you may not be able to return to full activity for up to twelve weeks. Consultation with your cardiologist will help you to determine the timing of your return to work.

Should I enroll in a rehabilitation program?

Although not essential, a formal cardiac rehabilitation program will help to monitor your progress and get you back to full activity sooner. In addition, you will receive advice and support regarding lifestyle changes, weight reduction, dietary management, and levels of exercise activity for which you should aim. Again, consultation with your cardiologist and surgeon will help you to determine if a cardiac rehabilitation program is appropriate for you and where you may find or enroll in such a program.

Will the bypass surgery cure my coronary artery disease?

No. Bypass surgery will improve blood supply to the heart, relieve symptoms, and in some instances prolong life. However, with time, further disease in the coronary arteries or grafts can develop. Therefore, it is essential that you control the risk factors that can lead to coronary artery disease. These measures include weight reduction (if overweight), smoking cessation, reduction of cholesterol (if elevated), maintenance of normal blood pressure, and control of diabetes (if applicable). Almost all patients should take aspirin (81 mg) indefinitely after surgery. You may be prescribed other medications such as beta-blockers, angiotensin-converting enzyme (ACE) inhibitors, medications to control heart rate irregularities, and cholesterol-lowering agents.

What follow-up care will I need?

You should be seen at regular intervals by your local doctor to monitor the control of risk factors, particularly cholesterol, blood pressure, and diabetes, and at least annually by your cardiologist to monitor your coronary artery disease. After bypass surgery, most people enjoy many

Table 76.1. Management of Patients after Coronary Bypass Surgery

A	Aspirin
	Abstain from smoking
	ACE inhibitors (for poor heart function)
B	Blood pressure control beta-blockers
C	Cholesterol management
D	Diet
	Diabetic control
E	Exercise
F	Follow-up

years of excellent health with relief of symptoms and are able to return to work with full activities.

References

1. Ornato JP, Hand MM. Warning signs of a heart attack. Cardiology Patient Page. *Circulation*. 2001; 104: 1212–13.

2. Gotto AM Jr. Statins: powerful drugs for lowering cholesterol: advice for patients. Cardiology Patient Page. *Circulation*. 2002; 105: 1514–16.

3. Jorenby DE. Smoking cessation strategies for the 21st century. Cardiology Patient Page. *Circulation*. 2001; 104: e51–e52.

Chapter 77

Valve Replacement and Repair

Heart Valve Replacement

Heart valve replacement refers to procedures aimed at replacing your own heart valve, rather than repairing your own valve. If a surgeon cannot repair a heart valve, the valve is removed and replaced with an artificial (prosthetic) valve by sewing it into the remaining tissue from the natural valve. Throughout the world, 95 percent of all valve replacements are performed for mitral or aortic valves. The mitral valve is positioned in the heart's left side, between the left upper chamber (left atrium) and the left lower chamber (left ventricle). The aortic valve separates the left ventricle from the aorta (which carries blood to the body).

Today, there are two types of prosthetic valves used for replacement: mechanical or tissue.

Mechanical Valves. A mechanical valve is carefully designed to mimic the native heart valve. It has a ring, like your own natural heart valve, to support the leaflets. Like your own heart valve, the mechanical valve opens and closes with each heartbeat, permitting proper blood flow through the heart. To prevent any blood clots from developing on the valve that can cause complications, a mechanical valve replacement requires you to take anticoagulation medicine (blood

"Heart Valve Replacement" and "Heart Valve Repair," © St. Jude Medical, Inc. 2004. Provided courtesy of St. Jude Medical, Inc. Visit: www.sjm.com.

thinners) daily. The dosage of this medication is different for each person, so you will be closely monitored to make sure you are on the correct dosage for you. Regular blood tests will be performed at the physician's office, an anticoagulation clinic, or at home with a specialized testing kit.

Tissue Valves. The tissue valve is a native valve taken from an animal. Once the tissue is explanted (removed), it is chemically treated and prepared for human use. Some tissue valves have a frame, or stent, that supports the valve, and some valves are stentless (no framework). A very thin polyester mesh cuff is sewn around the outside of the valve for easier implantation. Eliminating the stent makes it possible for the surgeon to implant a larger valve. Larger valves generally provide more surface area for blood flow; this allows more blood to flow through the valve to accommodate the body's needs.

Homografts or Allografts. A homograft or allograft is a human valve obtained from a donor. This type of valve is particularly beneficial for pregnant women and children, because it does not require long-term anticoagulation therapy. In addition, it can provide excellent hemodynamic performance, allowing for natural function of the surrounding structures. Because the availability of these valves depends on donors, supply is limited.

Heart Valve Repair

Heart valve repair involves a procedure to fix your own heart valve, as opposed to replacing it with a mechanical or tissue valve. Different techniques can be used to repair a heart valve depending upon the problem you have.

Valvuloplasty. Valvuloplasty is a technique aimed at making sure the flaps of the valves (or leaflets) close properly, preventing blood from backing up into the atrium. In the healthy heart, blood flows from the upper chamber (atrium) to the lower chamber (ventricle), and from the ventricle to the body.

Commissurotomy is a special form of valvuloplasty. Commissurotomy is used when the leaflets of the valve become stiff and actually fuse together at the base, which is the ring portion (or annulus) of the valve. Sometimes a scalpel is used to cut the fused leaflets (commissures) near the ring, which may help them open and close better. In other cases, a balloon catheter, similar to a catheter used during angioplasty, is inserted into the valve. The balloon is inflated, splitting the commissures and freeing the leaflets to open and shut fully. Unlike other valvuloplasty procedures, this procedure can be done in the cardiac catheterization lab, and the chest does not have to be opened.

Annuloplasty. Annuloplasty is a technique aimed at repairing the fibrous tissue at the base of the heart valve (the annulus). Sometimes, the annulus becomes enlarged, which enables blood to back up into the atrium. To repair this, sutures are sewn around the ring to make the opening smaller. This creates a purse string effect around the base of the valve and helps the leaflets meet again when the valve closes.

Sometimes when repairing the annulus, it is necessary for the surgeon to implant an annuloplasty ring. A ring is used to correct a problem, provide support for the valve, and reinforce other repair techniques or any combination of these.

What to Expect before Heart Valve Surgery

For your heart valve surgery, a highly qualified team of medical personnel works together to ensure the safest possible procedure. An anesthesiologist will examine and talk to you about the surgery and medications that will be used during the procedure. A perfusionist will operate the heart-lung machine that keeps oxygenated blood circulating through the body while the heart is stilled so that surgery can be performed on it. There are other specialized surgical assistants and nurses that assist and closely monitor your condition.

Before the surgery, you will receive an intravenous (IV) line in your arm or hand. This will enable your doctor to administer medications and fluids. You will be asked to remove any jewelry, contact lenses or eyeglasses, hearing aids, and dentures. Your doctor will probably give you a mild sedative in your IV prior to the procedure.

Complications and Risks

With improvement in technology and surgical techniques, there has been continued reduction in complications associated with open-heart surgery. Still, every open-heart surgery entails some risk. Though rare, some of the potential complications include infection, bleeding, stroke, and heart attack.

Ask your physician if you have any questions about potential risks or if you have more questions about heart valve repair.

What to Expect during Heart Valve Surgery

First, you will be fully anesthetized. To access the heart, the surgeon will make an incision down the center of the chest, separating the breastbone. In order to operate on the heart, it must be still. To accomplish this, the heart-lung machine is used to take over the job of the heart and the lungs. The right atrium is accessed with a special tube that will carry blood from the body to the machine, which oxygenates the blood. The machine then pumps the oxygenated blood through another tube that has been placed into the aorta to circulate the blood back through the body. The term bypass is often used to describe this method of bypassing the heart and lungs. (This is not to be confused with a coronary artery bypass or CABG procedure, which is also nicknamed bypass.)

Heart Valve Repair: The procedure depends on the nature of the valve disease (valvuloplasty or annuloplasty). Once the repair is made, the heart-lung machine is withdrawn; and the heart is started again to circulate blood through the lungs and body. The breastbone is rejoined with wires and the incision closed.

Heart Valve Replacement: The surgeon then makes another incision in the heart or aorta and removes the damaged valve. The new replacement valve is properly positioned and sewn into place. The incisions in the heart are then closed (sewn); the heart-lung machine is withdrawn; and the heart is started again to circulate blood through the lungs and body. The breastbone is rejoined with wires and the incision closed.

The procedure outlined here is a conventional, open-chest procedure for valve replacement or repair surgery. Recent technology has allowed surgeons to perform valve replacement or repair with less invasive techniques. This is not always an option for all people and may depend on whether the facility has the technology available. In some cases, the specific nature of the repair needed cannot be performed using the less invasive technology, and conventional surgery is required. The less invasive the approach, the more likely a shorter procedure time, reduced hospital stay, and quicker recovery will be involved.

What to Expect after Heart Valve Surgery

After surgery, you will be placed in the intensive care unit (ICU) where you can be continuously monitored. Breathing during surgery, and for a while afterward, is assisted through a tube that has been placed down your throat and positioned in your lungs. You will probably wake up with this tube still in position. It is removed as soon as you are stable and awake enough to breathe on your own. You will not be able to talk while this tube is in place. Other tubes will protrude from your chest near the heart to drain extra blood and fluid from the surgical area. Intravenous lines give fluid, blood, and medications as needed. A bladder catheter drains urine. A monitor shows the heart rate, heart rhythm, blood pressure, and other special pressures and waves that the nursing staff watches closely to assess how the recovery is going. Medications are given as needed to ease pain and anxiety.

Every patient recovers at a different rate. Tubes are removed as recovery progresses. The ICU stay is usually a day or two. Then you will be moved to a cardiac medical-surgical floor where your heart is still continually monitored, but you can be more independent and active. The health care team continues to support and instruct you in recovery care, rehabilitation, medications, nutrition, and other needs.

Returning Home. Just as the recovery from surgery in the hospital differs for each patient, so will your recovery at home. Upon discharge, you will not feel fully recovered. It will take, on average, six to eight weeks at home before you can return to your normal routine. You will gain more energy and strength each day during these weeks. Some days will be better than others. This is normal. Be sure to rest when you get tired.

During those first weeks, you will visit your surgeon or physician to monitor your recovery. You may undergo tests to assess how your new valve is working (electrocardiogram, echocardiogram, or chest x-ray). Blood work may also be performed to assess your medication levels.

Incision Care. It is normal to have some discomfort, bruising, numbness, and itching at your incision site for several weeks after the surgery. Follow the instructions from your physician for proper incision care. A shower or gentle washing of the incision is usually all that's recommended. Tub baths are typically not allowed because they can affect your circulation. To help prevent infections, avoid using creams or lotions around your incision, until your physician allows it.

Exercise Program. A progressive increase in activity over time will improve your strength and endurance. The goal is a well-conditioned heart muscle that pumps more effectively. Walking is one of the simplest and most effective forms of exercise you can do. More aerobic exercise, such as a brisk walk, swimming, or bicycle riding, will provide cardiovascular conditioning. Talk with your physician and follow his or her advice about the best exercise program for you.

Some activities, especially lifting, will be limited in the beginning to allow adequate healing of your breastbone. As healing continues, your physician will no longer find these restrictions necessary.

Fluid Retention. After surgery, some people experience fluid retention that can overload the heart and make it work inefficiently. To prevent fluid retention, your physician may recommend dietary changes or medications.

You can help monitor this at home by weighing yourself every morning. Report any sudden weight gain of three pounds or more in one day, or five pounds in one week. Also, contact your physician if you experience unusual shortness of breath or observe swollen hands, ankles, or stomach.

Infection. Bacteria can enter the bloodstream during dental and some surgical procedures, causing an infection, known as bacterial endocarditis, in the tissue surrounding the artificial heart valve. Although this occurs infrequently, antibiotics taken before and after medical procedures are the best defense. Consult your physician before you have any dental or surgical procedures done so that antibiotics can be prescribed. Be sure to tell your dentist and any other physicians that you have had heart valve surgery.

Anticoagulants. If you received a mechanical heart valve, your physician may prescribe an anticoagulant medication (blood thinner) to prevent blood clots from forming on or around your new valve. The level of anticoagulation will be closely monitored by blood tests. Your physician will determine the level of anticoagulant that is right for you based on the guidelines and your medical situation.

To maintain proper levels, take your medication as prescribed and follow up with blood tests as scheduled.

Other medications can affect your anticoagulation level, including over-the-counter products. Tell your physician about any medications that you take daily or use as needed for pain or other discomforts. Aspirin and aspirin-containing products should be avoided because they greatly impact the anticoagulation levels. Follow your physician's advice about taking other medications with anticoagulant therapy.

Food and alcohol may also affect your anticoagulation level. Consult with your physician about your dietary habits. He or she will let you know what specific dietary guidelines to follow.

Before any medical procedure you are scheduled to have, notify your dentist and any other physicians that you are on an anticoagulant. Adjustments in your medication may be needed prior to any procedure.

When taking anticoagulant medication, consult your physician if any of the following occur:

- Excessive bruising
- Excessive bleeding
- Blood in your urine
- Bloody or black, tarry stools
- Unusual nosebleeds
- Bleeding gums
- Pregnancy or planned pregnancy
- Fever or other illness, including vomiting, diarrhea, or infection

Emergency Identification. In an emergency situation, an identification bracelet, necklace, or wallet card can alert hospital personnel to your specific medical needs. If you are interested in registering for such a service, your physician will give you information on the agencies and services available. Or, you can purchase a medical identification bracelet or necklace from a jeweler or pharmacy. One of the best-known bracelets comes from Medic Alert. In the United States, you can reach Medic Alert at 800-432-5378.

Follow-Up. Long-term management of your health requires your active participation. Your physician will follow your progress, but only if you visit him or her as recommended and scheduled so that you receive the proper follow-up care. Consult your physician about any concerns or questions you have. Work as a team toward a healthy recovery.

Frequently Asked Questions

How many other people have heart valve replacement surgery annually?

If you need to have valve replacement surgery, remember that you are not alone. There are approximately 225,000 heart valve procedures performed worldwide each year.

Will I need to take antibiotics before surgery or dental work?

Bacteria may enter the bloodstream during dental and some medical procedures. These bacteria may then cause an infection, known as bacterial endocarditis, in the tissue surrounding an artificial heart valve. Although this does not happen frequently, it can have serious consequences. The easiest and best defense is simply taking antibiotics before and after dental work and other medical procedures. Check with your physician before having any dental or medical procedures performed. Inform your dentist and any other physicians that you have an artificial heart valve.

Will I need to take medications after the surgery?

During your hospital stay, you will most likely be given several medications. If you undergo heart valve replacement, one medication you will receive is an anticoagulant, warfarin (brand name Coumadin®). Anticoagulants are given to help keep your new heart valve free from blood clots, which could adhere to the valve if the blood is not anticoagulated (thinned) enough. While tissue valves may require several months of anticoagulant treatment following surgery, mechanical valves require lifelong treatment with anticoagulants.

Your physician will determine the level of anticoagulant that is right for you based on the guidelines and your medical situation.

How much anticoagulation will I need?

According to the American College of Cardiology/American Heart Association Guidelines for the Management of Patients With Prosthetic Heart Valves[1], the following International Normalized Ratios (INR) are recommended for bileaflet valves. For the first three months after valve replacement:

- INR = 2.5–3.5

Three or more months after valve replacement:

- INR = 2.0–3.0 (aortic valve replacement [AVR])

- INR = 2.5–3.5 (AVR with risk factors, such as atrial fibrillation, left ventricular dysfunction, previous thromboembolism, or hypercoagulable condition)

- INR = 2.5–3.5 (mitral valve replacement)

To maintain proper levels of anticoagulation, take your medication as prescribed and follow up with blood tests as scheduled. The blood tests performed indicate the anticoagulation level of the blood are the PT, or prothrombin time, and the INR, international normalized ratio. Always wear or carry patient identification with you that indicates the medications you are taking, their dosages, your PT and INR levels, and the fact that you have received a new heart valve.

Check with your physician if you are on anticoagulants and experience any of the following: excessive bleeding; excessive bruising; blood in your urine; bloody or black, tarry stools; unusual nosebleeds; bleeding gums; possible pregnancy; and fever or other illnesses that include vomiting, diarrhea, or infection.

Remember, take only those medications that are prescribed by your physician. Anticoagulants may be affected by many other medicines, so always check with your physician or pharmacist before taking any other medication, including over-the-counter products such as aspirin.

Certain foods and alcohol may also affect how your anticoagulant works, so it is important to discuss your diet with your physician. Some slight modifications may be necessary.

Will my artificial heart valve or ring set off an airport metal detector?

The amount of metal used in mechanical heart valves and heart valve rings is very small. It is usually not enough to set off the metal detectors; however, if it does, simply show security personnel your patient identification card. Passing through a metal detector will not hurt your heart valve.

How can I get an identification bracelet?

It is important to have some type of identification that indicates you have had a heart valve replaced. Additionally, if you are on anticoagulant medication, this information should be included on the identification. A bracelet, a necklace, or a wallet card are all good ways of identifying this important information.

You may purchase a medical identification bracelet or necklace from a jeweler or pharmacy. One of the best-known bracelets comes from Medic Alert. In the United States, you can reach Medic Alert at 800-432-5378.

What should I be eating?

A heart-healthy diet is recommended for everyone, but especially for people who have any type of heart disease, including heart valve disease, or for those who have had valve surgery. Surgery for heart valve replacement or repair does not eliminate the possibility of developing further heart disease.

What is a heart-healthy diet?

Use fats and oils sparingly, avoiding saturated fats such as butter, cream, cheese, fatty meats, and bakery products. Try to prepare your food by grilling, microwaving, and baking. Choose low-fat foods, such as lean meats, poultry, fish, fresh fruits, and vegetables, plus whole-grain breads and cereals. Ask your physician to help you develop a heart-healthy diet.

Is it okay for me to undergo diagnostic tests, such as MRI or CT scans?

Mechanical heart valves are made of materials that are compatible with magnetic resonance imaging (MRI), computed tomography (CT) scans, and x-rays. Yet it is important to check with your physician before any diagnostic testing is done, even if the test is for a health problem that is not heart-related.

How often will my valve need to be checked?

Long-term management of your health requires active participation. Your physician will tell you how often to return for regularly scheduled follow-up visits.

During these visits, blood tests may be done to monitor your medication levels, especially your anticoagulation levels. To check healing, your physician may also order chest x-rays, echocardiograms (to check valve function), or electrocardiograms (to show any abnormal heart rhythms).

Your physician will also discuss other factors affecting your health during these visits. Follow your physician's advice and guidelines regarding diet, exercise, and medications. Always keep your scheduled appointments.

What is the sound I hear coming from my chest? What does it mean?

Some patients have indicated that they hear a clicking sound during quiet or restful times. If you hear this sound, rest assured; it just means that everything is working fine. This clicking is actually the sound of the mechanical valve leaflets closing.

Not all people will even hear the clicking. Your individual anatomy and physiology affects the sound. Mechanical valves also sound differently in different people.

If your valve is new and you are noticing this different sound, understand that many patients grow accustomed to the sound with time. It becomes like "white noise" in the background that grows unnoticeable. There is some comfort in knowing that if you hear the sound, you can be assured that the valve is working properly and keeping you alive.

How long will the valve last?

The St. Jude Medical mechanical heart valve is made of graphite and coated with pyrolytic carbon. Studies have shown that the valve will not wear out during the patient's lifetime. However, if there are problems with blood clot formation, the valve may need to be replaced.

A tissue valve, which is composed of living tissue, may have a shorter life span than a mechanical valve. The symptoms of valve failure may be the same symptoms you experienced before surgery, such as shortness of breath, dizziness, chest pain, fatigue, and fluid retention. If one or more of these symptoms occur, notify your physician.

Reference

1. ACC/AHA Practice Guidelines, Guidelines for the Management of Patients with Valvular Heart Disease. *Circulation*; 98:1949–84.

Chapter 78

Other Types of Corrective Heart Surgery

Minimally Invasive Heart Surgery

Minimally invasive surgical techniques have been widely used in a variety of surgical specialties for years. Until recently, however, limitations in equipment had delayed their application to heart surgery. Technological advancements, including the revolutionary breakthrough of computerized robotic systems, now enable complex heart surgery to be performed without having to open a patient's chest.

What Is Minimally Invasive Heart Surgery?

Minimally invasive heart surgery entails operating on the heart (2–3 inches) with long-handled, tiny surgical instruments inserted through small incisions in the chest as opposed to traditional open-heart surgery, which requires a sternotomy (a 10–12 inch incision through the sternal bone) to access the heart. Because the minimally invasive approach "invades" the body less than a standard open-heart procedure, you experience significant benefits as a result.

Surgeons perform the following procedures using minimally invasive techniques:

"Minimally Invasive Heart Surgery" reprinted with permission from the website of PENN Cardiac Care at the University of Pennsylvania Health System. © 2004 The Trustees of the University of Pennsylvania. All rights reserved. For additional information, visit http://www.pennhealth.com/cardiac/. Additional text under "Transmyocardial Revascularization" reprinted with permission from www.americanheart.org © 2004, American Heart Association.

- Aortic valve replacement
- Atrial septal defects
- Coronary bypass
- Mitral valve repair and replacement
- Patent foramen ovale (hole in the heart)

What Is Robotic Cardiac Surgery?

Robotic surgery refers to procedures that are facilitated by surgeon-controlled robotic instruments. These devices provide extreme steadiness and wide range of motion, enabling access to areas inside the heart that were never possible before.

During heart surgery, a surgeon controls the robotic instruments, which are inserted through tiny incisions in the chest. The high-definition camera provides the operating surgeon a full view of the heart, virtually transporting his eyes and hands into the chest. The surgeon sits at the console with the controls, using his hands and wrists to manipulate the movements of the robotic instruments.

Using this technology, surgeons, anesthesiologists, nurses, and technicians are able to repair mitral valves, close atrial septal defects, and perform coronary artery bypass surgery.

What Are the Benefits of Minimally Invasive and Robotic Cardiac Surgery?

Minimally invasive surgery performed through a significantly reduced incision area provides less trauma and blood loss. Though each patient's experience may vary, minimally invasive surgery may result in the following benefits:

- Lower risk of infection
- Fewer medications
- Lessened pain and scarring
- Quicker recovery
- Shorter hospital stay

Is There Any Increase in Risk with These Procedures?

There is no increased risk with minimally invasive procedures. The operations within the heart are performed with the same techniques used in standard heart surgery, just via smaller, less painful incisions.

Beating Heart or Off-Pump Surgery

Using sophisticated technology, most coronary bypass procedures, including multivessel bypass operations, can be performed "off-pump" or while the heart is still beating. This avoids the need to stop and restart the heart, as is the case when one is placed on the heart-lung machine during standard heart surgery. Avoiding the heart-lung machine results in fewer blood transfusions and quicker recovery.

Coronary Artery Bypass Surgery

Our cardiothoracic surgeons are utilizing the latest research on arterial conduits for bypass grafts. Recent data has shown that arteries remain open longer than veins when used as bypass coronary vessels.

Recovery

Following surgery, all patients are closely monitored in the intensive care unit. Generally you will be awake shortly after surgery and can expect to sit up in bed the night of surgery, sipping fluids. Like most patients, you can move out of bed to a chair or take short walks the next day. Medication will be prescribed, adjusted, or discontinued depending on your condition. Patients receive physical rehabilitation while in the hospital and are usually ready to go home in three or four days after surgery. Although the speed of recovery varies, patients can expect to resume their lifestyle within two to four weeks of their operation.

Transmyocardial Revascularization

Reproduced with permission from www.americanheart.org © 2004, American Heart Association.

What Is Transmyocardial Revascularization?

Transmyocardial revascularization or TMR is a procedure used to relieve severe angina or chest pain in very ill patients who aren't candidates for bypass surgery or angioplasty.

How Is It Done?

In this procedure, a surgeon makes an incision on the left breast to expose the heart. Then, using a laser, the surgeon drills a series of holes from the outside of the heart into the heart's pumping chamber.

From 20 to 40 mm laser channels are placed during the procedure. Bleeding from the laser channels on the outside of the heart stops after a few minutes of pressure from the surgeon's finger.

In some patients TMR is combined with bypass surgery. In those cases an incision through the breastbone is used.

How Does It Work?

How TMR reduces angina still isn't fully understood.

- The laser may stimulate new blood vessels to grow, called angiogenesis.

- It may destroy nerve fibers to the heart, making patients unable to feel their chest pain.

How Does It Compare to Other Treatments?

Transmyocardial revascularization has received FDA approval for use in patients with severe angina who have no other treatment options. It has also produced early promising results in three large multicenter clinical trials. The angina of 80–90 percent of patients who've had this procedure has significantly improved (at least 50 percent) through one year after surgery. There's still limited follow-up data as to how long this procedure might last, however.

Transmyocardial revascularization won't replace coronary artery bypass or angioplasty as the most common method of treating coronary artery disease. These alternatives have been proven over time to be safe, effective ways to restore blood flow to the heart muscle. But TMR may be used for

- people who are high-risk candidates for a second bypass or angioplasty.

- people whose blockages are too diffuse to be treated with bypass alone.

- some patients with heart transplants who develop atherosclerosis after their transplant.

Check with a large medical center in your area to find locations in your region where this procedure is being done.

Chapter 79

Facts about Heart and Heart-Lung Transplants

In the time since the performance of the first human heart transplant in December 1967, the procedure has changed from an experimental operation to an established treatment for advanced heart disease. Approximately 2,800 heart transplants are performed each year in the United States.

In 1981, combined heart and lung transplants began to be used to treat patients with conditions that severely damage both these organs. This is a much less common operation than heart transplantation; less than 200 per year are performed worldwide.

There have been two main barriers to increasing the number of successful operations. In 1983, the first barrier to successful transplantations—rejection of the donor organ by the patient—was overcome. The drug cyclosporine was introduced to suppress rejection of a donor heart or heart-lung by the patient's body. Cyclosporine and other medications to control rejection have significantly improved the survival of transplant patients. About 80 percent of heart transplant patients survive one year. About 65 percent of heart-lung transplants live at least one year after surgery. Research is under way to develop even better ways to control transplant rejection and improve survival.

Today, the major remaining barrier to increasing transplantations is a shortage of donor organs. Hospitals and organizations nationwide

Reprinted from "Facts about Heart and Heart-Lung Transplants," NIH publication no. 97-2990, revised August 1997. Revised by David A. Cooke, M.D., August 15, 2004.

are trying to increase public awareness of this problem and improve organ distribution.

What happens during a heart or heart-lung transplant?

A transplant is the replacement of a patient's diseased heart or heart and lungs with a normal organ(s) from someone—called a donor—who has died. The donor's organ(s) is completely removed and quickly transported to the patient, who may be located across the country. Organs are cooled and kept in a special solution while being taken to the patient.

During the operation, the patient is placed on a heart-lung machine. This machine allows surgeons to bypass the blood flow to the heart and lungs. The machine pumps the blood throughout the rest of the body, removing carbon dioxide (a waste product) and replacing it with oxygen needed by body tissues. Doctors remove the patient's heart except for the back walls of the atria, the heart's upper chambers. The backs of the atria on the new heart are opened and the heart is sewn into place. A similar process is followed in heart-lung transplants, except doctors remove the heart and lungs as a unit from the donor; the new lungs are attached first, followed by the heart.

Surgeons then connect the blood vessels and allow blood to flow through the heart and lungs. As the heart warms up, it begins beating. Sometimes, surgeons must start the heart with an electrical shock. Surgeons check all the connected blood vessels and heart chambers for leaks before removing the patient from the heart-lung machine.

Patients are usually up and around a few days after surgery, and if there are no signs of the body immediately rejecting the organ(s), patients are allowed to go home within two weeks.

Why are transplants done?

A transplant is considered when the heart is failing and does not respond to all other therapies, but health is otherwise good. The leading reasons why people receive heart transplants are:

- **Cardiomyopathy:** a weakening of the heart muscle.

- **Severe coronary artery disease:** a condition in which the heart's blood vessels become blocked and the heart muscle is damaged.

- **Birth defects of the heart.**

Heart-lung transplants are performed on patients who will die from end-stage lung disease that also involves the heart. Alternative therapies for these patients have been tried or considered. Leading reasons people receive heart-lung transplants are:

- Severe pulmonary hypertension: a large increase in blood pressure in the vessels of the lungs that limits blood flow and delivery of oxygen to the rest of the body.

- A birth defect of the heart that results in Eisenmenger's complex—another name for acquired pulmonary hypertension.

Who can have a transplant?

Patients under age sixty are the most likely heart transplant candidates. Patients under age forty-five are generally accepted for heart-lung transplants. In both cases, patients must be suffering from end-stage disease and be in good health otherwise. The doctor, patient, and family must address the following four basic questions to determine whether a transplant should be considered:

- Have all other therapies been tried or excluded?

- Is the patient likely to die without the transplant?

- Is the person in generally good health other than the heart or heart and lung disease?

- Can the patient adhere to the lifestyle changes—including complex drug treatments and frequent examinations—required after a transplant?

Patients who do not meet the above considerations or who have additional problems—other severe diseases, active infections, or severe obesity—are not good candidates for a transplant.

How are donors found?

Donors are individuals who are brain dead, meaning that the brain shows no signs of life while the person's body is being kept alive by a machine. Donors have often died as a result of an automobile accident, a stroke, a gunshot wound, suicide, or a severe head injury. Most hearts come from those who die before age forty-five. Donor organs are located through the United Network for Organ Sharing (UNOS).

Not enough organs are available for transplant. At any given time, 3,500 to 4,000 patients are waiting for a heart or heart-lung transplant. A patient may wait months for a transplant. More than 25 percent do not live long enough. Yet, only a fraction of those who could donate organs actually do.

Does a person lead a normal life after a transplant?

After a heart or heart-lung transplant, patients must take several medications. The most important are those to keep the body from rejecting the transplant. These medications, which must be taken for life, can cause significant side effects, including hypertension, fluid retention, tremors, excessive hair growth, and possible kidney damage. To combat these problems, additional drugs are often prescribed.

A transplanted heart functions differently from the old one. Because the nerves leading to the heart are cut during the operation, the transplanted heart beats faster (about 100 to 110 beats per minute) than the normal heart (70 beats per minute). The new heart also responds more slowly to exercise and doesn't increase its rate as quickly as before.

A patient's prognosis depends on many factors, including age, general health, and response to the transplant. Recent figures show that 73 percent of heart transplant patients live at least three years after surgery. Nearly 30 percent of patients return to work. Many patients enjoy swimming, cycling, running, or other sports.

As noted, 65 percent of patients who receive combined heart-lung transplants survive at least one year. Fifty percent live at least three years.

What are the risks from transplants?

The most common causes of death following a transplant are infection or rejection of the heart. Patients with transplants must take drugs to prevent transplant rejection. Unfortunately, these same drugs may cause kidney damage, high blood pressure, osteoporosis (a severe thinning of the bones, which can cause fractures), and lymphoma (a type of cancer that affects cells of the immune system). They also increase risk of serious infections.

Coronary artery disease (atherosclerosis) is a problem that develops in about 40 percent of the patients who receive transplants. Normally, patients with this disease experience chest pain or other symptoms when their hearts are under stress. This is called angina and is an early warning sign of a blocked heart artery. However, transplant patients may have no early pain symptoms of a blockage building up because they have no sensations in their new hearts.

Thirty to fifty percent of patients who receive a heart-lung transplant develop bronchiolitis obliterans, in which there are obstructive changes in the airways of the lungs.

What does rejection mean?

The body's immune system protects the body from infection. Cells of the immune system move throughout the body, checking for anything that looks foreign or different from the body's own cells. Immune cells recognize the transplanted organ(s) as different from the rest of the body and attempt to destroy it—this is called rejection. If left alone, the immune system would damage the cells of a new heart and eventually destroy it. In a heart-lung transplant, immune cells may also destroy healthy lung tissue.

To prevent rejection, patients receive immunosuppressants, drugs that suppress the immune system so that the new organ(s) is not damaged. Because rejection can occur anytime after a transplant, immunosuppressive drugs are given to patients the day before their transplant and thereafter for the rest of their lives. To avoid complications, patients must strictly adhere to their drug regimen. The main drugs now being used are cyclosporine, azathioprine, mycophenolate, tacrolimus, sirolimus, and prednisone. Researchers are working on safer, more effective immunosuppressants for future testing.

Unfortunately, even with multiple drug therapy, rejection cannot always be prevented. Many experts believe that the widespread coronary artery disease seen in many heart transplants, and the bronchiolitis obliterans seen in many lung transplants, are a form of slow rejection that is not completely controlled by current medications.

Doctors must balance the dose of immunosuppressive drugs so that a patient's transplanted organ(s) is protected, but his or her immune system is not completely shut down. Without an active enough immune system, a patient can easily develop severe infections. For this reason, medications are also prescribed to fight any infections. During the period immediately after transplantation, when antirejection drugs are given at very high doses, transplant patients may need to remain in isolation to prevent them from catching infections from other people. Even when the doses of immunosuppressive drugs are later tapered down, patients remain unusually susceptible to infection, and must seek medical care if any sign of illness occurs.

To carefully monitor transplant patients for signs of heart rejection, small pieces of the transplanted organ are removed for inspection under a microscope. Called a biopsy, this procedure involves advancing a thin tube called a catheter through a vein to the heart. At the end of the catheter is a bioptome, a tiny instrument used to snip off a piece of tissue. If the biopsy shows damaged cells, the dose and kind of immunosuppressive drug may be changed. Biopsies of the heart muscle are usually performed weekly for the first three to six weeks after surgery, then every three months for the first year, and then yearly thereafter.

How much do transplants cost?

The estimated first-year cost for a heart transplant is $391,800. In most cases these costs are paid by private insurance companies. More than 80 percent of commercial insurers and 97 percent of Blue Cross/Blue Shield plans offer coverage for heart transplants. Medicaid programs in thirty-three states and the District of Columbia also reimburse for transplants. Heart transplants are covered by Medicare for Medicare-eligible patients if the operation is performed at an approved center.

Approximately 70 percent of commercial insurance companies and 92 percent of Blue Cross/Blue Shield plans cover heart-lung transplants. Medicaid coverage for heart-lung transplants is available in twenty states. Estimated first-year cost for a heart-lung transplant is $504,400.

What will transplants be like in five to ten years?

Hospitals nationwide are trying to set up a better system for distributing organs to patients in need. Researchers are looking for easier methods to monitor rejection to replace the regular biopsies that are needed now. Work is progressing to find immunosuppressive drugs with fewer long-term side effects so that coronary artery disease development and lung destruction may be prevented.

Chapter 80

Total Artificial Heart

The total artificial heart (TAH) is still in its early stages of development. It is being designed to replace the failing hearts of patients, as there are not enough donor hearts for everyone who needs a heart transplant. According to the American Heart Association, there are at any given time about 4,000 patients in the United States waiting for a heart transplant. Only about 2,200 donor hearts become available each year.

What is a total artificial heart?

Still being developed, a total artificial heart (TAH) is an experimental device designed to replace a patient's own failing heart. By eliminating the need for a heart transplant, TAHs could solve the problem of 4,000 people in the United States for whom a suitable heart donor cannot be found in time. There are two types of TAHs: a pneumatic total artificial heart, which uses a pneumatic (air-based) motor, and an electrical total artificial heart, which uses an electrical motor.

Currently, a TAH would be considered for patients meeting the following criteria:

- Has end-stage heart failure with a life expectancy of no more than thirty days

- Is ineligible for a donor heart transplant

- Has no available treatments remaining

What is the history and status of the total artificial heart?

The first total artificial heart kept an animal alive for ninety minutes in 1957. Pioneering attempts were made with human patients by the Texas Heart Institute in 1969 and then again in 1982. Unfortunately, the human patients survived for only a limited period of time, particularly because the TAHs required tubes to remain connected through the skin. As a result, there was a greater risk of infection and blood clots.

Researchers went back to the drawing board to improve on the TAH model. On July 2, 2001, a human patient received the first self-contained, fully implantable artificial heart. The device, about the size of a grapefruit, had no tubes or wires going through skin. The patient died on November 30, 2001. However, the patient's progress during those four months exceeded physicians' expectations. As of October 2002, seven individuals had received a TAH. One patient is alive and making progress six months after the implantation.

Researchers are optimistic that the total artificial heart will one day be as common as pacemakers are today, and the results of both laboratory studies and animal studies have been promising.

About HeartCenterOnline

HeartCenterOnline is a cardiovascular specialized health care website providing tools to help patients and their families better understand the complex nature of heart-related conditions, treatments, and preventive care. The website includes a library of physician-edited patient education information, interactive health-tracking tools, and an online cardiovascular community for patients, their families and other site visitors.

HeartCenterOnline
One South Ocean Boulevard, Suite 201
Boca Raton, FL 33432
http://www.heartcenteronline.com

Part Seven

Cardiovascular Concerns for Women

Chapter 81

Facts about Women and Heart Disease

Women and Heart Attack

If you're a woman, you may not believe you're as vulnerable to a heart attack as men—but you are. Women account for nearly half of all heart attack deaths. Heart disease is the number one killer of both women and men.

There are differences in how women and men respond to a heart attack. Women are less likely than men to believe they're having a heart attack and more likely to delay in seeking emergency treatment.

Further, women tend to be about ten years older than men when they have a heart attack. They are more likely to have other conditions, such as diabetes, high blood pressure, and congestive heart failure—making it all the more vital that they get proper treatment fast.

Heart Attack Warning Signs

Women should learn the heart attack warning signs. These are:

* Pain or discomfort in the center of the chest.

"Women and Heart Attack" is reprinted from "Women and Heart Attack," National Heart, Lung, and Blood Institute, 2001. "Heart Disease Statistics for Women" is reprinted from "Women and Heart Disease Fact Sheet," © 2004 National Coalition for Women with Heart Disease. Reprinted with permission. For additional information, visit www.womenheart.org.

- Pain or discomfort in other areas of the upper body, including the arms, back, neck, jaw, or stomach.

- Other symptoms, such as a shortness of breath, breaking out in a cold sweat, nausea, or lightheadedness.

As with men, women's most common heart attack symptom is chest pain or discomfort. Yet women are somewhat more likely than men to experience some of the other common symptoms, particularly shortness of breath, nausea or vomiting, and back or jaw pain.

If you feel heart attack symptoms, do not delay. Remember, minutes matter! Do not wait for more than a few minutes—five minutes at most—to call 9-1-1. Your family will benefit most if you seek fast treatment.

Heart Disease Statistics for Women

Prevalence

- 8,000,000 American women are currently living with heart disease—10 percent of women ages 45–64 and 25 percent age 65 and over.

- 6,000,000 of women today have a history of heart attack or angina or both. Nearly 13 percent of women age 45 and over have had a heart attack.

- 435,000 American women have heart attacks each year; 83,000 are under age 65 and 9,000 are under age 45. Their average age is 70.4.

- 4,000,000 women suffer from angina, and 47,000 of them were hospitalized in 1999.

Mortality

- Heart disease is the leading cause of death of American women and kills 32 percent of them.

- 43 percent of deaths in American women, or nearly 500,000, are caused by cardiovascular disease (heart disease and stroke) each year.

- 267,000 women die each year from heart attacks, which kill six times as many women as breast cancer.

- 31, 837 women die each year of congestive heart failure, or 62.6 percent of all heart failure deaths.

At-Risk

- The age-adjusted rate of heart disease for African American women is 72 percent higher than for white women, while African American women ages 55–64 are twice as likely as white women to have a heart attack and 35 percent more likely to suffer from coronary artery disease.

- Women who smoke risk having a heart attack 19 years earlier than nonsmoking women.

- Women with diabetes are two to three times more likely to have heart attacks.

- High blood pressure is more common in women taking oral contraceptives, especially in obese women.

- 39 percent of white women, 57 percent of black women, 57 percent of Hispanic women, and 49 percent of Asian/Pacific Islander women are sedentary and get no leisure time physical activity.

- 23 percent of white women, 38 percent of black women, and 36 percent of Mexican American women are obese.

Compared with Men

- 38 percent of women and 25 percent of men will die within one year of a first recognized heart attack.

- 35 percent of women and 18 percent of men heart attack survivors will have another heart attack within six years.

- 46 percent of women and 22 percent of men heart attack survivors will be disabled with heart failure within six years.

- Women are almost twice as likely as men to die after bypass surgery.

- Women are less likely than men to receive beta-blockers, ACE inhibitors, or even aspirin after a heart attack.

- More women than men die of heart disease each year, yet women receive only:
  - 33 percent of angioplasties, stents, and bypass surgeries
  - 28 percent of implantable defibrillators and
  - 36 percent of open-heart surgeries
- Women comprise only 25 percent of participants in all heart-related research studies.

Sources

National Center on Health Statistics; National Heart, Lung and Blood Institute; and American Heart Association's 2002 Heart and Stroke Statistical Update, which may be viewed online at: http://www .americanheart.org/downloadable/heart/1014832809466101319099 0123HS_State_02.pdf.

Chapter 82

Effects of Heart Disease
on Childbearing

Mitral Valve Prolapse

This is a valve abnormality that occurs in about 10 percent of "normal" young adults, especially young women. You may have mitral valve prolapse (MVP) that's first recognized during pregnancy. Most cases of this disorder in young women are mild, and there should be no increased risk to you or your baby. However, in some cases of MVP where the valve leaks, the strain that pregnancy adds to your heart could cause problems. That's why regular checkups by your cardiologist during pregnancy are important.

Congenital Heart Disease

Women who have congenital heart disease are born with a defect in the structure of the heart or the large blood vessels that carry blood to and from the heart. In general, most women with a congenital heart defect (especially those who've had corrective surgery) can look forward to having children. However, the outcome of pregnancy can be affected by many factors including the type of heart defect, the severity of symptoms, the presence of high blood pressure in the lungs (pulmonary hypertension), and the type of prior surgery and any remaining heart or lung disease. All risk factors must be carefully weighed for a woman with congenital heart disease who is considering pregnancy; each case must be individually evaluated.

If you have congenital heart disease, you should have a full evaluation by a pediatric cardiologist or internal medicine cardiologist who is very familiar with your condition. It's important to determine the nature and severity of your heart defect before becoming pregnant. Usually this will include a physical examination, electrocardiogram (ECG), chest x-rays, an echocardiogram, and possibly other tests such as an exercise test. Before you have these tests, tell your doctor if there's any chance that you're already pregnant. After a full evaluation, your cardiologist can advise you of the risk that you and your baby might encounter during and after the pregnancy. If you have a correctable defect, you might be advised to have surgery before becoming pregnant.

Pregnancy isn't advised if there's very high blood pressure in the lung blood vessels (pulmonary hypertension). There's a high risk of maternal death. Other heart defects that carry a high risk of maternal or fetal death during pregnancy include:

- severe unoperated aortic valve stenosis (a narrowed valve that prevents blood from being pumped out of the heart into the aorta),

- severe unoperated coarctation of the aorta (a narrowed area in the aorta that prevents blood from flowing from the upper body to the lower body), and

- cyanotic heart defects (unrepaired defects that cause blueness).

If you have congenital heart disease, once you become pregnant you'll require careful attention from a team of physicians skilled in prenatal care, including cardiologists and obstetricians. This attention, with more frequent visits and often more frequent diagnostic testing, is designed to decrease the risks to you and your baby during pregnancy. With this kind of management, most women with congenital heart disease can expect to safely deliver a healthy baby. You may be asked to deliver your baby at a hospital that specializes in complex pregnancy and newborn care.

Rheumatic Heart Disease

Rheumatic fever results from a streptococcal infection. The effects of rheumatic fever in some cases cause lasting damage to one or more of the heart valves (rheumatic heart disease). This damage might not be apparent for several years. Later, however, the inflammation of the heart valves that occurred during the earlier illness produces scarring. This scarring prevents the valves from opening or closing properly, and the normal flow of blood through the heart is hindered. When there's additional strain on the heart, such as during pregnancy, special medical care is necessary.

Prosthetic Heart Valves

If you have an artificial (prosthetic) heart valve, you and your baby have an increased risk during pregnancy. Discuss these risks with your doctor before you become pregnant. If you have a mechanical valve (made of metal or plastic with a moving ball or disc), and it's necessary for you to take blood-thinning medicine such as Coumadin or Dicumarol to prevent blood clots from forming on the valve, this medicine can cause damage to your baby. Before you become pregnant, your physician may want to change your medicine to one called heparin. Heparin doesn't affect the baby and works well as a blood-thinning medicine. It's given by injection. You or your family may have to learn how to give it twice a day.

If you have a nonmechanical or tissue valve, blood-thinning medicines usually aren't required. However, as with mechanical valves, a regular follow-up by your doctor during the pregnancy is necessary.

Marfan Syndrome

The Marfan syndrome is an inherited disorder of connective tissue that can affect many parts of the body, including the heart. The degree of heart involvement varies in this condition. Many doctors feel that if you have the Marfan syndrome with a dilated aortic root, you should avoid pregnancy. The reason is that the aortic root could rupture during the stress of labor, posing a high risk to both you and your baby. Any woman with the Marfan syndrome who does become pregnant should be watched closely by her cardiologist.

Other Conditions

If you have high blood pressure, certain kinds of irregular heartbeats, cardiomyopathy (a dilated heart), or other cardiac ailments, your risk of developing heart problems during pregnancy is greater than that of a woman with no heart disease. Also, some medications used to treat these disorders can affect your baby. Consult your doctor about your own and your baby's care during pregnancy.

Chapter 83

Birth Control Pill Linked to Heart Disease Protein

Birth control pills appear to be associated with increased levels of a protein linked to heart disease. In a newly reported study, young women who took birth control pills had twice as much C-reactive protein in their blood as a similar group of women who did not use birth control pills.

The findings, while preliminary, could help explain a reported increase in heart disease among birth control pill users. C-reactive protein (CRP) is produced in the liver in response to inflammation. Chronically high CRP has been linked to heart disease, and inflammation is believed to play a key role in narrowing and hardening of the arteries.

"It is possible that oral contraceptive use promotes inflammation," researcher Darlene M. Dreon, DrPH, of Galileo Pharmaceuticals, tells WebMD. "Hormone replacement therapy has also been linked to higher CRP levels in postmenopausal women." All of this suggests that estrogen hormones may increase inflammation, she adds.

Dreon and colleagues measured CRP levels in blood samples from thirty premenopausal women. Eighteen of the women were taking birth control pills and twelve were not. All of the women were healthy nonsmokers who were not obese. Those on birth control pills took low-dose progestin preparations similar to those most often prescribed today. The findings were reported in San Diego at the annual meeting of the American Physiological Society.

Plasma CRP levels were twice as high among the birth control pill users, even though other risk factors for heart disease were similar to those seen in the women not on birth control pills. However, CRP levels in both groups were considered in the normal range, leading the researchers to conclude that more research is needed to determine the clinical significance of the findings.

"We know nothing about what CRP levels mean in younger populations that aren't at risk for coronary artery disease," Dreon says. "This was a small study, and it certainly doesn't prove cause and effect."

Gynecologist and contraceptive specialist Trent MacKay, MD, agrees. He says the fact that both groups had normal CRP levels suggests that, for younger women at least, birth control pill use is of little clinical significance in terms of heart disease risk. MacKay is special assistant for obstetrics and gynecology in the Contraception and Reproductive Health Branch of the National Institutes of Health.

The only women who clearly need to worry about birth control pill use and heart disease risk, he says, are those who are over the age of thirty-five and are also heavy smokers.

"For everyone else, the association between oral contraceptive use and heart disease is weak, at best," he tells WebMD. "Women under the age of thirty-five are not at particularly increased risk, even if they smoke. The fact is, cardiovascular disease is a disease of aging, and aging women do not use oral contraceptives."

Chapter 84

Hormone Therapy and Coronary Heart Disease

Estrogen Plus Progestin and Risk of Coronary Heart Disease

In the August 7, 2003, issue of the *New England Journal of Medicine*, WHI [Women's Health Initiative] published the final coronary heart disease (CHD) results for the Estrogen plus Progestin (E+P) study. The findings suggest that E+P does not protect the heart and may even increase the risk of coronary heart disease (CHD).

In final analyses, E+P use was associated with:

- A 24 percent overall increase in the risk of CHD

- An 81 percent increase in the risk of CHD in the first year after starting E+P

Women who had higher baseline low-density lipoprotein (LDL) cholesterol levels at the beginning of the study were at particularly

"Estrogen Plus Progestin and Risk of Coronary Heart Disease" and "Frequently Asked Questions," Women's Health Initiative (WHI), August 2003. WHI was established by National Institutes of Health (NIH) to address the most common causes of death, disability, and impaired quality of life in postmenopausal women. The WHI Program Office is located within the Office of the Director of the National Heart, Lung, and Blood Institute (NHLBI). The WHI website, coordinated by the Fred Hutchinson Cancer Research Center (FHCRC), is available online at www.whi.org.

high risk of CHD with E+P use. No other factors significantly changed the risk of CHD while using E+P.

In conclusion, E+P does not protect the heart and may increase the risk of CHD among postmenopausal women, especially during the first year after beginning hormones.

Frequently Asked Questions

How are the latest results on coronary heart disease (CHD) different from the July 2002 report?

The present report (*New England Journal of Medicine*, August 7, 2003 issue) provides updated analyses of CHD-related health events through July 7, 2002 (the earlier report included health events through April 2002). It includes a detailed review of individual health events, including CHD-related health problems like heart attack, angina, acute coronary syndrome, and congestive heart failure. It also presents findings for smaller groups of women with different health characteristics.

What are the primary findings of this report?

Estrogen plus progestin (E+P) does not protect the heart and may even increase the risk of CHD in generally healthy postmenopausal women. Overall, there was a 24 percent higher risk of CHD among women in the E+P study compared to women taking placebo (six extra cases of CHD per ten thousand women per year). The greater risk of CHD was highest during the first year after starting hormone therapy (an 81 percent increase). E+P had no major effect on the risk of angina, coronary bypass surgery, angioplasty, or congestive heart failure.

Which women are at particularly high or low risk of CHD on E+P?

Women with higher LDL cholesterol levels at the beginning of the study had a particularly high risk of CHD with E+P, but no other factors significantly changed the risk of CHD while using E+P.

What is the conclusion of the study in terms of E+P and CHD?

E+P should not be started or continued for the prevention of heart disease. Women should consider this information when making decisions about E+P use.

Do these results apply to women in Estrogen-Alone study?

We do not yet know to what extent these findings may apply to Estrogen-Alone study participants. That part of the study (for women who have had a hysterectomy) is continuing as the balance of risks and benefits is not yet clear. This study is scheduled to be complete in 2005.

What type of hormone treatment did women in the E+P study take?

Women randomized (assigned by chance) to active hormones were taking one tablet containing conjugated equine estrogens (0.625 mg) and medroxyprogesterone acetate (2.5 mg) each day (Prempro™). When WHI first began, this was the most commonly prescribed menopausal hormone therapy in the United States for women with a uterus.

Chapter 85

Research on Women and Heart Disease

Coronary heart disease (CHD) is the number one cause of death among U.S. women. The survival rate following a heart attack is lower among women than men. Recent research indicates several possible reasons, including differences in diagnosis, treatment, symptoms, reaction to drugs, and age at the onset of the disease.

Introduction

Coronary heart disease (CHD) was responsible for one of every five deaths in the United States in 1997. Long thought of as primarily affecting men, we now know that CHD also affects a substantial number of women. More U.S. women die from heart disease than any other cause. Experts estimate that one in two women will die of heart disease or stroke, compared with one in twenty-five women who will die of breast cancer.

Current statistics reveal significant differences between men and women in survival following a heart attack. For example, 42 percent of women who have heart attacks die within one year, compared with 24 percent of men.

The reasons for this are not well understood. The explanation accepted by many is that women tend to get heart disease later in life than do men and are more likely to have coexisting, chronic conditions. However, research also has shown that women may not be diagnosed or

Reprinted from "Women and Heart Disease," Agency for Healthcare Research and Quality, AHRQ Publication No. 01-P016, September 2001.

treated as aggressively as men, and their symptoms may be very different from those of men who are having a heart attack. In addition, new studies indicate that men and women react to drugs prescribed for heart disease and other conditions quite differently—and that drugs that may help men can have serious adverse effects in women.

Research on Women and Heart Disease

The Agency for Healthcare Research and Quality (AHRQ) supports a vigorous women's health research program, including research focused on CHD in women.

AHRQ-supported projects are addressing women's access to:

- Quality health care services
- Accurate diagnoses
- Appropriate referrals for procedures
- Optimal use of proven therapies

AHRQ researchers also are concerned about CHD in vulnerable populations, including racial and ethnic minorities. Many studies have found that there are disparities along racial and ethnic lines in the care received by patients with CHD, particularly women. For example, data show CHD death rates are 34 percent higher for black women than for white women, and that death rates have declined more rapidly for white women than for black women.

Following are examples of current and completed research projects focused on CHD and women.

Research in Progress

Data are being gathered for an evidence report on differences between men and women in response to procedures to diagnose and manage heart disease. A research team at the University of California, San Francisco-Stanford Evidence-Based Practice Center is undertaking a two-part review of the current literature assessing whether there are sex-based differences in response to standard practices and procedures for diagnosis and management of CHD in men and women. (The evidence report topic was nominated by a coalition of organizations led by the American Heart Association and is cosponsored by the National Institutes of Health's Office of Research on Women's Health.)

Researchers are investigating the reasons for differences related to race and sex in the use of cardiac tests and procedures. Researchers at Boston's Brigham and Women's Hospital are conducting a study of 3,400 patients (about half are women) with chest pain. They are identifying reasons for previously documented differences related to race and sex in the use of tolerance tests, coronary angiography, bypass surgery, and coronary angioplasty. (Paula A. Johnson, Principal Investigator [AHRQ grant HS08302].)

Researchers are using historical data to compare the clinical characteristics and treatment of men and women who suffer a heart attack. These researchers are examining medical record data to compare the duration of coronary heart disease, symptoms, diagnostic evaluations and referrals, and the assessment and treatment of modifiable risk factors for coronary disease for ten years prior to the first heart attack in men and women. (Barbara P. Yawn, Principal Investigator [AHRQ grant HS10239].)

Recent Findings

Researchers find an association between heart attack outcomes and a woman's age. Heart attack mortality is higher for women than men before age sixty, but the opposite is true for women and men older than age seventy-nine. Age was a significant predictor of death even after adjustment for numerous demographic and clinical characteristics of patients and the treatments they received. Nonbiological factors may play a role, including behavioral, psychological, and social factors such as smoking, adherence to medication regimens, depression, social isolation, low income, and emotional stress. (Ayanian JZ. *Ann Intern Med* 2001;134[3]:239–41.)

Women and minorities often have atypical symptoms when suffering a heart attack or angina. Emergency room doctors miss diagnosing about 2 percent of patients with heart attacks or unstable angina because they do not have chest pain or other symptoms typically associated with a heart attack. When these patients are mistakenly sent home from the ER, they are twice as likely to die from their heart problems as similar patients who are admitted to the hospital. The patients in this study who were misdiagnosed tended to be women under the age of fifty-five or minorities who reported shortness of breath as their chief symptom—instead of chest pain—and to have apparently normal electrocardiograms. (Pope JH, Aufderheide TP,

Ruthazer R et al. *New Engl J Med* 2000;342[16]:1163–70 [AHRQ grant HS07360].)

Black women are much less likely than men or white women to receive life-saving therapies for heart attacks. Most of the one million U.S. patients who suffer a heart attack each year are candidates for reperfusion therapy—either thrombolytic (clot-busting) drugs or primary angioplasty. In a study of nearly twenty-seven thousand Medicare beneficiaries who met the strict criteria for reperfusion therapy between February 1994 and July 1995, only 44 percent of eligible black women received the treatment, compared with 59 percent of white men, 50 percent of black men, and 56 percent of white women. (Canto JG, Allison JJ, Kiefe CI et al. *New Engl J Med* 2000;342[15]:1094–1100 [AHRQ grants HS08843 and HS09446].)

Men and women differ in their reports of angina and symptoms of heart disease. Coronary artery disease risk is higher in certain women with angina, according to researchers who examined correlates of angina in men and women aged thirty-five to fifty-five. This is particularly true for women who have a poor cardiovascular risk profile and symptoms such as shortness of breath. (Nicholson A, White IR, Macfarlane P et al. *J Clin Epidemiol* 1999;52[4]:337–46 [AHRQ grant HS06516].)

Black women are less likely than men or other women to be referred for cardiac catheterization. In this study, blacks and women, particularly black women, had statistically significant lower odds for being referred for cardiac catheterization than whites and men. The study involved 720 primary care doctors and eight patient actors (two each black men, black women, white men, and white women) who used the same scripts to report the same symptoms, wore identical gowns, used similar hand gestures, and had the same insurance and professions. (Schulman KA, Berlin JA, Harless W et al. *N Engl J Med* 1999;340:618–26 [AHRQ grant HS07315].)

Women are 20 percent more likely than men to die in the hospital following a heart attack. This study of over twelve thousand women and men treated for heart attack in Seattle area hospitals between 1988 and 1994 found that even after accounting for differences between men and women in cardiac procedures, age, and health factors, the women were still 20 percent more likely to die than the men. Women also were less likely than men to receive clot-busting (thrombolytic) therapy promptly or undergo coronary angiography, angioplasty, or bypass surgery. (Maynard C, Every NR, Martin JS et al. *Arch Intern Med* 1997;157:1379–84 [Cardiac Arrhythmia Patient Outcomes Research Team (PORT), HS08362].)

Women receive less aggressive treatment than men after a heart attack and are more likely to die while in the hospital. This study found that women continue to lag behind men in both treatment received and outcomes. Differences in age and severity of illness did not explain the variations seen in this study, which involved more than fourteen thousand patients admitted for heart attacks to one hundred U.S. hospitals in 1991. (Iezzoni LI, Ash AS, Schwartz M, and Mackierman YD. *Med Care* 1997;35[2]:158–71 [AHRQ grant HS06742].)

Many patients with heart attack symptoms delay going to the hospital. In this study, 40 percent of patients arrived at the hospital more than six hours after the onset of heart attack symptoms. The first six hours after symptoms begin are critical,. It is during this time that thrombolytic therapy can be most effective in preventing further heart damage. Women, older patients, and those with a history of hypertension were most likely to wait. Time of day also made a difference; the highest risk of delay was from 6 P.M. to 6 A.M. (Gurwitz JH, McLaughlin YJ, Willison DJ et al. *Ann Intern Med* 1997;126[8]: 593–99 [AHRQ grant HS07357].)

Likelihood of heart attack in symptomatic patients who go to the ER is twice as great for men as for women. Generally, women who arrive at ER with chest pain or other heart attack symptoms are much less likely than men with similar symptoms to actually be having a heart attack. (Zucker DR, Griffith JL, Beshansky JR, and Selker HP. *J Gen Intern Med* 1997;12:79–87 [AHRQ grants HS07360 and HS00060].)

Among patients who go to the ER with heart attack symptoms, women usually are older and have more coexisting illnesses than men. In this study of nearly eleven thousand older patients (about half women) who arrived at the ER with acute cardiac symptoms, women had more hypertension (55 percent vs. 46 percent) and diabetes (23 percent vs. 17 percent) than men but had suffered fewer previous heart attacks (21 percent vs. 29 percent). The women also had more heart damage than men. (Coronado BE, Griffith JL, Beshansky JR, and Selker HP. *J Am Coll Cardiol* 1997;29:1490–96 [AHRQ grants HS00060 and HS07360].)

Women and the elderly are less likely than men to receive life-saving drugs for heart attacks. Medications recommended by the American Heart Association for treating heart disease are underused in elderly patients and women. After adjusting for age and hospital type, women in this study were less likely than men to be treated with aspirin, thrombolytic agents, beta blockers, or lidocaine. (McLaughlin TJ, Soumerai SB, Willison DJ et al. *Arch Intern Med* 1996;156:799–805 [AHRQ grant HS07357].)

Women are more likely than men to die or require follow-up bypass surgery after coronary angioplasty. Although angioplasty is nearly 90 percent successful in opening blocked arteries for both men and women, women have a 1.6 times greater risk of dying than men, and more women (5.3 percent) than men (4.5 percent) undergo bypass surgery or suffer a heart attack following angioplasty. The researchers examined data on 12,232 angioplasty patients treated between 1989 and 1993. (*Circulation* 1996;94[5] [Suppl II]:99–104 [Ischemic Heart Disease PORT, AHRQ grant HS06503].)

Women do not fare as well as men in some treatments for coronary artery disease. Significant clinical manifestations of coronary artery disease (CAD) are seen in one of every ten women by age sixty. CAD is the culprit in most cases of ischemic heart disease, a condition in which there is an insufficient flow of blood to the heart and, consequently, a high risk of heart attack. This five-year project studied the effectiveness of various surgical and nonsurgical treatments for ischemic heart disease in both men and women. (Outcome Assessment Program for Ischemic Heart Disease: Final Report of the Patient Outcomes Research Team [NTIS PB98-156557], Elizabeth R. DeLong, Ph.D., Principal Investigator [AHRQ grant HS06503]. This item may be purchased from the National Technical Information Service [NTIS]. Call 800-553-6847 for more information.)

Chapter 86

New Marker Linked with Heart Disease in Women

A protein called serum amyloid alpha (SAA) has been linked with existing heart disease in women, and higher protein levels were associated with severe coronary artery disease, according to today's issue of *Circulation: Journal of the American Heart Association*.

Researchers compared the predictive value of SAA to that of C-reactive protein (CRP). They found that while high levels of either can predict a woman's risk for future heart attack, only SAA was linked to existing heart disease.

This is one of several reports from the Women's Ischemia Syndrome Evaluation (WISE) study published today. The WISE study, partly funded by the National Heart, Lung, and Blood Institute, examined the nature and scope of gender differences in symptoms, detection, and treatment of chronic and acute cardiac ischemia. CRP and SAA are inflammatory markers, so they rise when inflammation is present. Inflammation has been associated with more of a heart attack, said B. Delia Johnson, Ph.D., lead author of the paper.

"Serum amyloid alpha and C-reactive protein strongly and independently predicted future cardiovascular events," said Johnson, an epidemiologist and research associate at the University of Pittsburgh's Graduate School of Public Health. "However, CRP did not predict whether a woman had existing significant coronary disease, while SAA showed a moderate association."

Johnson and her colleagues studied angiography results from 705 of the WISE women. An angiography is a video, taken through a catheter, which shows how an injected dye flows through the vessels of the heart. It detects blocked coronary arteries. Participants' median age was fifty-eight; and all had CRP and SAA levels measured when they entered the WISE study.

Women were split into three groups, or terciles, based on their SAA or CRP levels. The researchers found that the following had coronary artery disease (CAD): 29 percent of the women with the lowest SAA levels; 36 percent of women with SAA levels in the middle tercile; and 44 percent in the highest tercile. The average severity of CAD also increased as SAA levels increased. Average severity score was 12.8 in the lowest SAA tercile, 14.2 in the middle tercile, and 15.6 in the highest tercile.

CRP levels did not show differences in CAD prevalence or severity across terciles. SAA levels were more strongly related to the presence of significant artery disease than CRP.

The women were followed for about three years. Among the 686 women for whom outcome data were available, 117 (17 percent) suffered a cardiovascular event, which included heart attacks, strokes, and congestive heart failure. Forty-one of these women died. The three-year risk of a cardiovascular event increased 3.2 percent for each increase of 1 milligram per deciliter (mg/dL) of SAA. Johnson said they found a similar relationship between CRP levels and risk of a cardiovascular event.

As people age, heart arteries develop fatty deposits in their walls called plaques. These plaques can eventually narrow vessels to the point where significant coronary artery disease exists. Most heart attacks result when a blood clot forms at a plaque or a plaque ruptures, both of which can block a vessel and shut off blood flow entirely.

Johnson speculated that the two inflammation markers might be a warning of unstable plaques—ones that might soon form clots or rupture, leading to a heart attack or stroke. "The plaque may be loosening, and SAA and CRP may reflect the inflammation associated with the eroding plaque. These proteins may partly contribute to plaque erosion."

In another report from WISE, researchers found that a collection of heart risk factors called the metabolic syndrome predicted an unusually high risk of a major cardiovascular event during the next four years in women who also had significant coronary artery disease.

"It is clear that, in patients with significant coronary artery disease, the metabolic syndrome puts patients at high risk of having bad cardiac outcomes," said Oscar C. Marroquin, M.D., an assistant professor of medicine at the University of Pittsburgh Medical Center and a co-author.

Metabolic syndrome includes five disorders: abdominal obesity, low HDL ("good") cholesterol, high triglycerides, high blood pressure, and high fasting blood sugar. A diagnosis of metabolic syndrome means a person has three or more of the five symptoms.

Marroquin and his colleagues reviewed data on 755 participants to determine the risk imposed by having both metabolic syndrome and severe coronary artery disease. Women with both conditions had five times the risk of dying within four years compared to women with normal metabolism. "The metabolic syndrome put these women at very high risk—as high as if they had diabetes and coronary heart disease," he said.

In a separate analysis of 780 WISE women, Marroquin and his colleagues found that metabolic syndrome was a stronger predictor of future cardiovascular problems than obesity.

"Patients with the metabolic syndrome did the worst, regardless of their degree of obesity," he said. "Obesity alone did not carry the same risk."

However, this does not mean that obesity is irrelevant to heart health, he said. "Obesity appears to be the precursor to many of the abnormalities that make up the metabolic syndrome."

Co-authors include Kevin E. Kip, Ph.D.; Leslee J. Shaw, Ph.D.; Steven E. Reis, M.D.; Paul M. Ridker, M.D.; Sheryl F. Kelsey, Ph.D.; Carl. J. Pepine, M.D.; Barry L. Sharaf, M.D.; C. Noel Bairey Merz, M.D.; George Sopko, M.D.; Marian B. Olson, M.S.; David E. Kelley, M.D.; and William J. Rogers, M.D.

Part Eight

Cardiovascular Research

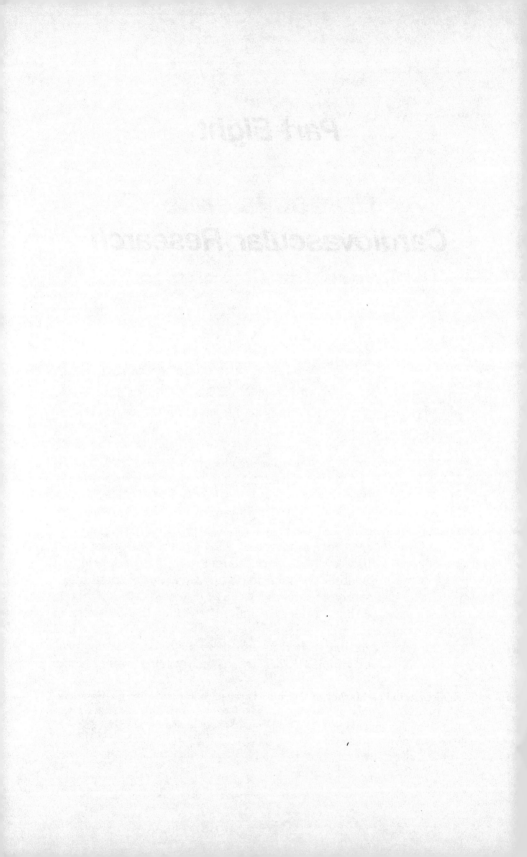

Part Eight

Cardiovascular Research

Chapter 87

Homocysteine:
The New "Bad Boy" of
Vascular Diseases

Homocysteine as Marker of Vascular Disease

A decade ago, only a handful of laboratories worldwide were studying homocysteine. Now this amino acid is rivaling the reputation of elevated blood cholesterol as a major contributor to heart disease and stroke—and to other maladies as well. Early studies at the Jean Mayer USDA Human Nutrition Research Center on Aging (HNRCA) at Tufts University in Boston have greatly contributed to bringing homocysteine research into the mainstream.

"Our work on the role of nutrition in regulating homocysteine had a big impact," says Paul F. Jacques, who heads nutritional epidemiology studies at the center, which is funded by ARS. Before 1993, most cases of high circulating homocysteine were thought to be of genetic origin.

Then Jacques, together with Jacob Selhub, who heads the center's vitamin metabolism research laboratory, center director Irwin Rosenberg, and others, reported that most cases of mildly elevated homocysteine in an elderly population were linked to low vitamin B status. They had looked for an association with B vitamins because the body requires folate, vitamin B_6, and vitamin B_{12} to convert homocysteine to other amino

"Homocysteine as Marker of Vascular Disease" is reprinted from "Homocysteine: The New 'Bad Boy' of Vascular Disease," in the May 2002 issue of *Agricultural Research* magazine, U.S. Department of Agriculture. "DASH Diet Reduces Homocysteine" is reprinted from "Blood Pressure–Lowering DASH Diet Also Reduces Homocysteine," National Heart, Lung, and Blood Institute, National Institutes of Health, August 2000.

acids that aren't toxic to the lining of blood vessels. Blood folate levels appeared to have the most influence on homocysteine levels.

Earlier this year, Jacques, Selhub, and colleagues with the Framingham (Massachusetts) Offspring Study reported on other diet and lifestyle factors that appear to contribute to elevated homocysteine. Their results supported findings by other researchers that high homocysteine concentrations were related to low vitamin B_6 and riboflavin (B_2) intake, to high alcohol and caffeine intake, and to smoking and hypertension.

"Smoking was one of the most noteworthy findings," says Jacques, "because it was so strongly associated with high homocysteine concentrations." He says the study was important because it established that other factors besides low folate influence blood homocysteine concentrations. Since 1998, virtually all grain products sold in the United States have been fortified with folate to prevent spinal abnormalities in fetuses. That has dramatically improved folate status in the U.S. population and halved the prevalence of high homocysteine, Jacques notes. He and colleagues reported this impact of folate fortification in 1999 after analyzing data from the Framingham Offspring Study.

Hard on the Heart and Brain

Meanwhile, evidence had been steadily growing that elevated circulating homocysteine increases the risk of vascular diseases, especially heart attack and stroke. However, a few studies hadn't found an association. So nutritional epidemiologist Martha S. Morris joined HNRCA to look for a link among the vast amount of data collected in the third National Health and Nutrition Examination Survey, NHANES III. She and Selhub's laboratory collaborated with the Centers for Disease Control and Prevention.

The researchers excluded all participants whose medical condition or use of nutritional supplements or estrogen might directly influence homocysteine levels, and they adjusted the analysis to account for differences in age, race, smoking, blood pressure, and other risk factors for vascular disease among participants aged forty years and over.

The result: Men and women who had blood homocysteine levels over 12 micromoles per liter were more than twice as likely to have experienced a heart attack or stroke.

"The new finding," says Morris, "was that blood homocysteine concentrations were not related to heart attack or stroke in women who had not reached menopause, whereas the relationship was strong in men of the same age group." Conversely, the relationship faded among the older men and surfaced among postmenopausal women, Jacques adds. This may explain why some studies found no association. It may differ depending on gender and age.

"The findings support the idea that women may be protected from heart attack and stroke by their high estrogen status," says Morris.

The Helpful Hormone

There was already evidence that estrogen helps keep blood homocysteine concentrations down. Premenopausal women, those who use oral contraceptives, and pregnant women all have lower blood homocysteine than men and postmenopausal women—except those who take estrogen replacement. Yet Morris, Jacques, and their HNRCA colleagues wanted to confirm the thesis by again using data from NHANES III.

"The data provides a unique opportunity to explore the variation of homocysteine concentration with estrogen status in a large, representative sample of the U.S. population," Morris says. She noted that previous studies compared old and young women, so age alone could have accounted for their homocysteine differences.

The researchers analyzed data from nearly 8,400 people ranging in age from seventeen to over seventy years. Last year, they reported that higher estrogen status is associated with a decreased mean serum homocysteine concentration—independent of nutritional status or muscle mass. Muscle mass is a possible contributor because homocysteine is created during production of a substance that aids energy flow in muscle tissue.

"It's a dramatic demonstration of the relationship between estrogen status and homocysteine concentrations," says Morris. "Estrogen may explain the previously reported differences in homocysteine concentrations between males and females."

Brain Function and Folate

Morris, Jacques, and colleagues again turned to NHANES III data on the over-sixty participants to tease out a possible association between elevated homocysteine and memory loss. The amino acid increases risk of stroke, which is a major player in the loss of cognitive function. But the researchers wanted to see if homocysteine or B vitamin status had a more subtle influence on memory.

The B vitamins are involved in the synthesis of chemicals crucial to brain function, explains Morris. Or homocysteine itself might be toxic to nerve cells. Fortunately, the NHANES III included a sensitive test of recall after a short delay—one that can identify individuals with a mild loss of recall.

She says others had found evidence that elevated homocysteine was related to Alzheimer's disease, as well as to poor cognitive function in elderly both with and without dementia. The difference, she explains, is that "people without dementia sometimes can't remember where they left their keys; people with dementia can't remember what keys are for." Perhaps 75 percent of dementia is due to stroke or Alzheimer's disease—which is now thought to develop from minor strokes, Morris says. So the researchers excluded data from people who had reported having a stroke.

While they did find an association between memory loss and elevated homocysteine levels, the survey subjects in the upper half for blood folate levels appeared to be protected from memory loss even if their homocysteine levels were high.

"The take-home message," says Morris, "is to keep your folate levels up." That's easy to do now that grain products are being fortified with the vitamin.

DASH Diet Reduces Homocysteine

The blood pressure-lowering DASH diet also reduces levels of the amino acid homocysteine, according to a National Heart, Lung, and Blood Institute (NHLBI)-funded study. A high level of homocysteine appears to increase the risk of heart disease, stroke, and peripheral vascular disease.

The study appears in the August 22 [2003] issue of *Circulation: Journal of the American Heart Association*.

DASH stands for Dietary Approaches to Stop Hypertension. This new report is based on data from the DASH trial, which found that a diet rich in fruits, vegetables, and low-fat dairy foods and low in saturated fat, total fat, and cholesterol significantly and quickly lowers blood pressure. The diet also included whole grains, poultry, fish, and nuts.

The DASH trial involved four sites and a coordinating center. The homocysteine results come from the Johns Hopkins University site in Baltimore, Maryland.

Homocysteine levels are affected by various factors, including intake of folic acid (or folate) and vitamins B_6 and B_{12}. In the trial, participants followed one of three diets—a control diet similar to what most Americans eat, a diet rich in fruits and vegetables, and the DASH diet. Compared with homocysteine levels of those on the control diet, homocysteine levels of those on the DASH diet were significantly lower, with levels of those on the fruits and vegetables diet being intermediate. Changes in the homocysteine levels were significantly associated with changes in folate levels.

Chapter 88

C-Reactive Protein as a Predictor of Cardiovascular Disease

A simple blood test that could predict risk for heart disease has been getting a lot of hype lately: "A new test could save the lives of millions who don't even know they're in danger," announced *U.S. News & World Report* in a November 2002 cover story. Other reports were equally glowing: "New Test for Risk of Heart Disease; Study Shifts Focus from Cholesterol" said the *Washington Post* in a nationally distributed story; the Associated Press declared, "Researchers Find a New Enemy of the Heart."

What's creating all the buzz is a test for a substance called C-reactive protein, or CRP. It's not a new test; C-reactive protein was first identified in the 1930s. Nor is it yet the definitive breakthrough in diagnosing risk for coronary artery disease in every patient, says cardiologist David S. Marks, MD, associate professor of medicine at the Medical College of Wisconsin and director of the Cardiac Catheterization Laboratory at Froedtert & Medical College Clinics. Dr. Marks has been ordering the CRP test on selected patients for several years.

The CRP test, which has been used to detect areas of acute inflammation from diseases such as rheumatoid arthritis and rheumatic fever, is increasingly being utilized in cardiac care. "Patients should know that the C-reactive protein test is not actually a diagnostic test for coronary artery disease but rather a nonspecific marker for inflammation," he says. Even if the test results are positive for inflammation, he notes, the inflammation could be triggered by other factors such as arthritis or an infection; or it could signal the potential for future heart disease.

Some researchers think inflammation can trigger heart attacks by affecting the walls of diseased blood vessels. "There's no question that C-reactive protein has moved beyond a test for the presence of rheumatic disease," says Dr. Marks. "We keep learning more about the impact of inflammation and heart disease, but we still don't know if the C-reactive protein mechanism has a causative effect."

Cautious Guidelines for Testing

Based on current information, Dr. Marks says not every middle-aged patient should be tested for CRP, "but they should ask their cardiologist or primary care doctor about it."

In a January 2003 article published in the medical journal *Circulation*, the American Heart Association (AHA) and the Centers for Disease Control and Prevention (CDC) cautiously recommended limited, optional testing for C-reactive protein for patients at some risk for heart disease over the next ten years based on such factors as age, high cholesterol, and high blood pressure—but only if test results will help doctors decide whether the patients need treatment. Treatment typically includes drugs to lower blood pressure and cholesterol, plus lifestyle changes—quitting smoking, eating better diets, exercising, and achieving and maintaining an appropriate weight. Dr. Marks has been following those recommendations with his patients.

"If I'm with a patient who has few risk factors for coronary artery disease but has a strong family history for the disease, I might order the C-reactive protein test." If the results are positive, he might start the patient on a preventive program that could include a low-dose aspirin regimen and possibly other drugs, as well as encouraging them to maintain a healthy weight through diet and exercise. "However, if I'm with a patient I already know has coronary artery disease and is taking medication for it and following preventive steps, the CRP test has a different implication.

"It's always a challenge whenever we introduce a new screening test," Dr. Marks says. "The AHA and CDC report was cautious, which reflects the fact that physicians still aren't unanimous in their opinions of the test's value." Some fear that widespread use of the test could result in false positive readings, which could raise patients' anxiety and cost money.

A recent study by Dr. Paul Ridker of Brigham and Women's Hospital in Boston found that half of all heart attacks and strokes occurred in women with seemingly safe cholesterol levels, and that those with high CRP had double the risk of women with low levels.

Prevention Is Still Best

Research into the link between inflammation and heart disease continues. Regardless of the outcome of the research, however, Dr. Marks emphasizes a familiar refrain:

"There's no substitute for good preventive care. We already know a lot about the risks for heart disease—smoking, high blood pressure, obesity, sedentary lifestyle, diabetes. We don't need a test to tell us people with these conditions are at risk. These are all modifiable risks that can be managed through lifestyle changes and medication.

"One risk factor that can't be modified, though, is a family history for heart disease, and the C-reactive protein test can be useful for those patients."

Furthermore, he adds, for patients with established heart disease, the CRP test "may be helpful in showing that the medications those patients are using are effective."

"The important thing is this," Dr. Marks says, "the test for C-reactive protein is definitely part of the armamentarium of the physician, and doctors will be using it more and more. It's not appropriate to test everyone for it right now, but that may change. It doesn't alter what we already know about risks that can be modified by the patient and by medication."

Chapter 89

Can Vitamin E Supplements Help Prevent Cardiovascular Disease?

Antioxidants are natural substances that exist as vitamins, minerals, and other compounds in foods. They are believed to help prevent disease by fighting free radicals, substances that harm the body when left unchecked. Free radicals are formed by normal bodily processes such as breathing, and by environmental contaminants like cigarette smoke. Without adequate amounts of antioxidants, these free radicals travel throughout the body, damaging cells.

Part of this cellular damage leads to one of the major known factors in the development of heart disease, oxidation of cholesterol. Oxidation, meaning the addition of oxygen to low-density lipoproteins (LDL or "bad" cholesterol), contributes to the buildup of fatty plaque on artery walls (atherosclerosis), which can eventually slow or block blood flow to the heart.

Studies Disagree

The potential link between LDL oxidation and antioxidants has led investigators to explore the role of antioxidants and heart disease. Over the years, many studies have been done. However, the designs of some of the studies left their results open to question. For example, some of the studies used too few participants to obtain valid results. Some used doses of vitamin E that were later thought too low. Some had a limited duration of treatment, and others could not determine whether the beneficial results were from the antioxidants or other lifestyle factors.

On the other hand, some of the studies were well designed. Nonetheless, their results differed from one another. Some found benefit in antioxidants. Some didn't. Still others found potential harm from one of the antioxidants, beta carotene.

The media has announced the findings of these conflicting studies with great fanfare. "Take vitamin E to fight heart disease." Or : "Don't take vitamin E," leaving consumers confused about the best way to support their cardiac health.

Clearing the Confusion

Researchers at the Cleveland Clinic decided to clear up the confusion by doing a meta-analysis, an overview study of the best designed, largest studies of antioxidants. A meta-analysis allows investigators to combine the results of many studies, thereby allowing small benefits or harm to be seen that may not have been appreciated in any one study. Their findings were recently published in the prestigious British medical journal *The Lancet*. Here's what they found.

The researchers analyzed results from seven large randomized trials of vitamin E, alone or in combination with other antioxidants, and eight of beta carotene. The doses of vitamin E ranged from 50–800 international units (IU); for beta carotene, the doses were 15–50 milligrams (mg).

Overall, 81,788 patients were included in the vitamin E portion of the meta-analysis and 138,113 in the beta carotene portion. The Cleveland Clinic Foundation (CCF) researchers looked for the effect of antioxidant vitamins on death rates, either from cardiovascular disease or from any other cause ("all-cause mortality").

The Bottom Line

Vitamin E did not provide any benefit in lowering mortality compared to control treatments, and it did not significantly decrease the risk of cardiovascular death or stroke ("cerebrovascular accident"). The lack of any beneficial effect was seen consistently regardless of the doses of vitamins used and the diversity of the patient populations.

Therefore, the CCF researchers conclude that this study does "not support the routine use of vitamin E."

Beta carotene led to small but statistically significant increase in all-cause mortality and a slight increase in cardiovascular death. The researchers call their findings "especially concerning" because beta carotene doses are commonly included in over-the-counter vitamin supplements and multivitamin supplements that have been advocated for widespread use.

The study says that using vitamin supplements that contain beta carotene should be "actively discouraged" because of the increase in the risk of death. They also recommend discontinuing study of beta carotene supplements because of their risk.

Researchers further stated that they do not support the continued use of vitamin E treatment, and they discourage the inclusion of vitamin E in further studies of patients who are known to be at high risk of heart disease.

These findings further strengthen the contention that diet supplements are no substitute for good eating habits, exercise, weight loss, and smoking cessation as a means of minimizing the risk of heart disease.

Antioxidant Foods: A Different Story

Even though supplements did not prove beneficial in avoiding heart problems, foods that are sources of antioxidants are still recommended. There are benefits to getting vitamins in food that don't necessarily occur in supplement form. For example, foods rich in antioxidants may have nutrients such as flavonoids and lycopenes that are not necessarily included in standard oral vitamin supplements. Eating a diet rich in antioxidant-containing foods, such as fruits, vegetables, and whole grains, is linked to a reduced risk of cardiovascular (heart and blood vessels) disease.

Good Food Sources of Antioxidants

Sources of Vitamin E

Best: green leafy vegetables, legumes, nuts, papaya, seeds, and whole grains.

Good: brown rice, oatmeal, soybeans, sweet potatoes, watercress, wheat and wheat germ.

Sources of Beta Carotene

Best sources are dark orange, red, and dark green vegetables and fruits.

National and international dietary recommendations are to eat between five and ten servings of fruit and vegetables daily to ensure adequate intake of disease-fighting antioxidant nutrients.

Reducing Your Risk of Heart Disease

To reduce your risk of heart disease, it remains important to decrease your risk factors using more proven methods than vitamin supplementation. Some of the best methods include:

- Quit smoking and using tobacco products

- Have your doctor check your lipid profile

- Get treatment, if necessary, to reach a lipid goal of LDL less than 100 (those at high risk should reach a goal of less than 70) and HDL greater than 45

- Eat foods low in saturated fat and cholesterol and rich in fiber and nutrients (including antioxidants)

- Be active and exercise regularly

- Control high blood pressure and diabetes

- Achieve and maintain an appropriate weight

- Ask your doctor to do a blood test to detect high-sensitivity c-reactive protein, a general marker of arterial inflammation an indicator of heart disease

- Have regular checkups with your doctor

- Ask your doctor about taking aspirin (between 80 and 160 mg once a day)

Resources

Vivekananthan DP, Penn MS, Sapp SK, Hsu A, Topol EJ. Use of antioxidant vitamins for the prevention of cardiovascular disease: meta-analysis of randomised trials *Lancet* 2003 June 14; 361: 2017–23. http://www.thelancet.com

Yusuf S, Davaenis G, Pogue J, Bosch, J, Sleight P. Vitamin E supplementation and cardiovascular events in high-risk patients. The Heart Outcomes Prevention Evaluation Study Investigators. *New England Journal of Medicine* 2000 Jan; 342(3):154–60.

Yusaf S. Vitamin E supplementation and cardiovascular events in high-risk patients. Correspondence. *New England Journal of Medicine* 2000 June; 342(5):1917–18.

Topol EJ and Califf RM. Clinical trial commentary: HPS. http://www.theheart.org

Vitamin E: The Little Heart Health Supplement that Couldn't, *Men's Health Advisor*, Vol 5/Number 4, April 2003.

Vitamin and Mineral Supplements, American Heart Association.

Chapter 90

Does Garlic Have an Effect on Cardiovascular Risks and Disease?

This chapter is a systematic review that summarizes clinical studies of garlic in humans. It addresses the following topics:

- Whether oral ingestion of garlic (fresh, cooked, or supplements) compared with no garlic, other oral supplements, or drugs lowers lipids, blood pressure, glucose, and cardiovascular morbidity and mortality.

- Whether garlic increases insulin sensitivity and antithrombotic activity.

- Types and frequency of adverse effects of oral, topical, and inhaled garlic dust.

- Interactions between garlic and commonly used medications.

Cardiovascular-Related Outcomes

Thirty-seven randomized trials, all but one in adults, consistently showed that compared with placebo, various garlic preparations led to small, statistically significant reductions in total cholesterol at one month (range of average pooled reductions 1.2 to 17.3 milligrams per deciliter [mg/dL]) and three months (range of average pooled reductions

Excerpted from "Garlic: Effects on Cardiovascular Risks and Disease, Protective Effects against Cancer, and Clinical Adverse Effects," Summary, Evidence Report/Technology Assessment: Number 20, Agency for Healthcare Research and Quality, AHRQ Publication No. 01-E022, October 2000.

12.4 to 25.4 mg/dL). Garlic preparations that were studied included standardized dehydrated tablets (Kwai®, Pure-Gar®, or noncommercial enteric-coated tablets, dehydrated tablets), "aged garlic extract™," oil macerates, distillates, raw garlic, and combination tablets. Eight placebo-controlled trials reported total cholesterol outcomes at six months; pooled analyses showed no significant reductions of total cholesterol with garlic compared with placebo. It is not clear if statistically significant positive short-term effects—but negative longer term effects—are due to: systematic differences in studies that have longer or shorter follow-up durations; fewer longer term studies; or time-dependent effects of garlic. Statistically significant reductions in low-density lipoprotein levels (LDL) (range 0 to 13.5 mg/dL) and in triglycerides (range 7.6 to 34.0 mg/dL) also were found in pooled analyses at three months. No significant changes in high-density lipoprotein levels (HDL) were seen in pooled analyses at one and three months. One multicenter trial involving ninety-eight adults with hyperlipidemia found no differences in lipid outcomes at three months between persons who were given an antilipidemic agent and persons who were given a standardized dehydrated garlic preparation. Interpreting the lipid results is best tempered by recognizing that trials often had unclear randomization processes, short durations, and no intention-to-treat analyses.

Twenty-seven small, randomized, placebo-controlled trials, all but one in adults and of short duration, reported mixed but never large effects of various garlic preparations on blood pressure outcomes. Most studies did not find significant differences between persons randomized to garlic compared with those randomized to placebo. The one small trial (n = 40) that directly compared a standardized dehydrated garlic preparation with an active antihypertensive agent found no differences in blood pressure between groups. Because of unclear randomization processes, lack of intention-to-treat analyses, missing data, and variability in blood pressure measurement techniques, no firm conclusions can be drawn from these trials.

Twelve small, randomized trials, all in adults, suggested that various garlic preparations had no clinically significant effect on glucose in persons with or without diabetes. Two small short trials, both in adults, reported no statistically significant effects of garlic compared with placebo on serum insulin or C peptide levels.

Ten small, randomized trials, all but one in adults and of short duration, showed promising effects of various garlic preparations on platelet aggregation and mixed effects on plasma viscosity and fibrinolytic activity. Because the trials had only 409 participants, short follow-up periods, unclear randomization processes, no intention-to-treat analyses, missing data, and variability in techniques used to assess outcomes, no firm conclusions can be drawn.

There were insufficient data to confirm or refute effects of garlic on clinical outcomes such as myocardial infarction and claudication. One three-year randomized trial with 492 participants found no statistically significant decreases in numbers of myocardial infarctions and deaths when placebo was compared with 6 to 10 grams of garlic ether extract. This trial was not published in peer-reviewed literature; details confirming its randomization process and follow-up were not obtained, despite requests to the author.

Two double-blind trials in participants with atherosclerotic lower extremity disease evaluated whether garlic increased pain-free walking distance at twelve to sixteen weeks compared with placebo. In one trial, sixty-four of eighty (80 percent) participants completed follow-up. Pain-free walking increased by approximately forty meters with standardized dehydrated garlic (Kwai®) compared with approximately thirty meters with placebo. In the other trial, with one hundred participants, the maximum walking distance increased significantly (114 percent) among persons randomized to a combination treatment of garlic oil macerate/soya lecithin/hawthorn oil/wheat germ oil compared with those randomized to placebo (17 percent) ($p < 0.05$).

Randomized controlled trials did not establish whether garlic effectiveness varies across preparations or dosages. Limited data not derived from head-to-head comparisons, suggest, but do not prove, that standardized dehydrated preparations may result in greater short-term (one- to three-month) drops in total cholesterol than other preparations.

Adverse Effects

Adverse effects of oral ingestion of garlic are "smelly" breath and body odor. Other possible, but not proven, adverse effects include flatulence, esophageal and abdominal pain, small intestinal obstruction, contact dermatitis, rhinitis, asthma, bleeding, and myocardial infarction. There are two reports of patients taking warfarin who experienced increases in International Normalized Ratio (INR) when taking garlic pearls or tablets. The content and method of preparation of the pearls and tablets were not given. The frequency of adverse effects with oral ingestion of garlic and whether they vary by particular preparations are not established. Adverse effects of inhaled garlic dust include allergic reactions such as asthma, rhinitis, urticaria, angioedema, and anaphylaxis. Adverse effects of topical exposure to raw garlic include contact dermatitis, skin blisters, and ulcero-necrotic lesions. Frequency of reactions to inhaled garlic dust or topical exposures of garlic is not established.

Conclusions

There are insufficient data to draw conclusions regarding garlic's effects on clinical cardiovascular outcomes such as claudication and myocardial infarction. Garlic preparations may have small, positive, short-term effects on lipids; whether effects are sustainable beyond three months is unclear. Consistent reductions in blood pressure with garlic were not found, and no effects on glucose or insulin sensitivity were found. Some promising effects on antithrombotic activity were reported, but few data are available for definitive conclusion.

Multiple adverse effects, including smelly breath and body odor, dermatitis, bleeding, abdominal symptoms, and flatulence, have been reported. Whether adverse effects occur more commonly with certain preparations than others was not established. Furthermore, the causality of the adverse effects was not clear, except for breath and body odor, and the expected frequency of adverse effects was not determined.

Future Research

Cardiovascular-Related Effects

Before undertaking future trials that evaluate the efficacy of garlic, the equivalency and the amount of release of the main constituents of various garlic preparations must be established. Placebos designed to simulate garlic odor should be developed, and adequacy of blinding should be assessed in trials. Well-designed randomized trials that are longer than six months in duration and that are powered to assess morbidity and mortality outcomes, as well as lipid and thrombotic outcomes, are needed. Appropriate analyses that are intention-to-treat and two-tailed should be used.

Adverse Effects and Interactions

The frequency and severity of adverse effects related to garlic should be quantified. Whether adverse effects are specific to particular preparations, constituents, or doses should be elucidated. In particular, adverse effects related to bleeding and interactions with other drugs such as aspirin and warfarin warrant study.

Chapter 91

Study Finds Possible New Indicator of Heart Disease Risk

Levels of a type of adult stem cell in the bloodstream may indicate a person's risk of developing cardiovascular disease, according to a study supported by the National Heart, Lung, and Blood Institute (NHLBI), part of the National Institutes of Health in Bethesda, Maryland.

The study looked at the blood level of endothelial progenitor cells, which are made in the bone marrow and may help the body repair damage to blood vessels. Scientists from NHLBI and Emory University Hospital in Atlanta, Georgia, found that cardiovascular disease risk was higher in persons with fewer endothelial progenitor cells. The cells of those at higher risk also aged faster than those at lower risk, as determined by the Framingham Heart Study risk factor score, a standard measurement of cardiovascular risk. Additionally, the study found that blood vessels were much less likely to dilate and relax appropriately in persons with low levels of the cells.

Results of the study, which involved forty-five healthy men aged twenty-one and older, some of whom had standard cardiovascular risk factors, appear in the February 13, 2003, issue of the *New England Journal of Medicine*. The two main forms of cardiovascular disease are heart disease and stroke. Standard heart disease risk factors are age, family history of early heart disease, smoking, high blood pressure, high blood cholesterol, overweight/obesity, physical inactivity, and diabetes.

Reprinted from "NHLBI Study Finds Possible New Indicator of Heart Disease Risk," National Institutes of Health, NIH News, February 12, 2003.

"Past research on cardiovascular disease has often focused on what causes the damage to the blood vessels," said Dr. Toren Finkel, chief of NHLBI's Cardiology Branch and coauthor of the study. "We looked at the other part of the equation: How does the body repair damaged blood vessels? What does that tell us about the cause of the disease?

"We believe that these endothelial progenitor cells patch damaged sites in blood vessel walls," he continued. "When the cells start to run out, cardiovascular disease worsens. We don't yet know what causes their depletion but it may be related to the fact that the risk of cardiovascular disease increases as people age. For instance, the cells may be used up repairing damage done by other risk factors, or those risk factors could directly affect the survival of the endothelial cells themselves.

"Much more research needs to be done to better understand this finding," Finkel added. "But it's possible that, some day, doctors may be able to test a person's risk of cardiovascular disease by taking a blood sample and measuring these cells. If the level is too low, an injection of endothelial cells might boost the body's ability to repair itself and prevent more blood vessel damage."

Chapter 92

Is There an Association between Periodontal Disease and Cardiovascular Disease?

Scientists have hypothesized that people with chronic gum, or periodontal, disease may be predisposed to heart disease and stroke. However, supporting this hypothesis has been difficult, in part because researchers have yet to identify a molecule or some other telltale biological marker that is somehow linked to these conditions.

Now, a team of scientists reports that it may have found a possible marker. As published online in the journal *Stroke*, the researchers found in a large, racially mixed group of adults that the more teeth a person has lost, the more likely he or she is to have both advanced periodontal infections and potentially clogging plaques in the carotid artery, the vessel that feeds the brain.

"There is no way to look into the mouth and know why a tooth was lost a year or two after the fact," said Moise Desvarieux, M.D., Ph.D., lead author on the study and an assistant professor of Epidemiology at the University of Minnesota School of Public Health. "But, in our study, we could ask: In middle-aged and older people with periodontal disease, is there a measurable association between tooth loss, severity of their oral infections, and subclinical cardiovascular disease? In this population at least, the answer was most definitely yes."

Desvarieux said he and his colleagues also found that the association held true in a large subgroup of people with periodontal disease

Reprinted from "Scientists Report Important Lead in Studying Possible Association between Periodontal and Cardiovascular Disease," National Institute of Dental and Craniofacial Research, National Institutes of Health, August 2003.

who had never smoked. He said this finding is especially noteworthy, because results from several related studies have been questioned on the grounds that a large percentage of the participants smoked. Smoking is a major risk factor for both periodontal infections and heart disease, raising the possibility that the smoking, not the gum disease, might be responsible for the reported effect in these studies.

The Theory

The Desvarieux et al. paper builds on the broader idea that disease-causing bacteria shed from periodontal infections, enter the circulatory system, and contribute to disease in other parts of the body, such as the heart or brain. The more chronic and severe a person's periodontal infections are, the thinking goes, the greater the risk for secondary infections.

What particularly intrigues researchers is, if the theory proves to be correct, it may be possible to help prevent or control the development of vascular disease in some people by treating their periodontal disease. Over the past decade, however, researchers have yielded mixed results to support the theory. According to some, these variable results do not necessarily disprove the hypothesis. Rather, they show how difficult research on complex biological problems can be without the needed specificity of biomarkers and other necessary research tools to simplify the process.

Among the published studies in the scientific literature are a few that have looked at the possible association between tooth loss, periodontal disease, and cardiovascular disease. Most notable is a retrospective analysis of data from a large national health survey, known by the acronym NHANES, that compared the rate of heart disease among people who were edentulous (lost their teeth) and those who had severe periodontal disease. The researchers hypothesized that, because people without teeth do not develop periodontal disease, their rate of heart disease would be lower than those with active periodontal infections. That was not the case, however, as the researchers found the rate of heart disease was similar in both groups.

Desvarieux and colleagues reasoned there might be an alternative explanation. "While one certainly can interpret these results as there is no association between periodontal disease and cardiovascular disease, the other possible explanation is the edentulous patients lost their teeth, in part, because of previous periodontal disease," said Desvarieux, who is also an assistant professor of medicine at the University of Minnesota Medical School. "The fact that the teeth are gone doesn't necessarily mean that the possible effect of the previous periodontal infections hasn't already occurred."

The Study

To begin testing this idea, Desvarieux and colleagues collected baseline data on 711 randomly selected participants enrolled in the Oral Infections and Vascular Disease Epidemiology Study (INVEST). The study, which is supported by NIH's National Institute of Dental and Craniofacial Research and whose principal investigator is Dr. Desvarieux, will monitor the oral and cardiovascular health of a large, racially mixed group of people for at least three years. All people enrolled in the study live in a northern section of Manhattan in New York City and are age fifty-five or older. Participants also must have no previous history of heart disease or chronic inflammatory conditions, such as Lyme disease. All enrollees are also members of the Northern Manhattan Study (NOMAS), a prospective cohort study supported by NIH's National Institute of Neurological Disorders and Stroke.

During the baseline dental examination, the researchers defined periodontal disease as oral infections that have created a pocket depth between a tooth and the surrounding gum that is 5 millimeters or greater and a loss of a tooth's normal attachment to bone that is 4 millimeters or greater. Both of these values are slightly higher than several previously reported studies, which typically have defined severe periodontal disease using a pocket depth of 4 millimeters or more and an attachment loss of 3 millimeters or greater. "If we had used the common standards for periodontal disease, about 90 percent of those in the study would have been classified as having serious disease," said Panos Papapanou, D.D.S., Ph.D., an author on the study and professor and director of the Division of Periodontics at Columbia University School of Dental and Oral Surgery. "That wouldn't have given us enough discriminatory power to see differences in disease progression."

Papapanou and his collaborators also counted and categorized the number of missing teeth in their participants. The categories were: zero to nine teeth missing, ten to nineteen teeth missing, twenty to thirty-one teeth missing, and edentulous.

Results

After completing the oral examinations and analyzing the data, the scientists determined that the greater the number of teeth that a person had lost, the greater the proportion of their remaining teeth that were riddled with deep pockets and severe attachment loss. For instance, in the people with zero to nine missing teeth, on average, 28 percent of their remaining teeth had severe attachment loss and 8 percent had deep pocket depths. For those missing twenty to thirty-one teeth, the average rates were 60 percent attachment loss and 15 percent deep pocket depths.

This still left open the question of whether tooth loss correlated with cardiovascular disease. To get their answer, clinicians performed high-resolution ultrasound on the carotid arteries of the participants to detect the presence or absence of potentially clogging plaques. Using the standard measures of periodontal disease—attachment loss and pocket depth—the scientists found no relation between those with severe gum disease and the development of carotid plaques. "That was not the case when they compared levels of tooth loss to carotid plaques," said Ralph Sacco, M.D., M.S., senior author on the paper and professor of neurology and epidemiology at Columbia University College of Physicians and Surgeons and principal investigator of the companion Northern Manhattan Study. "Among participants who had lost zero to nine teeth, 45 percent had plaques, while among those who had lost ten to nineteen teeth, 62 percent had plaques. For people who were edentulous, 57 percent had plaques.

"Interestingly, when the researchers examined their data in non-smokers, the correlation held. Carotid plaques were present in 39 percent of those missing zero to nine teeth, 52 percent of people missing ten to nineteen teeth, and 58 percent of edentulous volunteers. "We made extensive adjustments for smoking in our data analysis," said David Jacobs, Ph.D., an author on the paper and professor in the Division of Epidemiology at the University of Minnesota School of Public Health. "Irrespective of all of the variables that we factored into our analysis, the relationship remained.

"The study is titled, "Relationship between periodontal disease, tooth loss, and carotid artery plaque," and it was published online in the journal *Stroke* on July 31, 2003. The authors are: Moise Desvarieux, Ryan T. Demmer, Tatjana Rundek, Bernadette Boden-Albala, David R. Jacobs, Panos Papapanou, and Ralph L. Sacco.

Chapter 93

Treadmill Testing, EKG, and CT Scans Not Recommended for Screening Patients at Low Risk for Heart Disease

The U.S. Preventive Services Task Force said today that it does not recommend using treadmill exercise testing, resting electrocardiograms (EKG; ECG), or electron beam computerized tomography (EBCT) to screen for heart disease in low-risk adults who don't have any symptoms of heart disease. For adults at increased risk for heart disease, the Task Force found insufficient evidence for or against using these three tests for screening.

The recommendations are published in the February 17, 2004 issue of *Annals of Internal Medicine*, and further information about the three screening tests can be found on the Agency for Healthcare Research and Quality (AHRQ) website at http://www.ahrq.gov/clinic/uspstf/uspsacad.htm.

An estimated twenty-two million Americans have heart disease, and more than seven hundred thousand die from it each year. Heart disease is the leading killer of both men and women and is estimated to cost more than $350 billion annually in medical care, time lost from work and other expenses.

Men under age fifty and women under age sixty who have normal blood pressure and cholesterol levels, do not smoke, and do not have diabetes are at low risk of heart disease. A simple calculator to estimate risk of heart disease can be found at http://hin.nhlbi.nih.gov/atpiii/calculator.asp?usertype=pub.

Reprinted from "Treadmill Testing, EKG, and CT Scans Not Recommended for Screening Patients at Low Risk for Heart Disease," Agency for Healthcare Research and Quality, February 2004.

Concerns about Testing in Low-Risk Individuals

The Task Force recommends screening for many of the risks for heart disease, such as high blood pressure, obesity, diabetes, and high cholesterol. The Task Force found that while treadmill testing, EKG, and EBCT could identify persons at higher risk of heart disease, no studies to date have examined whether or not using these tests to screen adults improves health outcomes. Furthermore, the Task Force concluded that using these three technologies to screen for heart disease in low-risk adults could cause more harm than good because of the frequency of false-positive and false-negative results.

False-positive results, in addition to causing a patient psychological stress and anxiety, often lead to invasive tests, such as coronary angiography or treatment with unnecessary medications. Although coronary angiography—a test in which a catheter is inserted into the patient and a dye injected—is considered generally safe, complications, such as internal bleeding, stroke, or infection, and even death, can occur. False-negative results can mislead those with heart disease and result in delayed treatment.

The Task Force said that the evidence is inadequate to determine how test results would change the course of treating patients and noted concern that potential harms, such as false-positive findings, unnecessary invasive procedures, and overtreatment could outweigh any benefit of the tests in lower risk persons.

"These recommendations can help clinicians and their patients make more informed decisions about use of these tests to screen for heart disease and may help guide employers and insurers as well," said Task Force chair, Ned Calonge, M.D., chief medical officer and state epidemiologist for the Colorado Department of Public Health and Environment. "The most important thing individuals at low risk can do is to work with their clinician to monitor their blood pressure, cholesterol, and weight, and to be physically active."

The Task Force

The Task Force, sponsored by the Agency for Healthcare Research and Quality, is the leading independent panel of private-sector experts in prevention and primary care and conducts rigorous, impartial assessments of the scientific evidence for a broad range of preventive services. Its recommendations are considered the gold standard for clinical preventive services. The Task Force based its conclusions on a report from a research team led by Michael Pignone, M.D., M.P.H., assistant professor of medicine at the University of North Carolina-Chapel Hill School of Medicine and the RTI [Research Triangle Institute] International-University of North Carolina Evidence-based Practice Center.

Recommendations

The Task Force recommends against routine screening with resting electrocardiogram, exercise treadmill test, or electron beam computerized tomography scanning for coronary calcium, for either the presence of severe coronary artery stenosis or the prediction of coronary heart disease (CHD) events in adults at low risk for CHD events. For adults at increased risk for CHD events, the Task Force found insufficient evidence to recommend for or against routine screening with EKG, treadmill testing, or EBCT scanning for coronary calcium, for either the presence of severe coronary artery disease or the prediction of CHD events.

Chapter 94

"Polypill" and Heart Disease Prevention

"Polypill" Hints at Future Heart Disease Prevention

Taking a single combination pill daily could reduce the incidence of cardiovascular (heart and blood vessel) disease by over 80 percent, U.K. researchers have found.

The researchers present the concept of combining six active components in one pill (the 'Polypill') taken every day from age fifty-five, or sooner if people have a diagnosis of cardiovascular disease or diabetes (*British Medical Journal* 326 [2003]: 1427–31).

The Polypill would contain the combination of:

- a statin (a cholesterol-lowering medication);

- a thiazide (a diuretic or "fluid" tablet);

- a beta blocker (used to lower blood pressure, treat angina, and some other heart conditions);

- an angiotensin converting enzyme inhibitor (a blood pressure–lowering medication);

- folic acid (a vitamin); and

- aspirin (a nonsteroidal anti-inflammatory medication).

The radical strategy is based on analysis of over 750 trials involving 400,000 participants.

Each component of the Polypill would reduce one of four cardiovascular risk factors:

- low density lipoprotein (LDL) cholesterol (so-called bad cholesterol);

- blood pressure;

- serum homocysteine (elevated levels of this blood chemical are linked to an increased risk of blood vessel disease); and

- the function of platelets (cells involved in forming blood clots).

The researchers say the pill need not be expensive and should be safe with minimal side effects. Trials of the Polypill are planned, to see if the combination is safe and effective, and may take several years to complete.

The authors suggest that the pill would be taken without a medical examination or measurement of risk factors, as treatment would be effective whatever initial levels of cardiovascular risk factors were present.

A Closer Look at the Polypill Proposal

Introduction

Two British professors of medicine have recently made what appears to be a revolutionary proposal—a "Polypill" with six ingredients that everyone fifty-five and older would take, cutting their risk of heart attack and stroke by over 80 percent. Of course, changes in lifestyle (improved diet, no smoking, more exercise) could probably produce similar benefits, but it's harder to get people to undertake them within a reasonable time frame. So let's look at the pill proposal carefully.

The Idea

The plan involves attacking four major cardiovascular risk factors—low density lipoprotein (LDL) cholesterol, blood pressure, serum homocysteine, and platelet function—using medications that are widely accepted as safe and effective. Yet which drugs to choose, and how effective are they in lowering the risks?

Low density lipoprotein (LDL) cholesterol. Statins are the best sort of drug to lower LDL cholesterol levels. Out of six statins analyzed in over two hundred studies, three—atorvastatin, simvastatin, and lovastatin—were selected as candidates for inclusion in the Polypill. In normally prescribed doses, they reduce LDL cholesterol by roughly 70 mg/dL (1.8 mmol/L), and cut coronary heart events (i.e., a heart attack or angina) at age sixty by 61 percent, and strokes by 17 percent.

Blood pressure. Five sorts of blood pressure medication were studied, using analyses of 350 clinical studies. They were: thiazide diuretics (water pills), beta-blockers, ACE inhibitors, angiotensin II receptor blockers (ARBs), and calcium channel blockers. All five types of drug produce similar blood pressure reductions. Using half the standard recommended dose, blood pressure lowering is about 80 percent of that obtained with the full standard dose. On the other hand, combining three drugs at half-dose strength is calculated to cause a reduction of 20 mm Hg in the top (systolic) number, and 10 mm Hg in the lower (diastolic) number.

Using a three-drug combination would reduce heart attack and angina by 46 percent and strokes by 63 percent. While these "good" effects of high blood pressure drugs can be added together when drugs are combined (as there is only one target—raised blood pressure), the side effects reported are those of the individual drugs used, and usually different for each type of drug, and cannot be added together.

Serum homocysteine. Raised homocysteine levels are known to be associated with an increased risk of heart attack and stroke. Taking 0.8 mg/day of folic acid reduces homocysteine levels by about 25 percent, and is associated with a reduction in heart attacks and angina of 16 percent, and in strokes of 24 percent.

Platelet function. Platelets are likely to clump together if there is any underlying artery wall damage, producing a heart attack (coronary thrombosis, myocardial infarction or MI) or a stroke (cerebral thrombosis). Analyses of fifteen clinical trials have shown that a 75 mg/day dose of aspirin is associated with a reduction in heart attacks and angina of 32 percent and in strokes of 16 percent.

The Polypill Approach

We've outlined the reductions in cardiovascular events by medications acting on the four risk factors. The British professors calculated the effect of taking a pill containing the six drugs necessary to influence all four risk factors by multiplying the relative risks associated with each. (This approach has been shown to be valid in previous studies.) In this way, they calculated a theoretical reduction in heart attacks and angina of 88 percent, and in stroke of 80 percent.

Taking the Polypill from the age of fifty-five up to eighty-five would mean that thirty out of one hundred men would avoid a heart attack, angina, or stroke, and would have an estimated thirteen extra years of life. Out of one hundred women, twenty-four would avoid these cardiovascular events, and would gain an average of fourteen years of life.

The side effects produced by the Polypill would vary slightly, depending on which blood pressure–lowering drugs were used. The three types with the lowest risk of side effects (thiazides, ARBs, and calcium blockers) would cause symptoms in about 8 percent of people on the Polypill. If, on the other hand, the three cheapest types of blood pressure–lowering drugs were selected (thiazides, beta-blockers, and ACE inhibitors), side effects would be reported in about 15 percent of those taking the pill.

Comment

This is an exciting proposal. Millions of people are already taking different combinations of the various drugs that have been proposed, but doing so in response to a recognized increased risk, such as high blood pressure, high LDL cholesterol, and so on. However, the two professors believe that everyone over fifty-five, as well as younger people with known arterial disease, should take the Polypill. They say that there's no need to measure the cholesterol, blood pressure, homocysteine, or platelet function before or during treatment, as the benefits have been calculated for whatever the initial levels of risk. Taking the Polypill should reduce heart attacks and strokes by over 80 percent, and only 1–2 percent of those taking it would need to stop because of side effects.

The size of the predicted benefits is remarkable. Only large reductions in smoking and obesity could achieve similar results. Furthermore, using generic drugs throughout would keep the cost down to less than that of screening regularly for the four risk factors. In summary, if the project proves to be feasible (and there are many "ifs" and "buts"), the chances of making a big dent in cardiovascular disease look quite bright.

Source

A strategy to reduce cardiovascular disease by more than 80%. NJ Wald, MR Law. *BMJ*, 2003, vol. 326, pp. 1419–23.

Chapter 95

Light-to-Moderate Drinking May Reduce Heart Disease Risk in Men

A twelve-year study of 38,077 male health professionals found that men who drank alcohol three or more days per week had a reduced risk of heart attack compared with men who drank less frequently. Men who drank less than one drink a day had similar risk reduction to those who drank three.

Many epidemiologic studies have reported that moderate drinking— for men two drinks a day—is associated with a reduced risk of heart disease. This study looked at the relationship between quantity and frequency and found that it was the frequency of drinking—not the amount, the type of alcohol, or whether or not it was consumed with a meal—that was the key factor in lowered heart disease risk. Compared with men who drank less than once a week, men who consumed alcohol three or four days a week had approximately two-thirds (68 percent) the risk of heart attack, and men who consumed alcohol five to seven days per week had slightly less (63 percent) risk. Study data suggested no additional cardiac benefit to drinking more than two drinks a day. Also, the study authors point out that the small number of study participants who drank roughly three and a half or more drinks (fifty or more grams of alcohol) per day limited their ability to study the harmful effects of heavy drinking. However, heavy drinking has well-documented adverse health effects.

Reprinted from "Frequency of Light-to-Moderate Drinking Reduces Heart Disease Risk in Men," National Heart, Lung, and Blood Institute, National Institutes of Health, January 8, 2003.

The Study

The study, published in the *New England Journal of Medicine*, was based on an analysis of data from the Health Professionals Follow-up Study, which has followed a population of male dentists, veterinarians, optometrists, osteopathic physicians, and podiatrists, ages forty to seventy-five, for twelve years. Kenneth J. Mukamal, M.D., M.P.H., at Beth Israel Deaconess Medical Center, was lead author for the project, which included scientists from the University of Sydney, Sydney, Australia; the Harvard School of Public Health, Boston; Brigham and Women's Hospital, Harvard Medical School, Boston; and the Massachusetts General Hospital, Boston. The National Institute on Alcohol Abuse and Alcoholism (NIAAA), the National Heart, Lung, and Blood Institute (NHLBI), and the National Cancer Institute (NCI), all components of the federal government's National Institutes of Health, supported the study.

NIAAA director Ting-Kai Li, M.D., said, "This rigorously conducted observational study adds to the epidemiologic evidence of a strong association between light-to-moderate alcohol consumption and reduced risk of heart disease. Only by research on the mechanisms of alcohol's effects on the cardiovascular system, and perhaps the liver, and the genetic background of how individuals respond to alcohol, will we provide a scientifically informed means for assessing the risks and benefits of alcohol use on a person-to-person basis."

NHLBI director Claude Lenfant, M.D., said, "There are well-proven ways to prevent cardiovascular disease and reduce its risks, including lowering cholesterol levels and blood pressure, maintaining a healthy weight, being physically active, and stopping smoking. These preventive measures do not have the risks associated with alcohol consumption. Therefore, we do not advise the public to begin drinking alcohol to prevent heart disease. However, those who already drink alcohol should be aware that current evidence suggests that moderate drinking may reduce the risk of heart disease in some individuals."

At entry into this study, all participants had to be free of heart disease. Participants in the study completed questionnaires on diet every four years. Investigators confirmed the validity of the questionnaire responses by comparing them with seven-day dietary records in 127 participants. The investigators controlled for numerous health and dietary factors, including smoking, exercise, diet, and family history of premature heart attack. Also, because alcohol use changes over time, and the effects of alcohol may be short-term, the study tracked the effect of recent versus baseline alcohol consumption, and found that the level of risk was more strongly related to recent, rather than past, consumption.

Study Results

By the end of the twelve-year follow-up, the investigators had documented 1,418 heart attacks. Men who consumed alcohol three or more times a week had a reduced risk of fatal or nonfatal heart attack, even when the amount consumed was only 10 grams of alcohol a day or less. A standard drink—a 12-ounce bottle of beer, a 5-ounce glass of wine, or 1.5 ounces of 80-proof distilled spirits—has between 11 and 14 grams of alcohol. Dr. Mukamal, the study's lead author, said, "We found little difference among different alcoholic beverage types in our study. This further emphasizes the role of frequent intake, rather than any specific beverage type, in the link between moderate drinking and heart attack risk."

In an accompanying editorial, Ira J. Goldberg, M.D., of the Columbia University College of Physicians and Surgeons, New York, points out that some studies show a reduction in cardiovascular disease, but not overall mortality, in patients who drink alcoholic beverages (this study did not report on overall mortality). He notes that alcohol has toxic effects that are well established and that additional research is needed to inform physicians on how to advise their patients.

The paper, "Roles of Drinking Pattern and Type of Alcohol Consumed in Coronary Heart Disease in Men," appears in the January 9, 2003, issue of the *New England Journal of Medicine* 348(2): 109–18. An accompanying editorial appears on pages 163–64.

The Dietary Guidelines for Americans, issued jointly by the U.S. Department of Agriculture and the U.S. Department of Health and Human Services, defines moderate drinking for men as no more than two drinks per day.

Chapter 96

A Plan to Prevent Brain Damage after Cardiac Arrest

Lowering the body temperature of a person who has been resuscitated after suffering cardiac arrest can help prevent brain damage, according to an international advisory statement published in *Circulation: Journal of the American Heart Association*.

The American Heart Association and resuscitation councils around the world helped craft the advisory from the Advanced Life Support Task Force of the International Liaison Committee on Resuscitation (ILCOR).

Cardiac arrest is the abrupt loss of heart function in a person who may or may not have diagnosed heart disease. No statistics are available for the exact number of sudden cardiac arrests that occur each year. But the American Heart Association estimates that about 250,000 people a year die of coronary heart disease without being hospitalized. That's about half of all deaths from coronary heart disease—more than 680 Americans each day. Cardiac arrest results from the extremely rapid, chaotic quivering of the heart's lower chambers, a disorder called ventricular fibrillation. It's often reversible if treated within a few minutes with an electric shock to the heart from a defibrillator, a device that can allow a normal rhythm to resume.

Because the supply of oxygen-rich blood to the brain is cut off when the heart stops pumping, people who survive a cardiac arrest lasting more than a few minutes often suffer brain damage. Now, two major studies have shown that cooling the body temperature to below normal—mild therapeutic hypothermia—can help prevent that damage, says Jerry P. Nolan, M.D., lead author of the statement and co-chairman of the International Liaison Committee on Resuscitation's Advanced Life Support Task Force.

The procedure, which aims to lower the body temperature to between 89.6 degrees F and 93.2 degrees F, should be started as soon as possible after successful resuscitation and continued for twelve to twenty-four hours, says Nolan, a consultant in anesthesia and critical care medicine at the Royal United Hospital in Bath, England.

Doctors have known for some time that reducing a person's body temperature before the heart stops—such as when open-heart surgery is performed—can help prevent brain damage.

"What is so exciting about these new studies is that they showed that even if we cooled the brain after the oxygen supply had been cut off, people did better," Nolan says.

In both studies, cardiac arrest survivors whose bodies were cooled were less likely to sustain neurological damage, compared with survivors who were not cooled.

A study in Europe used a special mattress with a cover that blew air over the body and used ice bags if necessary to cool the victims for twenty-four hours once they arrived at the critical care unit. In an Australian study, paramedics applied ice packs to patients' heads and torsos, with ice applications continuing in the hospital for twelve more hours.

When a patient is successfully resuscitated and the supply of oxygen-rich blood to the brain is restored, it sets off a series of chemical reactions that can continue for up to twenty-four hours and can cause significant inflammation in the brain, Nolan says.

"Cooling slows down the chemical reactions, thereby lowering inflammation," he says.

Many more questions remain to be answered—including how to best cool patients, how long they should be chilled, whether paramedics should be taught the procedure, and when it's too late to help. Cooling therapy carries a slightly increased risk of bleeding, infection, and abnormal heart rhythms.

In addition, the cooling studies enrolled less than 10 percent of all cardiac arrest patients initially considered for treatment. Researchers studied only patients who met certain strict criteria—such as those with relatively known times of cardiac arrest, good blood pressure, and evidence of coma after arrest. Further studies are needed to determine what other groups of cardiac arrest patients might benefit from cooling.

Nevertheless, the task force says the evidence that cooling prevents brain damage is compelling enough to recommend therapeutic hypothermia for some out-of-hospital cardiac arrest patients.

The American Heart Association urges people to call 9-1-1 and begin cardiopulmonary resuscitation (CPR) immediately if someone suffers cardiac arrest. If an automated external defibrillator (AED) is available and someone trained to use it is nearby, involve him or her.

However, grabbing a blanket and trying to warm up a cardiac arrest victim could do more harm than good, Nolan adds.

"The sooner the patient is successfully resuscitated and we can start cooling, the better," he says.

Co-authors are Peter T. Morley; Terry L. Vanden Hoek, M.D.; and Robert W. Hickey, M.D.

The advisory is also supported by the European Resuscitation Council, Resuscitation Council of Southern Africa, Australia and New Zealand Council on Resuscitation, Japanese Resuscitation Council, Latin American Resuscitation Council, and the Heart and Stroke Foundation of Canada.

Chapter 97

Recent Research on Stroke

Angioplasty Clears Clogged Brain Arteries

Angioplasty opened narrowed brain arteries, preventing strokes in patients for whom standard medication had failed, according to a study presented at the American Stroke Association's 29th International Stroke Conference.

"Angioplasty improves the outcome over what we would expect to see with medication alone," said study author Michael P. Marks, M.D., associate professor of radiology and neurosurgery and chief of interventional neuroradiology at Stanford University Medical Center in Palo Alto, California. Additionally, "Stent treatment may not be necessary."

The study was not a head-to-head comparison of angioplasty and medical therapy. Researchers used data from other studies to make risk comparisons.

Angioplasty uses a tiny balloon threaded into the area of blockage. Once in this area, the balloon is inflated. As it expands, it forces the

---

This chapter includes the following American Heart Association press releases: "Angioplasty Clears Clogged Brain Arteries," February 5, 2004; "Cooling Helmets May Provide Innovative Stroke Treatment," February 5, 2004; "Corkscrew Device Retrieves Clots, Quickly Reverses Stroke Damage," February 5, 2004; "Blood-Diverting Catheter Holds Promise for Stroke Treatment," February 5, 2004; "Cholesterol Drugs May Lower Risk for Mental Impairment after Stroke," February 6, 2004; and "Metabolic Syndrome May Be an Important Link to Stroke," February 6, 2004. Reproduced with permission from www.american heart.org © 2004, American Heart Association.

fatty plaque against the artery wall, opening the vessel. Balloon angioplasty is widely used to open blocked heart arteries but is not as commonly used for clearing neck and brain arteries. In some cases, a miniature wire tube called a stent is left behind after angioplasty to keep the artery propped open.

Blood thinners such as aspirin and anticoagulants such as warfarin are standard medical therapy for clogged brain vessels. Anticoagulants interfere with the blood's ability to clot.

The study examined both the overall rate of stroke and the rate of stroke in areas supplied by the treated vessel in patients with symptomatic intracranial stenosis (narrowing of a brain blood vessel) undergoing angioplasty.

Researchers studied thirty-six patients with significant intracranial stenosis, all of whom had unsuccessful medical therapy. Before angioplasty stenosis averaged 84.2 percent. After angioplasty, stenosis averaged 43.3 percent.

One ischemic stroke occurred during angioplasty but the patient recovered. No other ischemic strokes occurred within one month of angioplasty, the periprocedural period.

Two deaths occurred in the periprocedural period, one due to reperfusion hemorrhage and one due to vessel perforation. Follow-up was available in thirty-four patients and varied between 4 and 128 months (average follow-up 53 months) with twenty-nine patients (or 85.3 percent) having greater than 24 months follow-up. The annual stroke rate in the area of the angioplasty was 3.36 percent. The annual rate for all strokes was 5.38 percent.

"One would expect 8 percent to 10 percent of these patients to have suffered a stroke in the territory of angioplasty annually had they been treated with medication," Marks said.

The researchers then looked at the subgroup of patients at high risk of stroke after angioplasty, which "has been used as an argument to use stents," he said. High-risk patients include those who still have significant vessel narrowing (residual stenosis) after angioplasty and those in whom the angioplasty caused a small tear, or dissection, in the vessel.

For patients with residual stenoses, some argue that the stent will open the vessel wider, Marks said. Some also believe stenting can help repair tears.

The subgroup of eighteen patients with moderate but significant residual stenosis (50 percent to 75 percent) had an annual stroke rate of 3 percent—just as low as when there was no residual stenosis, Marks said. "So by opening the vessel even a small amount, we had a favorable effect on clinical outcome."

There does not appear to be any advantage to adding a stent to help prop the artery open after angioplasty for patients with symptomatic intracranial stenosis compared to angioplasty alone, he said.

Also, none of the eleven patients with evidence of a tear in their vessel after angioplasty had a stroke at follow-up. "The tear heals itself. Stenting is not necessary for these patients either," he said.

Co-authors are Mary L. Marcellus, R.N.; Huy M. Do, M.D.; Gary K. Steinberg, M.D., Ph.D.; David C. Tong, M.D.; and Gregory A. Albers, M.D.

Cooling Helmets May Provide Innovative Stroke Treatment

Reproduced with permission from www.americanheart.org © 2004, American Heart Association.

Helmets that cool the brain may minimize stroke damage, according to two small studies presented at the American Heart Association's 29th International Stroke Conference.

In a Japanese study, a "helmet-type cooling apparatus" was tested on seventeen patients with severe ischemic stroke. An American study tested a "NASA-spinoff" helmet on six patients with severe ischemic stroke.

Ischemic strokes are caused by blood clots in blood vessels of the brain or leading to it.

The helmets may improve patient outcomes and lengthen the time treatment window for ischemic strokes.

Hypothermia—low temperature—is known to protect the brain from ischemic injury. However, overall surface cooling is associated with various adverse effects, said Kentaro Yamada, M.D., of the National Cardiovascular Center in Osaka, Japan.

"The largest problem of systemic surface cooling is the requirement of general anesthesia, which increases risks of respiratory and circulatory diseases," he said. "Systemic surface cooling is commonly associated with severe infections, arrhythmia, hypopotassemia (low potassium), or decrease of platelet counts, which may countervail protective effects of hypothermia."

He also noted that "in our experience of hypothermia therapy in acute stroke patients using systemic surface cooling, excellent functional recovery was obtained in 83 percent of younger patients under age sixty but only in 20 percent of elderly patients."

Scientists have tried various methods to cool the brain, including cooling the entire body, using dry ice, and blowing cool air on the head. However, methods were unable to selectively cool the brain rapidly and maintain such preferential cooling over the rest of the body, said Huan Wang, M.D., assistant and resident of neurosurgery at the University of Illinois, College of Medicine, Peoria, Illinois.

He said it is well known that "brains like to be cold." Stroke and head trauma patients fare worse when they are running fevers. However, the same is not true for the rest of the body, including the heart and immune system, which do better at normal temperatures, Wang said.

Yamada and colleagues tested the helmet on patients (average age sixty-eight) three to twelve hours after stroke onset. The helmet was attached to the head and neck. The cooling of the head continued nonstop for three to seven days without anesthesia.

Researchers evaluated functional outcome three to ten months after stroke. The surface cooling was performed successfully in all patients.

Tympanic temperature, which measures surface brain temperature, was lowered 4.0 degrees Fahrenheit, and jugular temperature, which reflects deep brain temperature, was lowered 1.4 degrees Fahrenheit. In hypothermia with a helmet, such a temperature gradient in the brain results because of the local nature of the cooling method, Yamada said. Some patients experienced mild shivering, elevated potassium levels, mild skin damage, and infections, but none had serious adverse effects.

After ten months of follow-up, only one patient (6 percent) had died. Six patients (35 percent) had "good" functional outcome three to ten months after stroke.

The American study evaluated patients average age sixty-eight and used liquid cooling technology developed by NASA scientist William Elkins, "father of the American spacesuit," Wang said.

In animal studies, researchers have determined that cooling the brain can reduce the damage that stroke does to the brain tissue by as much as 70 percent, Wang said. "The goal with this therapy, therefore, is to try to improve neurological outcomes by minimizing stroke's effect," Wang said. "The first step in that direction was to find a therapy that effectively cooled the brain and, judging by this study, we have."

In this study, researchers gauged brain temperature via tiny fiberoptic probes inserted in the brain. These probes are often used to monitor vital brain functions of stroke patients in intensive care. The patients had neurological deterioration despite being treated for brain swelling.

Researchers took patients' brain temperatures at the start of the study (before patients put on the helmets) and throughout the next forty-eight to seventy-two hours. They found that the helmet preferentially cools the brain much more rapidly and profoundly than it does the body. The patients' brains cooled an average of 6 degrees Fahrenheit the first hour, without dropping body temperature significantly. Then, the helmet continued cooling the brain, while cooling body temperature at a much slower rate. Researchers were able to use the technology an average of six to eight hours before body temperature dropped below 97 degrees F. Five patients tolerated the helmet cooling well. One eighty-five-year-old woman with a previous heart arrhythmia experienced an abnormal heart rate but responded promptly to treatment.

The study did not report patient outcomes, but Wang said the treatment has great potential. If EMS personnel can use the helmet in the field, they theoretically can lengthen the time that a stroke patient is eligible for clot-busting therapy. "We believe that if you keep the brain tissue cool, you will have a longer tissue survival time. Then, when we open the artery, we could salvage much more brain tissue and hopefully avoid adverse neurological effects," Wang said.

"Rapid and selective brain cooling is a simple but elegant strategy that has been shown to limit injury in stroke, brain trauma, and cardiac arrest," said Vinay Nadkarni, M.D., immediate past chair of the American Heart Association's emergency cardiovascular care committee. "Building upon space-age technology, this novel technique is a good example of how bright scientists and innovative industry technologists can collaborate to speed the delivery of emergency cardiovascular care interventions. This device, and others like it, may have wide applicability in the field."

Yamada's co-authors are Hiroshi Moriwaki, M.D.; Hiroshi Oe, M.D.; Takemori Yamawaki, M.D.; Kazuyuki Nagatsuka, M.D.; Masahiro Oomura, M.D.; Kenichi Todo, M.D.; Kotoro Miyashita, M.D.; and Hiroaki Naritomi, M.D.

Wang's co-authors are David Wang, D.O.; William Olivero, M.D.; Giuseppe Lanzino, M.D.; Debra Honings, R.N.; Mary Rodde, R.N.; Janet Burnham, R.N.; Joe Milbrandt, Ph.D.: and Jean Rose, R.N., M.S.

Corkscrew Device Retrieves Clots, Quickly Reverses Stroke Damage

Reproduced with permission from www.americanheart.org © 2004, American Heart Association.

A revolutionary tiny corkscrew that captures blood clots from vessels deep inside the brain can "almost instantly" reverse damage caused by ischemic stroke, according to the first report on the safety and efficacy of the device presented at the American Stroke Association's 29th International Stroke Conference.

Ischemic strokes are caused by a blood clot that blocks blood supply to the brain. Each year, about seven hundred thousand Americans suffer a stroke and 88 percent of those strokes are ischemic, according to the American Stroke Association.

Blood clots causing stroke can be dissolved using the FDA-approved clot-busting drug tissue plasminogen activator (tPA) as standard therapy. But, it must be initiated intravenously within three hours (the earlier the better) of stroke onset to be effective. Moreover, it "typically takes one to two hours for tPA to dissolve a clot and open a vessel, if at all," said Sidney Starkman, M.D., professor of emergency medicine and neurology at the University of California, Los Angeles and co-director of the UCLA Stroke Center.

The investigational device, the Concentric MERCI® Retrieval System, restored blood flow in 61 of 114 patients (54 percent) in Phase I and II of the Mechanical Embolus Removal in Cerebral Ischemia (MERCI I /II) trials, which studied patients up to eight hours after initial stroke symptoms who were not eligible for standard tPA therapy, said principal investigator Starkman.

Restoring blood flow in these trials reversed paralysis and other stroke symptoms, Starkman said.

"How often do we get a chance to reverse a patient's stroke on the table? We have had patients completely paralyzed on one side of their body, who were made normal almost instantaneously when the clot was retrieved," he said.

Of the sixty-one patients whose arteries were unblocked with the device, "twenty-three have no disability or have minor disability, such as handwriting problems," Starkman said.

The MERCI® Retrieval System is inserted into an artery in the groin, and then carefully guided via standard angiography into the brain until it reaches the blood clots. The device is made from a combination of nickel and titanium, "which is unique in that it allows the device to have a 'memory.' So in this case, when it is deployed, it 'remembers' to form itself into a helical shape, like a corkscrew," Starkman said.

Starkman says the corkscrew-shaped MERCI Retriever is the only device specifically designed to remove clots from all major cerebral vessels.

Once the device "captures" the blood clot, the device and clot are withdrawn into a larger catheter with a balloon. During the evacuation process, the balloon is briefly inflated to momentarily stop blood flow so the clots can be safely removed. Starkman added that the re-trieval procedure can be performed only by a highly trained team at specialized centers.

The results presented today are based on 114 patients from twenty-five centers, (average age seventy, 46 percent women), whose average National Institutes of Health baseline stroke score was 19, which indicates severe impairment.

"Thus far, we have seen that the MERCI® Retrieval System is quite safe and we believe it holds great promise, but more research is needed to refine the device and study its effectiveness," Starkman said.

Concentric Medical, Inc., of Mountain View, California, funded the studies. The Food and Drug Administration is reviewing the device.

Blood-Diverting Catheter Holds Promise for Stroke Treatment

Reproduced with permission from www.americanheart.org © 2004, American Heart Association.

A new catheter device that diverts some blood from the lower body to the brain appears safe for treating acute stroke and may significantly reduce stroke complications—even after a critical treatment window has lapsed.

The results of this experimental study were reported at the American Stroke Association's 29th International Stroke Conference.

"The device treats stroke by a unique approach that increases blood flow to the brain," said lead author Morgan S. Campbell III, M.D., director of interventional neurology at the Alabama Neurological Institute, in Birmingham. "Ten of the fifteen patients who were conscious when they arrived at the hospital improved during the procedure, which is very impressive."

Campbell and his colleagues tested the safety and effectiveness of the device, called NeuroFlo, on patients who suffered ischemic strokes. Ischemic strokes occur when a blood clot blocks an artery, reducing blood flow and oxygen to part of the brain. Using two balloons attached to a catheter, NeuroFlo diverts some blood from the lower extremities and sends it to the upper body.

Not all the brain cells affected by an ischemic stroke die immediately, Campbell said. A large number of cells in the stroke area initially have the potential to recover if their blood supply is restored. In theory, increasing the volume of blood to these damaged brain cells should preserve some of them even more than three hours after a stroke onset.

Ischemic stroke patients who arrive within three hours of symptom onset can often be treated with clot-busting drugs. However, these clot busters are not recommended for use more than three hours after stroke onset.

"The blood volume theory has been studied before but no one had really shown that it actually works and makes a difference," Campbell said. "So it is very encouraging that the device can divert more oxygenated blood to the brain and that patients get better."

Campbell conducted the study while he was an assistant professor of neurology and radiology at the University of Texas Health Science Center at Houston. He and colleagues at eight medical centers in the United States, Turkey, Germany, and Argentina studied seventeen patients whose strokes had been in progress for 3 to 12 hours. The average time between stroke onset and the beginning of treatment was 7.5 hours.

Each patient had a NeuroFlo device inserted into an artery in the groin. The device was then threaded up to the abdominal aorta and positioned with collapsed balloons above and below the renal arteries. The balloons were then inflated to partially obstruct the aorta. The device was left in place for one hour.

"By blowing up these balloons and limiting the blood flow to the lower extremities, we shifted more of the blood flow up to the head," Campbell explained.

This greater volume of blood increased collateral flow, the flow of blood through smaller vessels in the brain. The collateral flow bypassed the blocked section of the artery that was causing the patient's stroke, and brought needed oxygen to the cells downstream from the blockage.

The study's primary intent was to test the device's safety. Although two study participants died, their deaths were attributed to their strokes and not adverse effects of the device. Nor did people treated with the device suffer damage to their kidneys, heart, or blood vessels.

The research team also evaluated the patients' treatment response.

Twelve of sixteen patients monitored with ultrasound had a 15 percent increase or more of their cerebral blood flow velocity, with an average boost of 25 percent. Ultrasound waves passing into the skull can measure blood flow velocity. Velocity is an indirect measure of blood flow volume.

The blood pressure in the arteries increased an average of only 6 percent overall and did not increase in five patients. "This shows the increased blood flow did not simply result from an increase in blood pressure but from an increase in blood volume," Campbell said. "This is the desired effect of the device."

The researchers also assessed the degree of deficit of the stroke patients. While undergoing their hour-long treatment, ten of the fifteen conscious patients (67 percent) showed significantly higher scores on the National Institutes of Health Stroke Scale, the most commonly used assessment tool in acute stroke. Thirty days after treatment, six of the fifteen survivors had "good" physical function, on the modified Rankin scale, which rates disability.

The second phase of the study has begun enrollment. CoAxia, Inc., the device's maker, will seek approval from the U.S. Food and Drug Administration to conduct a larger clinical trial.

Co-authors are James C. Grotta, M.D.; Camilo R. Gomez, M.D.; and Gazi Ozdemir, M.D.

Cholesterol Drugs May Lower Risk for Mental Impairment after Stroke

Reproduced with permission from www.americanheart.org © 2004, American Heart Association.

High cholesterol may increase the risk of stroke, but cholesterol-lowering drugs might reduce the risk of impaired brain function after a stroke, according to a study presented at the American Stroke Association's 29th International Stroke Conference.

Patients with a history of high cholesterol had a lower risk of cognitive impairment three to six months after stroke. However, the finding likely relates to high cholesterol treatment, rather than a protective or helpful effect of cholesterol. About 45 percent of the patients were being treated with cholesterol-lowering drugs known as statins before their stroke, said Eugenia Gencheva, M.D., a research fellow at the University of Illinois at Chicago (UIC) Center for Stroke Research. The research was conducted at Rush Medical College in Chicago.

"We're certainly not saying that the high cholesterol itself is protective," added David Nyenhuis, Ph.D., associate professor of neurology and rehabilitation at UIC. "Patients who had elevated cholesterol levels were more likely to be treated with statin drugs. We believe that perhaps statins were exerting the protective effect."

Elevated cholesterol is a risk factor for atherosclerotic vascular disease. In this observational study, hypercholesterolemia was determined by self-report and verification of current medication. Participants taking cholesterol-lowering drugs were defined as hypercholesterolemic, although their cholesterol levels might have been within acceptable limits as a result of their treatment.

Several observational studies have indicated that statin therapy is associated with a reduced risk of Alzheimer's disease and vascular dementia. However, the precise mechanisms by which statins might affect cognitive impairment are poorly understood, Gencheva said.

"Other research has shown that the effect of statins might be mediated by direct cholesterol-lowering properties, causing a reduction in cholesterol production and turnover in the brain," she said. "Statins also might reduce the concentration of proteins linked with dementia that accumulate in the brain in Alzheimer's patients."

Cognitive impairment—or loss of memory or other aspects of brain function—often occurs after stroke. Cardiovascular risk factors such as hypertension, diabetes, and obesity are widely assumed to influence cognitive impairment after stroke. But, the assumption hasn't been documented in medical literature, Gencheva said.

At the UIC Center for Stroke Research, an ongoing study led by Philip B. Gorelick, M.D, M.P.H., focuses on identifying markers for dementia after stroke through brain scans with magnetic resonance imaging. As an extension of that research, investigators evaluated demographic factors and cardiovascular risk factors as potential predictors of stroke-related cognitive impairment.

Ischemic strokes, which are caused by clots that disrupt blood flow to the brain, can result in various brain disorders known collectively as vascular cognitive impairment. The mildest disorder is vascular cognitive impairment-no dementia (VCIND); at the opposite end of the spectrum is vascular dementia, the most severe form of stroke-related brain dysfunction. The prevalence of VCIND is not known but vascular dementia may occur in up to one-third of stroke survivors, researchers said.

This study focused on VCIND. Researchers studied 103 consecutive ischemic stroke patients—41 diagnosed with VCIND and 62 who had no evidence of cognitive impairment after their strokes. All patients completed interviews that included questions about potential risk factors for cognitive impairment, and underwent neuropsychological testing. Information about cholesterol levels, blood pressure, and other vascular risk factors was self-reported and not based on actual measurement when patients were evaluated.

An initial analysis of different variables identified three statistically significant predictors of cognitive impairment: the patient's level of education, the presence of heart disease (defined as a history of heart attack, heart failure, disease of the heart muscle, disease of the heart valve, and abnormal heart rhythm), and a history of high cholesterol (hypercholesterolemia).

In a second analysis, heart disease and hypercholesterolemia remained significant predictors of cognitive impairment when results were not adjusted for education level. Increased education and hypercholesterolemia were associated with a reduced risk of cognitive impairment after stroke. When the researchers performed an analysis that controlled for the confounding effects of education, only hypercholesterolemia remained as a statistically significant predictor of the risk for cognitive impairment.

"Education is a well-known protective factor for cognitive impairment, and after adjusting for the effects of education, only hypercholesterolemia as defined in the study was statistically significant in the multivariate model," Gencheva said.

A major strength of the main study is that patients are being followed over time, including annual neurocognitive testing and MRI scans, Nyenhuis said. Continued evaluation of the patients eventually could lead to identification of changes in brain regions or structures that predict cognitive impairment.

Co-authors are Gorelick and Sally Freels, Ph.D. The National Institutes of Health supported the study.

Metabolic Syndrome May Be an Important Link to Stroke

Reproduced with permission from www.americanheart.org © 2004, American Heart Association.

Metabolic syndrome—the simultaneous occurrence of multiple cardiovascular risk factors—may almost double the risk of stroke, researchers reported at the American Stroke Association's 29th International Stroke Conference.

The findings suggest that treating the risk-factor components of metabolic syndrome might reduce stroke risk before the onset of Type 2 diabetes.

"Before it becomes necessary to begin aggressive treatment of diabetes and other predisposing factors for stroke, it might be possible to take steps that can prevent these serious conditions from developing," said the study's lead author, Robert M. Najarian, a third-year medical student at Boston University School of Medicine.

The U.S. National Cholesterol Education Program (NCEP) and the World Health Organization define the metabolic syndrome as the simultaneous presence of at least three of five metabolic abnormalities: abdominal obesity, high fasting levels of blood sugar, high triglycerides levels, low levels of HDL ("good" cholesterol) and high blood pressure.

This study found that compared to people without metabolic syndrome, men with the condition have a 78 percent greater risk of stroke, and women affected by the condition have more than double the stroke risk of women who do not have the syndrome. But, the overall stroke risk associated with metabolic syndrome remained below that of people with diabetes.

Metabolic syndrome greatly increases a person's chances of developing Type 2 diabetes. Because of its strong association with diabetes, metabolic syndrome often is considered a prediabetic condition. Both conditions increase the risk of coronary heart disease, and diabetes is a potent risk factor for stroke. However, the relative effect of metabolic syndrome and diabetes on stroke risk has not been studied extensively.

Najarian and his co-investigators compared the impact of metabolic syndrome and diabetes on the ten-year risk of stroke and transient ischemic attack (TIA), a temporary interruption in blood flow to the brain that often precedes a stroke. The study involved 1,881 diabetes-free participants (average age fifty-nine) of the offspring cohort in the Framingham Heart Study.

Men and women were evaluated for a current diagnosis of diabetes and the five metabolic syndrome components: abdominal obesity (waist circumference greater than thirty-five inches in women and greater than forty inches in men); low HDL (less than 40 mg/dL in men and less than 50 mg/dL in women); blood pressure 130/85 mm Hg or greater, or current treatment with antihypertensive medication; triglycerides 150 mg/dL or greater; and fasting blood glucose of 110–26 mg/dL (the definition of impaired fasting glucose). Participants were considered to have the metabolic syndrome if they met at least three of the five criteria.

Najarian found that 27.6 percent of the men and 21.5 percent of the women met the criteria for a diagnosis of metabolic syndrome without including diabetes. When the additional 216 participants with diabetes were included in the analysis, 30.3 percent of men and 24.7 percent of women met diagnosis criteria.

During a maximum follow-up of fourteen years, 5.6 percent of the men in the study and 4.3 percent of the women had a stroke or TIA. Diabetic patients had a significantly higher ten-year risk of stroke compared to people with metabolic syndrome: 14 percent vs. 8 percent in men and 10 percent vs. 6 percent in women.

Although metabolic syndrome is a less potent risk factor for stroke than diabetes, the condition occurs more often than diabetes, making it a major consideration for stroke risk and prevention, Najarian said. Interventions aimed at preventing or treating metabolic syndrome could have a major impact on overall stroke risk.

"Metabolic syndrome looks like the precursor for a number of health problems," Najarian said. "Because the prevalence of the syndrome is so high, we need to start thinking about how to prevent the condition, particularly since it appears to be a factor in the continuum that leads to outright diabetes and cardiovascular disease. The end result is a higher death rate from all causes, a higher death rate from vascular causes, and higher rates of cardiovascular disease."

Co-authors are Lisa M. Sullivan, Ph.D.; Ralph B. D'Agostino, Ph.D.; Peter F. Wilson, M.D.; William B. Kannel, M.D.; and Philip A. Wolf, M.D.

Najarian is a recipient of an American Stroke Association 2003 Student Scholarship in Cerebrovascular Disease.

Editor's note: The American Heart Association's *The Heart Of Diabetes: Understanding Insulin Resistance* is a free twelve-month program designed to educate people about the association between cardiovascular disease, diabetes, and insulin resistance. People with Type 2 diabetes are encouraged to control their heart disease risk through physical activity, nutrition and cholesterol management. To register for the program, call 1-800-AHA-USA1 or visit www.american heart.org/diabetes.

Chapter 98

Trial of
EDTA Chelation Therapy
for Coronary Artery Disease

The National Center for Complementary and Alternative Medicine (NCCAM) and the National Heart, Lung, and Blood Institute (NHLBI), both components of the National Institutes of Health (NIH), have launched the Trial to Assess Chelation Therapy (TACT). TACT is the first large-scale, multicenter study to determine the safety and efficacy of EDTA chelation therapy for individuals with coronary artery disease. The following questions and answers provide additional information on coronary artery disease, EDTA chelation therapy, and the study.

What is coronary artery disease?

Coronary artery disease (CAD) is the most common form of heart disease. In CAD the coronary arteries, the vessels that bring oxygen-rich blood to the tissues of the heart, become blocked by deposits of a fatty substance called plaque. As plaque builds, the arteries become narrower and less oxygen and nutrients are transported to the heart. This condition can lead to serious problems, such as angina (pain caused by not enough oxygen-carrying blood reaching the heart) and heart attack. In a heart attack, or myocardial infarction, there is such poor oxygen supply to the heart that part of the heart muscle dies. If

Reprinted from "Questions and Answers: The NIH Trial of EDTA Chelation Therapy for Coronary Artery Disease," National Center for Complementary and Alternative Medicine, National Institutes of Health, October 2003, updated February 2004.

a sufficiently large portion of the heart is affected, it may no longer be able to pump blood efficiently to the rest of the body, resulting in death or chronic heart failure.

Approximately seven million Americans suffer from CAD. It is the leading cause of death among American men and women; more than five hundred thousand Americans die of CAD-related heart attacks each year.

There are several factors that can each increase the risk of developing CAD:

- High blood pressure
- High cholesterol levels
- Smoking
- Obesity
- Physical inactivity
- Diabetes
- Family history of CAD
- Gender
- Age

A person with CAD may or may not have symptoms. Symptoms can include chest pain from angina, shortness of breath, lightheadedness, cold sweats, or nausea.

How is CAD diagnosed and treated?

Because the severity of CAD and its symptoms can vary from person to person, the way the disease is diagnosed and treated can also vary. CAD is often diagnosed through a series of tests that can include blood tests to see if protein has been released into the bloodstream from damaged heart tissues, electrocardiograms (EKG) to check the heart's electrical activity, "stress" tests to record the heartbeat during exercise, nuclear scanning to check for damaged areas of the heart, and angiography to see how blood flows.

Treatment of CAD depends on many factors, such as the patient's age, heart function, and overall health. Often, treatment begins with focusing on lifestyle—stopping smoking for patients who smoke, reducing fat in the diet, and engaging in a prescribed exercise program. Medications may also be prescribed, such as aspirin to prevent additional heart attacks, medications that decrease the workload on the heart, or medicines to reduce high blood cholesterol levels or high blood pressure. If these efforts are not effective, a patient may need to have the narrowed or blocked arteries re-opened through a procedure called balloon angioplasty, or bypassed through surgery. Balloon angioplasty involves threading a thin tube into the artery and expanding a balloon-like apparatus as a way to increase the size of the artery so more blood can flow. Bypass surgery is used to treat severe blockages by using veins or arteries from other areas of the body to divert blood flow around the blocked coronary arteries.

What is EDTA chelation therapy?

Chelation is a chemical process in which a substance is used to bind molecules, such as metals or minerals, and hold them tightly so that they can be removed from a system, such as the body. In medicine, chelation has been scientifically proven to rid the body of excess or toxic metals. For example, a person who has lead poisoning may be given chelation therapy in order to bind and remove excess lead from the body before it can cause damage.

In the case of EDTA chelation therapy, the substance that binds and removes metals and minerals is EDTA (ethylene diamine tetraacetic acid), a synthetic, or man-made, amino acid that is delivered intravenously (through the veins). EDTA was first used in the 1940s for the treatment of heavy metal poisoning. EDTA chelation removes heavy metals and minerals from the blood, such as lead, iron, copper, and calcium, and is approved by the U.S. Food and Drug Administration (FDA) for use in treating lead poisoning and toxicity from other heavy metals. Although it is not approved by the FDA to treat CAD, some physicians and alternative medicine practitioners have recommended EDTA chelation as a way to treat this disorder.

Does EDTA chelation therapy have side effects?

When used as approved by the FDA (at the appropriate dose and infusion rate) for treatment of heavy metal poisoning, chelation with EDTA has a low occurrence of side effects. The most common side effect is a burning sensation experienced at the site where the EDTA is delivered into the veins. Rare side effects can include fever, hypotension (a sudden drop in blood pressure), hypocalcemia (abnormally low calcium levels in the blood), headache, nausea, vomiting, and bone marrow depression (meaning that blood cell counts fall). Injury to the kidneys has been reported with EDTA chelation therapy, but it is rare.

Other serious side effects can occur if EDTA is not administered by a trained health professional.

How might EDTA chelation therapy work to clear blocked arteries?

Several theories have been suggested by those who recommend this form of treatment. One theory suggests that EDTA chelation might work by directly removing calcium found in fatty plaques that block the arteries, causing the plaques to break up. Another is that the process of chelation may stimulate the release of a hormone that in turn causes calcium to be removed from the plaques or causes a lowering of cholesterol levels. A third theory is that EDTA chelation therapy may work by reducing the damaging effects of oxygen ions (oxidative stress) on the walls of the blood vessels. Reducing oxidative stress could reduce inflammation in the arteries and improve blood vessel function. None of these theories has been well tested in scientific studies.

Is there evidence that EDTA chelation therapy works for CAD?

There is a lack of adequate prior research to verify EDTA chelation therapy's safety and effectiveness for CAD. The bulk of the evidence supporting the use of EDTA chelation therapy is in the form of case reports and case series. Some patients who have undergone chelation therapy and the physicians who prescribed it claim improvement in CAD. In addition, there are approximately twelve published descriptive studies and five randomized controlled clinical trials regarding the use of EDTA chelation for CAD. Although each descriptive study did report a reduction in angina, they were uncontrolled clinical observations or retrospective data, typically with a small number of participants. Of the five clinical trials in which patients were randomly selected to receive chelation therapy or a placebo (a dummy solution), the most rigorous way of assessing a new treatment, three trials involved so few people that only a dramatic improvement could have been detected. Studies need a larger number of participants to detect more mild benefits of a treatment. The fourth study was never published in final form, so its conclusions are uncertain. Finally, the fifth study reported that EDTA chelation was associated with an improvement in ability to exercise, but it had only ten participants.

How frequently is EDTA chelation therapy used?

It is estimated by the American College for Advancement in Medicine (ACAM), a professional association that supports the use of chelation therapy, that more than eight hundred thousand visits for chelation therapy were made in the United States in 1997 alone.

Why did NCCAM and NHLBI decide to study this therapy?

CAD is the leading cause of death among men and women in the United States. In spite of effective standard therapies, such as lifestyle modifications, medications, and surgical procedures, some patients with CAD seek out EDTA chelation therapy as a treatment option.

Therefore, NCCAM and NHLBI saw a public health need to conduct a large-scale, well-designed clinical trial that could determine more clearly whether EDTA chelation therapy is indeed an effective and safe alternative for treating CAD. However, there are professional organizations that are of the opinion that a large study of EDTA chelation therapy should not be carried out because of the lack of scientific evidence supporting its effectiveness.

How will the NIH study be conducted?

This placebo-controlled, double-blind study will recruit 2,372 participants aged fifty years and older with a prior myocardial infarction (heart attack) to test whether EDTA chelation therapy or high-dose vitamin therapy is effective for the treatment of CAD. This study, with a total cost of approximately $30 million, is over twenty times larger than any previous study of chelation therapy. It is designed to be large enough to detect if there are any mild or moderate benefits or risks associated with the therapy.

EDTA chelation therapy, as practiced in the community, often includes administration of high doses of antioxidant vitamin and mineral supplements. Thus, it is possible that effects of the therapy could be connected to these supplements. In order to test whether some of the therapy's effect may be attributable to vitamin or mineral supplements, or to the EDTA solution itself, the investigators will first randomly assign participants to receive either EDTA chelation solution or placebo. Then the patients in these two groups (about 1,186 in each) will again be randomly selected to receive either low-dose or high-dose vitamin or mineral supplements.

The EDTA chelation therapy or placebo solution will be delivered through forty intravenous infusions that are administered over a twenty-eight-month course of treatment. The first thirty infusions will be delivered on a weekly basis and the last ten will be delivered bimonthly. Following the infusion phase, participants will have contact with study staff at three-month intervals until the study is complete.

The protocol for the trial was developed using a model protocol for EDTA chelation therapy endorsed by the American College for Advancement in Medicine (ACAM). The ACAM protocol is used worldwide by chelation practitioners. It is the intent of this study to ensure that the most widely practiced method of delivering EDTA chelation is rigorously tested.

What will the study determine?

Overall, the investigators will assess whether EDTA chelation therapy or high-dose vitamin or mineral supplements are safe and effective in treating individuals with CAD. Specifically, they will determine if EDTA chelation or high-dose vitamin supplements improve event-free survival (length of time without another heart attack, etc.), are safe for use, improve quality of life, and are cost-effective.

The investigators will look at several markers of improvement, or endpoints, to make these determinations. The primary endpoint in the trial will be a composite of:

- All causes of death
- Heart attack
- Stroke
- Hospitalization for angina
- Coronary revascularization.

Secondary endpoints will include:

- Cardiac death, or nonfatal heart attack, or nonfatal stroke
- The individual components of the primary endpoint
- The safety of the therapy
- Health-related quality of life
- Cost-effectiveness.

Who is the study's principal investigator?

The principal investigator for the trial is Gervasio A. Lamas, M.D., director of cardiovascular research and academic affairs at Mount Sinai Medical Center-Miami Heart Institute, Miami Beach, Florida. Dr. Lamas is a board-certified cardiologist and an associate professor of medicine at University of Miami School of Medicine. He has extensive experience in the design, conduct, and analysis of randomized, multicenter trials of the treatment and management of cardiac diseases, including CAD.

What types of participants will be recruited?

Participants must be fifty years of age or older, have had a heart attack at least six weeks prior to evaluation, and have not had chelation therapy within the past five years. Other exclusion criteria include:

- History of allergic reactions to EDTA or any of the therapy's components
- Coronary or carotid revascularization procedures within the past six months or a scheduled revascularization
- History of cigarette smoking within the last three months
- Childbearing potential
- History of liver disease
- Diagnoses of additional medical conditions that could otherwise limit patient survival, such as cancer.

The goal is to recruit a patient study population of both men and women that is fairly typical of people with CAD. The study investigators also will recruit participants whose ethnic and racial makeup reflects the diversity of the United States population.

Where will the study take place?

The study will take place at more than one hundred research sites located across the country. The research sites will represent a mix of clinical settings—university or teaching hospitals, clinical practices or cardiology research centers, or chelation practices. The sites will be selected based on a thorough review of qualifications by the study team and require approval of the study by their local institutional (ethical) review boards.

How long will it take to complete the study?

Over the next several months, additional study sites will be identified. The investigators enrolled the first participants in September 2003. The study will take approximately five years to complete.

How can I learn more about the study?

Information about the study, locations, and enrollment will be available from the NCCAM Information Clearinghouse at 1-888-644-6226, NCCAM's Web site, and from ClinicalTrials.gov, the NIH Web site for clinical trials information.

Chapter 99

Cellular Therapy: Potential Treatment for Heart Disease

Introduction

As novel cellular therapies move from laboratory findings to clinical practice, medical researchers and regulators face new issues and uncertainties involving long-term safety and efficacy.

Currently, there are no effective drug therapies for many acquired and congenital diseases. Recent discoveries in cellular therapy research present new opportunities for cellular products to be used in disease areas with critical, unmet medical needs. The Food and Drug Administration (FDA) regulates cellular therapies to ensure that they are safe and effective, and that persons enrolled in clinical trials using cellular products are protected from undue risk.

Cellular products hold great potential for use in treating damaged or diseased tissues of the body. Cellular products come from a variety of sources, such as stem cells from bone marrow and peripheral blood, and myoblasts from skeletal muscle cells.[1, 2, 3]

There is still much to learn about how cellular products work, how to administer them safely, and whether, over time, the cells will continue to work properly in the body without harmful side effects. FDA is committed to supporting cellular therapy research and development, and future licensure of cellular products, and wants the public

Reprinted from "Cellular Therapy: Potential Treatment for Heart Disease," U.S. Food and Drug Administration, Center for Biologics Evaluation and Research, updated June 2004.

to understand both the promise and the challenges presented by this exciting new therapy.

Stem Cell Research

Stem cells, regardless of origin, have the remarkable potential to develop into many different cell types in the body. When a stem cell divides, each new cell has the potential to either remain a stem cell or become another type of cell with a more specialized function, such as the beating cells of the heart.[1, 2]

There are two characteristics that distinguish stem cells from other types of cells. First, stem cells can self-renew, and second, they can differentiate into other types of cells. Stem cells are unspecialized cells that renew themselves for long periods through cell division, and given certain conditions, can be induced to become cells with special functions.[2]

Stem cells have potential in many areas of medical research. One possible application is to make new cells and tissues for medical therapies. For example, donated organs and tissues are often used to replace those that are diseased or destroyed. Unfortunately, the number of people suffering from disorders that might benefit from stem cell therapy is much greater than the number of organs and tissues available for transplantation.

Stem cells offer the possibility of renewable sources of replacement cells and new tissues to treat many kinds of diseases, conditions, and disabilities.[1, 4]

Cellular Therapy to Treat Heart Disease

Despite many recent advances in medical therapy and interventional techniques, ischemic heart disease and congestive heart failure (CHF) remain the major causes of morbidity and mortality in the United States.[4, 5]

Cellular therapy for treating these and other heart conditions is a growing field of clinical research. Potential cell treatments for patients with congestive heart failure (CHF) and ischemic heart disease are of great interest to medical researchers and treating physicians.

Research to date has involved cells from autologous (donors who are also the recipients of the cellular therapy) skeletal muscle, hematopoietic stem cells from autologous peripheral blood, and unspecialized mesenchymal or hematopoietic stem cells from bone marrow. They have been administered through catheters into the coronary arteries, transendocardially through injection catheters into the left ventricular myocardium, or transepicardially through a needle during coronary artery bypass graft.[3] (Myoblasts are muscle precursor cells that come from differentiated skeletal muscle cells. Because they are easily obtained and capable of regeneration, researchers are attempting to use myoblasts as a source of cells to repair the heart.)

Issues

A diversity of opinion surrounds the feasibility of beginning clinical studies using human stem cells. Some scientists and medical researchers believe it is reasonable to expect that, within the next five years, human stem cells will be used to replace dead or dying cells within organs, such as the failing heart. Others argue that more information is needed about the basic biology of human stem cells before it is possible to assess their therapeutic potential.[4]

Before clinical studies involving cellular therapy can be done, it is essential to demonstrate that cellular products have the relevant biological activity—that the therapy does what it is supposed to do without being toxic.[4, 5]

Three important issues confronting the development of cellular products for the treatment of heart disease include manufacturing, catheter-cellular product interactions, and the nature and quantity of pre-clinical data needed to begin early phase clinical studies.[3]

Differences among individual cell donors can produce inconsistencies, even among products using the same manufacturing process. Different formulation and storage conditions may also have an effect on the cellular product.[3]

Many questions remain about the safety and mechanisms of action of stem cells for the treatment of heart diseases. Pre-clinical studies provide toxicity data, and may also provide useful data regarding the cellular product's mechanism of action.[3]

Certain in vitro studies have shown that non-heart cells may be manipulated to take on functional characteristics of heart cells. These transplanted cells may acquire the ability to revascularize, regenerate muscle, and conduct electrical impulses in the heart.[3]

Heart catheterization methods and devices are being investigated as a way to deliver cellular products. Current research in this area is focused on development of heart catheters and methods that can provide targeted delivery of high concentrations of cells to specific regions of the heart muscle.[3]

Issues related to the safety and effectiveness of the medical devices used to deliver stem cells to a patient are still under investigation. For example, more understanding is needed regarding the safety and effectiveness associated with the delivery of cells by coronary artery balloon catheter devices.[3]

Stem cells are hypothetically able to migrate into areas of muscle degeneration or injury, participate in the regeneration or repair process, and give rise to fully differentiated heart muscle fibers. These stem cells appear to be recruited by long-range, possibly inflammatory, signals originating from the degenerating or injured tissue. They appear to access the heart muscle from the blood circulation.[6]

Role of FDA

The Food and Drug Administration (FDA) has a long history of effectively safeguarding the public health and strong experience in regulating drugs and biological products. FDA's regulatory framework is based, in part, on manufacturing procedures, the use of investigational devices in some studies, the different use of cellular products, and safety concerns associated with administration of these products.[7, 8]

FDA has developed a framework that provides a tiered approach to both cell and tissue regulation. This regulation focuses on three general areas to: (1) prevent the use of contaminated tissues or cells with the potential for transmitting infectious diseases such as AIDS and hepatitis; (2) prevent improper handling or processing that might contaminate or damage tissues or cells; and (3) ensure that clinical safety and effectiveness is demonstrated for tissues or cells that are highly processed, are used for other than their normal function, are combined with nontissue components, or are used for metabolic purposes.[5]

FDA's main priority is to ensure safe human cellular therapy studies. FDA does not want to stand in the way of progress that may lead to effective treatments, but the Agency recognizes that new cellular therapies may have unknown risks, even as they provide benefits to patients.[9]

The regulatory pathway for cellular products is an evolving process and certain issues related to the licensure of cellular products are not resolved yet. FDA's Biological Response Modifiers Advisory Committee (BRMAC) continues to meet to discuss the scientific basis for clinical development of cellular products to be used in the treatment of heart diseases and to discuss the regulatory issues associated with late phase clinical development of these cellular products.

References

1. Stem Cell Basics. NIH website: http://stemcells.nih.gov/info Center/stemCellBasics.asp.

2. Stem Cells: Scientific Progress and Future Research Directions. NIH website: http://stemcells.nih.gov/stemcell/scireport.asp.

3. Briefing document: Cellular Products for the Treatment of Cardiac Disease. Biological Response Modifiers Committee Meeting #37. March 18–19, 2004.

4. Fink, DW. Assessing human stem cell safety. 2001 NIH Stem Cell Report.

5. Proposed Approach to Regulation of Cellular and Tissue-Based Products. February 1997. FDA website: http://www.fda. gov/cber/gdlns/celltissue.pdf.

6. Jensen GS and Drapeau C. The use of in situ bone marrow stem cells for the treatment of various degenerative diseases. *Med Hypotheses* 2002; 59(4): 422–28.

7. Guidance for Industry: Guidance for Human Somatic Cell Therapy and Gene Therapy. March 1998. FDA website: http:// www.fda.gov/cber/gdlns/somgene.pdf.

8. Draft Guidance for Reviewers: Instructions and Template for Chemistry, Manufacturing, and Control (CMC) Reviewers of Human Somatic Cell Therapy Investigational New Drug Applications (INDs). August 2003. FDA website: http://www.fda .gov/cber/gdlns/cmcsomcell.pdf.

9. Human Gene Therapy and the Role of the Food and Drug Administration. FDA website: http://www.fda.gov/cber/infosheets/ genezn.htm.

10. Scientists find new way to grow human embryonic stem cells. March 19, 2003. Science Daily website: http://www.science daily.com/releases/2003/03/030319081016.htm.

Part Nine

Additional Help and Information

Chapter 100

Glossary of
Cardiovascular Terms

Aneurysm: Circumscribed dilation of an artery or a cardiac chamber, usually due to an acquired or congenital weakness of the wall of the artery or chamber.[2]

Angina pectoris: Chest pain lasting a few seconds or minutes, usually brought on by stress or exertion and relieved by rest; considered an early sign of heart disease.[1]

Angioplasty: Reconstitution or recanalization (opening) of a blood vessel; may involve balloon dilation, mechanical stripping of intima, forceful injection of fibrinolytics, or placement of a stent.[2]

Angiotensin converting enzyme (ACE) inhibitor: A drug used to decrease pressure inside blood vessels.[1]

Aorta: A large artery of the elastic type that is the main trunk of the systemic arterial system, arising from the base of the left ventricle and ending at the left side of the body of the fourth lumbar vertebra

---

The terms in this glossary were excerpted from *Stedman's Electronic Medical Dictionary* v.5.0, © 2000 Lippincott Williams and Wilkins [marked 2], and from several documents produced by the National Heart, Lung, and Blood Institute [marked 1], including "Facts about Cardiomyopathy," NIH Publication No. 97-3082 (1997); "Facts about Heart Failure" (1997); and "Strong Heart Study Data Book: A Report to American Indian Communities," NIH Publication No. 01-3285 (2001).

by dividing to form the right and left common iliac arteries. The aorta is subdivided into: ascending aorta; aortic arch; and descending aorta, which is in turn, divided into the thoracic aorta and the abdominal aorta.[2]

Arrhythmia: An irregular heartbeat.[1]

Artery: A relatively thick-walled, muscular, pulsating blood vessel conveying blood away from the heart.[2]

Atherosclerosis: Cholesterol-containing deposits occurring in the inner layer of medium and large arteries; atherosclerosis can lead to heart attack and stroke if the blood vessels become clogged.[1]

Beta blocker: A drug used to slow the heart rate and reduce pressure inside blood vessels. It also can regulate heart rhythm.[1]

Blood pressure (BP): The pressure or tension of the blood within the systemic arteries, maintained by the contraction of the left ventricle, the resistance of the arterioles and capillaries, the elasticity of the arterial walls, as well as the viscosity and volume of the blood; expressed as relative to the ambient atmospheric pressure.[2]

Body mass index (BMI): A measure of body fat calculated as the ratio of weight to (height squared) measured in kilograms and meters.[1]

Bradycardia: Slowness of the heartbeat, usually defined as a rate under 50 beats/minute.[2]

Calcium channel blocker (or calcium blocker): A drug used to relax the blood vessel and heart muscle, causing pressure inside blood vessels to drop. It also can regulate heart rhythm.[1]

Carbohydrates: The component of food that includes starches, sugars, celluloses, and gums.[1]

Cardiac: Referring to the heart.[1]

Cardiac arrest: A sudden stop of heart function.[1]

Cardiomyopathy: A disease of the heart muscle (myocardium).[1]

Cardiomyoplasty: A surgical procedure that involves detaching one end of a back muscle and attaching it to the heart. An electric stimulator causes the muscle to contract to pump blood from the heart.[1]

Cardiovascular disease (CVD): Broad category of diseases of the heart and blood vessels. It includes coronary heart disease, stroke, and heart failure.[1]

Catheterization: A procedure in which a thin, hollow tube is inserted into a blood vessel. The tube is then advanced through the vessel into the heart, enabling a physician to study the heart and its pumping activity.[1]

Cholesterol: Fat-like substance found in animal foods—meat, milk, butter, cheese, and egg yolks; cholesterol is also measured in a person's blood.[1]

Computed tomography (CT): Imaging anatomic information from a cross-sectional plane of the body, each image generated by a computer synthesis of x-ray transmission data obtained in many different directions in a given plane.[2]

Congenital: Existing at birth, referring to certain mental or physical traits, anomalies, malformations, diseases, etc. which may be either hereditary or due to an influence occurring during gestation up to the moment of birth.[2]

Congestive heart failure: A heart disease condition that involves loss of pumping ability by the heart, generally accompanied by fluid accumulation in body tissues, especially the lungs.[1]

Coronary heart disease (CHD): Heart disease resulting from inadequate oxygen supply to the heart, usually because of atherosclerosis.[1]

Defibrillator: Any agent or measure, e.g., an electric shock, that arrests fibrillation of the ventricular muscle and restores the normal beat.[2]

Diastolic blood pressure (DBP): Blood pressure at the point when the heart is not pumping; the second (lower) of the two numbers used in blood pressure measurement.[1]

Diastolic heart failure: Inability of the heart to relax properly and fill with blood as a result of stiffening of the heart muscle.[1]

Digitalis: A drug used to increase the force of the heart's contraction and to regulate specific irregularities of heart rhythm.[1]

Dilated cardiomyopathy: Heart muscle disease that leads to enlargement of the heart's chambers, robbing the heart of its pumping ability.[1]

Diuretic: A drug that helps eliminate excess body fluid; usually used in the treatment of high blood pressure and heart failure.[1]

Dyspnea: Shortness of breath.[1]

Echocardiogram: Picture of the heart taken by using sound waves (ultrasonography).[1]

Echocardiography: A test that bounces sound waves off the heart to produce pictures of its internal structures.[1]

Edema: Abnormal fluid accumulation in body tissues.[1]

Electrocardiogram (ECG or EKG): Measurement of the electrical activity of the heart taken by placing electrodes on the chest of an individual.[1]

Endocarditis: Inflammation of the endocardium.[2]

Endocardium: The innermost tunic of the heart, which includes endothelium and subendothelial connective tissue; in the atrial wall, smooth muscle and numerous elastic fibers also occur.[2]

Folate: One of the B vitamins.[1]

Heart attack: See myocardial infarction.

Heart failure: Loss of pumping ability by the heart, often accompanied by fatigue, breathlessness, and excess fluid accumulation in body tissues.[1]

Holter monitor: A technique for long-term, continuous usually ambulatory, recording of electrocardiographic signals on magnetic tape for scanning and selection of significant but fleeting changes that might otherwise escape notice.[2]

Hypertension: term for high blood pressure; currently defined as systolic blood pressure of at least 140 mmHg or diastolic blood pressure of at least 90 mmHg.[1]

Hypertrophic cardiomyopathy: Heart muscle disease that leads to thickening of the heart walls, interfering with the heart's ability to fill with and pump blood.[1]

Idiopathic: Results from an unknown cause.[1]

Impaired glucose tolerance (IGT): Inability of the body to handle sugar properly following food intake; IGT may lead to diabetes.[1]

Intermittent claudication: A condition caused by ischemia of the muscles; characterized by attacks of lameness and pain, brought on by walking, chiefly in the calf muscles; however, the condition may occur in other muscle groups.[2]

Ischemia: Local anemia due to mechanical obstruction (mainly arterial narrowing or disruption) of the blood supply.[2]

Left ventricular assist device (LVAD): A mechanical device used to increase the heart's pumping ability.[1]

Left ventricular hypertrophy: Enlargement of the chamber of the heart that pumps blood throughout the body; sometimes an indication of pending heart disease.[1]

Lipid: Cholesterol or fats in the blood.[1]

Lipoprotein: Particle that allows fats to be carried in the blood; the particle is made up of a fat particle attached to a protein to make it soluble in blood.[1]

Low density lipoprotein (LDL): Lipoprotein particle; elevated levels have been linked to increased risk of heart disease.[1]

Mitral valve: The valve closing the orifice between the left atrium and left ventricle of the heart; its two cusps are called anterior and posterior.[2]

Mitral valve prolapse: Excessive retrograde movement of one or both mitral valve leaflets into the left atrium during left ventricular systole, often allowing mitral regurgitation; responsible for the click-murmur of Barlow syndrome, and rarely may be due to rheumatic carditis, a connective tissue disorder such as Marfan syndrome, or ruptured chorda tendinea ("flail mitral leaflet").[2]

Myocardial infarction: heart attack resulting from too little oxygen supply to the heart muscle.[1]

Myocardium: The middle layer of the heart, consisting of cardiac muscle.[2]

Nitroglycerin: An explosive yellowish oily fluid formed by the action of sulfuric and nitric acids on glycerin; used as a vasodilator, especially in angina pectoris; generates nitric oxide.[2]

Obesity: Excess body fat; may be measured in a variety of ways, such as body mass index (BMI); for BMI defined as BMI of 30 kg/m^2 or greater.[1]

Overweight: Amount of body fat between normal and obese; for BMI defined as BMI between 25 and 29.9 kg/m^2.[1]

Pericarditis: Inflammation of the pericardium.[2]

Pericardium: The fibroserous membrane, consisting of mesothelium and submesothelial connective tissue, covering the heart and beginning of the great vessels. It is a closed sac having two layers: the visceral layer (epicardium), immediately surrounding and applied to all the heart's surfaces, and the outer parietal layer, forming the sac, composed of strong fibrous tissue lined with a serous membrane. The phrenic nerves pass to the diaphragm through the anterior pericardium and divide the pericardium into antephrenic and retrophrenic portions; the pulmonary hilum divides both of these portions into suprahilar, hilar, and infrahilar portions.[2]

Pulmonary: Relating to the lungs, to the pulmonary artery, or to the aperture leading from the right ventricle into the pulmonary artery.[2]

Pulmonary congestion (or edema): Fluid accumulation in the lungs.[1]

Regurgitation: A backward flow, as of blood through an incompetent valve of the heart.[2]

Restrictive cardiomyopathy: Heart muscle disease in which the muscle walls become stiff and lose their flexibility.[1]

Risk factor: A personal characteristic that is associated with increased risk of disease.[1]

Saturated fat: Dietary fat that is unhealthy because of its link with high blood cholesterol and atherosclerosis.[1]

Septum: In the heart, a muscle wall separating the chambers.[1]

Silent ischemia: Myocardial ischemia without accompanying signs or symptoms of angina pectoris; can be detected by ECG and other lab techniques.[2]

Sinuatrial node: The mass of specialized cardiac muscle fibers that normally acts as the "pacemaker" of the cardiac conduction system; it lies under the epicardium at the upper end of the sulcus terminalis.[2]

Sinus node: See sinuatrial node.

Stroke: Damage to the brain resulting from too little oxygen.[1]

Sudden cardiac death: Cardiac arrest caused by an irregular heartbeat. The term "death" is somewhat misleading, because some patients survive.[1]

Systolic blood pressure (SBP): Blood pressure at the moment the heart has just finished a beat; the first (higher) of the two numbers used in blood pressure measurement.[1]

Systolic heart failure: Inability of the heart to contract with enough force to pump adequate amounts of blood through the body.[1]

Thrombosis: Formation or presence of a thrombus; clotting within a blood vessel which may cause infarction of tissues supplied by the vessel.[2]

Thrombus: A clot in the cardiovascular systems formed during life from constituents of blood; it may be occlusive or attached to the vessel or heart wall without obstructing the lumen (mural thrombus).[2]

Transplantation: Transfer of living tissue (kidney, blood, heart) from one individual to another to prolong or improve the quality of life of the recipient.[1]

Triglycerides: A fat-like substance found in the blood; higher levels of triglycerides have been linked to heart disease.[1]

Ultrasound/ultrasonography: A technique for imaging internal components of the body using sound waves that is without harm or discomfort to the patient.[1]

Valves: Flap-like structures that control the direction of blood flow through the heart.[1]

Varicose veins: Permanent dilation and tortuosity of veins, most commonly seen in the legs, probably as a result of congenitally incomplete valves; there is a predisposition to varicose veins among persons in occupations requiring long periods of standing, and in pregnant women.[2]

Vascular: Relating to or containing blood vessels.[2]

Vein: A blood vessel carrying blood toward the heart; postnatally, all veins except the pulmonary carry dark unoxygenated blood.[2]

Ventricles: The two lower chambers of the heart. The left ventricle is the main pumping chamber in the heart.[1]

Ventricular dysfunction: Inability of the ventricle to pump the blood adequately.[1]

Ventricular fibrillation: Rapid, irregular quivering of the heart's ventricles, with no effective heartbeat.[1]

Chapter 101

Cookbooks for Cardiovascular Health

Heart Healthy Cookbooks

American Heart Association Around the World Cookbook:
Low-Fat Recipes with International Flavor
Author: American Heart Association
Publisher: Times Books, 1996
ISBN: 0-812-92344-8

American Heart Association Low-Fat, Low-Cholesterol
Cookbook
Author: American Heart Association
Publisher: Ballantine Books, 2002
ISBN: 0-345-46182-7

American Heart Association Low-Salt Cookbook
Author: American Heart Association
Publisher: Clarkson N Potter Publishers, 2002
ISBN: 0-609-80968-7

Information in this chapter was compiled from various sources deemed reliable. This list is not intended to be comprehensive; inclusion does not constitute endorsement. Please check with your local library or bookstore, or contact the publisher for ordering information.

American Heart Association Kids' Cookbook
Author: American Heart Association
Publisher: Clarkson Potter Publishers, 1993
ISBN: 0-812-91930-0

American Heart Association Low-Fat and Luscious Desserts, Cakes, Cookies, Pies, and Other Temptations
Author: American Heart Association
Publisher: Clarkson N Potter Publishers, 2000
ISBN: 0-812-93336-2

Betty Crocker Healthy Heart Cookbook
Author: Betty Crocker Editors
Publisher: Betty Crocker, 2004
ISBN: 0-764-57424-8

Betty Crocker's New Low-Fat, Low-Cholesterol Cookbook
Author: Betty Crocker Editors
Publisher: John Wiley and Sons, 1996
ISBN: 0-028-60388-5

Choices for a Healthy Heart
Author: Joseph C. Piscatella and Bernie Piscatella
Publisher: Workman Publishing, 1987
ISBN: 0-894-80138-4

Delicious Heart Healthy Latino Recipes
Author: National Heart, Lung, and Blood Institute
(NIH Pub. No. 96-4049)
Website: www.nhlbi.nih.gov/health/public/heart/other/sp_recip.htm

Don't Eat Your Heart Out Cookbook, Second Edition
Author: Joseph C. Piscatella
Publisher: Workman Publishing, 1994
ISBN: 1-563-05558-9

Down Home Healthy: Family Recipes of Black American Chefs
Author: Leah Chase
Publisher: Diane Publishing Company, 1994
ISBN: 0-788-12063-8

Healthy Heart Cookbook:
300 Low-Sodium, Low-Salt Recipes
Author: Karin Caldwell, Edith Tibbetts, and Alvin F. Goldfarb
Publisher: Sterling, 2004
ISBN: 1-402-71681-8

The Healthy-Heart Cookbook:
Over 700 Recipes for Every Day and Every Occasion
Author: Joseph Piscatella and Bernie Piscatella
Publisher: Block Dog and Leventhal Publishers, 2003
ISBN: 1-579-12330-9

The Healthy Heart Cookbook for Dummies
Author: James M. Rippe
Publisher: For Dummies, 2000
ISBN: 0-764-55222-8

Healthy Mexican Cooking: Authentic Low-Fat Recipes
Author: Velda De La Garza, et al.
Publisher: Appletree Press, 1995
ISBN: 0-962-04715-5

Healthy Snacks for Kids
Author: Penny Warner
Publisher: Bristol Publishing Enterprises, 1999
ISBN: 1-558-67159-5

The New American Heart Association Cookbook,
Sixth Edition
Author: American Heart Association
Publisher: Clarkson Potter, 1998
ISBN: 0-812-92954-3

Quick and Easy Cookbook:
More than 200 Healthful Recipes You Can Make in Minutes
Author: American Heart Association
Publisher: Clarkson N Potter Publishers, 2001
ISBN: 0-609-80862-1

Cookbooks for People with Hypertension

**American Heart Association Low-Calorie Cookbook:
More Than 200 Delicious Recipes for Healthy Eating**
Author: American Heart Association
Publisher: Clarkson N Potter Publishers, 2003
ISBN: 0-8129-2854-7

American Heart Association Meals in Minutes Cookbook
Author: American Heart Association
Publisher: Clarkson Potter Publishers, 2002
ISBN: 0-6098-09776

**American Heart Association One-Dish Meals:
Over 200 All-New, All-in-One Recipes**
Author: American Heart Association
Publisher: Clarkson Potter Publishers, 2003
ISBN: 0-609-61085-6

American Medical Association Family Health Cookbook
Author: Brooke Dojny
Publisher: Atria, 1997
ISBN: 0-671-53667-2

Betty Crocker's Low-Fat, Low-Cholesterol Cooking Today
Author: Betty Crocker Editors
Publisher: Betty Crocker, 2000
ISBN: 0-028-63762-3

Cooking With Herbs and Spices: Easy, Low-Fat Flavor
Author: Judy Gilliard
Publisher: Adams Media Corporation., 1999
ISBN: 1-580-62219-4

**Dash Diet for Hypertension: Lower Your Blood Pressure in
14 days—Without Drugs**
Author: Thomas Moore and Mark Jenkins
Publisher: Pocket, 2003
ISBN: 0-743-41007-6

Get the Salt Out: 501 Simple Ways to Cut the Salt Out of Any Diet
Author: Ann Louise Gittleman
Publisher: Three Rivers Press, 1996
ISBN: 0-517-88654-5

Keep the Beat: Heart Healthy Recipes
Author: National Heart, Lung, and Blood Institute
Website: http://www.nhlbi.nih.gov/health/public/heart/other/
ktb_recipebk/index.htm

Lifeclinic Healthy Cookbook
Author: Lifeclinic.com
Website: http://www.lifeclinic.com/whatsnew/cookbook/cookbook.asp

Mediterranean Diet Cookbook: A Delicious Alternative for Lifelong Health
Author: Nancy Jenkins
Publisher: Bantam, 1994
ISBN: 0-553-09608-7

Mediterranean Heart Diet: How It Works and How to Reap the Health Benefits, with Recipes to Get You Started
Author: Helen V. Fisher, et al.
Publisher: Perseus Publishing, 2001
ISBN: 1-555-61281-4

No-Salt Cookbook: Reduce or Eliminate Salt Without Sacrificing Flavor
Author: David C. Anderson, Thomas D. Anderson
Publisher: Adams Media Corporation, 2001
ISBN: 1-580-62525-8

No-Salt, Lowest-Sodium Baking Book
Author: Donald A. Gazzaniga and Michael Fowler
Publisher: Thomas Dunne Books, 2003
ISBN: 0-312-30118-9

No-Salt, Lowest-Sodium Cookbook
Author: Donald A. Gazzaniga
Publisher: St. Martin's Griffin, 2002
ISBN: 0-312-29164-7

Stay Young at Heart Recipe Cards
Author: National Heart, Lung, and Blood Institute
Website: http://www.nhlbi.nih.gov/health/public/heart/other/syah/
index.htm

Cookbooks for Diabetics

American Diabetes Association Diabetes Cookbook
Author: Sally Mansfield, et al.
Publisher: DK Publishing, 2000
ISBN: 0-789-45175-1

The Art of Cooking for the Diabetic (3rd edition)
Author: Mary Abbott Hess and Jane Grant Tougas
Publisher: McGraw-Hill, 1996
ISBN: 0-809-23393-2

Betty Crocker's Diabetes Cookbook: Everyday Meals, Easy as 1-2-3
Author: Betty Crocker Editors
Publisher: Betty Crocker, 2003
ISBN: 0-764-56704-7

Brand-Name Diabetic Meals in Minutes
Author: American Dietetic Association, American Diabetes Association
Publisher: McGraw-Hill, 1997
ISBN: 0-945-44876-7

The Complete Step-by-Step Diabetic Cookbook
Author: Anne C. Chappell
Publisher: Oxmoor House, 1995
ISBN: 0-848-71431-8

The Diabetes and Heart Healthy Cookbook
Author: American Diabetes Association, American Heart Association
Publisher: American Diabetes Association, 2004
ISBN: 1-580-40180-5

Diabetic Meals In 30 Minutes—or Less!
Author: Robyn Webb
Publisher: McGraw-Hill, 1996
ISBN: 0-945-44860-0

The Diabetic's Innovative Cookbook: A Positive Approach to Living with Diabetes
Author: Joseph Juliano and Dianne Young
Publisher: Henry Holt and Company, 1994
ISBN: 0-805-02518-9

Get the Sugar Out: 501 Simple Ways to Cut the Sugar in Any Diet
Author: Ann Louise Gittleman
Publisher: Three Rivers Press, 1996
ISBN: 0-517-88653-7

Healthy & Hearty Diabetic Cooking
Author: Canadian Diabetes Association
Publisher: R.A. Rappaport Publishing, 1993
ISBN: 0-963-17012-0

Month of Meals: All-American Fare
Author: American Diabetes Association
Publisher: American Diabetes Association, 2002
ISBN: 1-580-40077-9

Month of Meals: Ethnic Delights
Author: American Diabetes Association
Publisher: McGraw-Hill, 1998
ISBN: 1-580-40015-9

Month of Meals: Meals in Minutes
Author: American Diabetes Association
Publisher: American Diabetes Association, 2002
ISBN: 1-580-40078-7

Month of Meals: Old-Time Favorites
Author: American Diabetes Association
Publisher: McGraw-Hill, 1998
ISBN: 1-580-40017-5

More Diabetic Meals in 30 Minutes—Or Less!
Author: Robyn Webb
Publisher: McGraw-Hill, 1999
ISBN: 1-580-40029-9

The New Diabetic Cookbook, Fifth Edition
Author: Mabel Cavaiani
Publisher: McGraw-Hill, 2002
ISBN: 0-071-39135-5

The New Family Cookbook for People with Diabetes
Author: American Dietetic Association
Publisher: Simon and Schuster, 1999
ISBN: 0-684-82660-7

One-Pot Meals for People with Diabetes
Author: Ruth Glick and Nancy Baggett
Publisher: McGraw-Hill, 2002
ISBN: 1-580-40066-3

The UCSD Healthy Diet for Diabetes: A Comprehensive Nutritional Guide and Cookbook (University of California at San Diego)
Author: Susan Algert, et al.
Publisher: Houghton Mifflin Company, 1990
ISBN: 0-345-49477-X

Chapter 102

Directory of Resources for Cardiovascular Patients

Cardiovascular Disease

Agency for Healthcare Research and Quality (AHRQ)
540 Gaither Road
Rockville, MD 20850
Phone: 301-427-1364
Website: http://www.ahrq.gov
E-mail: info@ahrq.gov

American Academy of Family Physicians (AAFP)
11400 Tomahawk Creek Parkway
Leawood, KS 66211-2672
Toll-Free: 800-274-2237
Phone: 913-906-6000
Website: http://www.aafp.org
E-mail: fp@aafp.org

American Academy of Pediatrics (AAP)
141 Northwest Point Blvd.
Elk Grove, IL 60007-1098
Phone: 847-434-4000
Fax: 847-434-8000
Website: http://www.aap.org
E-mail: kidsdocs@aap.org

American Association of Cardiovascular and Pulmonary Rehabilitation (AACVPR)
401 N. Michigan Ave.
Suite 2200
Chicago, IL 60611
Phone: 312-321-5146
Fax: 321-527-6635
Website: http://www.aacvpr.org
E-mail: aacvpr@sba.com

The information in this chapter was compiled from various sources deemed accurate. All contact information was verified and updated in August 2004. Inclusion does not imply endorsement. This list is intended to serve as a starting point for information gathering; it is not comprehensive.

American College of Cardiology (ACC)
Heart House
9111 Old Georgetown Road
Bethesda, MD 20814-1699
Toll-Free: 800-253-4636 x694
Phone: 301-897-5400
Fax: 301-897-9745
Website: http://www.acc.org
E-mail: resource@acc.org

American College of Chest Physicians (ACCP)
3300 Dundee Road
Northbrook, IL 60062
Toll-Free: 800-343-2227
Phone: 847-498-1400
Fax: 847-498-5460
Website: http://www.chestnet.org

American College of Physicians
190 N. Independence Mall West
Philadelphia, PA 19106-1572
Toll-Free: 800-523-1546 x2600
Phone: 215-351-2600
Website: http://
www.acponline.org

American Council on Exercise
4851 Paramount Drive
San Diego, CA 92123
Toll-Free: 800-825-3636
Phone: 858-279-8227
Fax: 858-279-8064
Website: http://
www.acefitness.org
E-mail: certify@acefitness.org

American Heart Association (AHA)
National Center
7272 Greenville Ave.
Dallas, TX 75231
Toll-Free: 800-242-8721
Website: http://
www.americanheart.org

American Lung Association
61 Broadway, 6th Floor
New York, NY 10006
Toll-Free: 800-LUNGUSA (800-586-4872)
Phone: 212-315-8700
Website: http://www.lungusa.org

American Medical Association (AMA)
515 N. State St.
Chicago, IL 60610
Toll-Free: 800-621-8335
Website: http://www.ama-assn.org

American Medical Women's Association (AMWA)
801 N. Fairfax St., Suite 400
Alexandria, VA 22314
Phone: 703-838-0500
Fax: 703-549-3864
Website: http://www.amwa-doc.org
E-mail: info@amwa-doc.org

Brain Aneurysm Foundation, Inc.
12 Clarendon Street
Boston, MA 02116
Phone: 617-723-3870
Fax: 617-723-8672
Website: http://bafound.org
E-mail: information@bafound.org

Centers for Disease Control and Prevention (CDC)
1600 Clifton Road
MS D-25
Atlanta, GA 30333
Toll-Free: 800-311-3435
Phone: 404-639-3311 or
404-639-3435
Fax: 404-639-7394
Website: http://www.cdc.gov
E-mail: ccdinfo@cdc.gov

Cleveland Clinic
Department of Patient
Education and Health
Information
9500 Euclid Avenue, NA31
Cleveland, OH 44195
Toll-free: 800-223-2273, ext. 43771
Phone: 216-444-2200
TTY: 216-444-0261
Website: http://
www.clevelandclinic.org
E-mail: healthl@ccf.org

HeartCenterOnline
1 S. Ocean Blvd., Suite 201
Boca Raton, FL 33432
Fax: 561-620-9799
Website: http://
www.heartcenteronline.com

Heart Failure Society of America
Court International, Suite 240 S
2550 University Avenue West
St. Paul, MN 55114
Phone: 651-642-1633
Fax: 651-642-1502
Website: http://www.hfsa.org
E-mail: info@hfsa.org

Heart Rhythm Society
Six Strathmore Road
Natick, MA 01760
Phone: 508-647-0100
Fax: 508-647-0124
Website: http://
www.hrspatients.org

Howard Gilman Institute for Valvular Heart Disease
Weill Medical College of Cornell
University
525 East 68th Street
New York, NY 10021
Phone: 212-746-2189
Fax: 212-746-8448
Website: http://
www.gilmanheartvalve.org
E-mail:
info@gilmanheartvalve.org

Johns Hopkins School of Medicine
720 Rutland Ave.
Baltimore, MD 21205
Phone: 410-955-5000
TTY: 410-955-6446
Website: http://
www.hopkinsmedicine.org/som/
index.html

KidsHealth
Nemours Center for Children's
Health Media
1600 Rockland Road
Wilmington, DE 19803
Phone: 302-651-4046
Fax: 302-651-4077
Website: http://kidshealth.org
E-mail: info@kidshealth.org

Mayo Clinic
Website: http://
www.mayoclinic.com
E-mail:
comments@mayoclinic.com

Mayo Foundation for
Medical Education and
Research
200 First St. SW
Rochester, MN 55905
Phone: 507-284-2511
TDD: 507-284-9786
Fax: 507-284-0161
Website: http://www.mayo.edu

Medical College of
Wisconsin
9200 West Wisconsin Ave.
Suite 2977
Milwaukee, WI 53226
Phone: 404-456-8296
Fax: 404-805-6337
Website: http://
healthlink.mcw.edu
E-mail: healthlink@mcw.edu

Minneapolis Heart Institute
Foundation
920 E 28th Street
Minneapolis, MN 55407
Toll-Free: 877-800-2729
Phone: 612-863-3833
Fax: 612-863-3801
Website: http://
www.mplsheartfoundation.org

National Center for
Chronic Disease Prevention
and Health Promotion
Centers for Disease Control and
Prevention
1600 Clifton Road
Atlanta, GA 30333
Phone: 404-639-3311
Website: http://www.cdc.gov/
nccdphp
E-mail: ccdinfo@cdc.gov

National Center for
Complementary and
Alternative Medicine
(NCCAM)
P.O. Box 7923
Gaithersburg, MD 20898
Toll-Free: 888-644-6226
Phone: 301-519-3153
TTY: 866-464-3615
Fax: 866-464-3616
Website: http://nccam.nih.gov
E-mail: info@nccam.nih.gov

National Center for Health
Statistics (NCHS)
3311 Toledo Road
Hyattsville, MD 20782
Phone: 301-458-4000
Website: http://www.cdc.gov/
nchs
E-mail: nchsquery@cdc.gov

National Heart, Lung, and Blood Institute (NHLBI)
NHLBI Health Information Center
P.O. Box 30105
Bethesda, MD 20824-0105
Phone: 301-592-8573
Fax: 301-592-8563
TTY: 240-629-3255
Website: http://www.nhlbi.nih.gov/index.htm
E-mail: nhlbiinfo@nhlbi.nih.gov

National Institutes of Health (NIH)
9000 Rockville Pike
Bethesda, MD 208920
Phone: 301-496-4000
Website: http://www.nih.gov
E-mail: nihinfo@od.nih.gov

National Library of Medicine
8600 Rockville Pike
Bethesda, MD 20894
Toll-Free: 888-346-3656
Phone: 301-594-5983
Fax: 301-402-1384
Website: http://www.nlm.nih.gov
E-mail: custserv@nlm.nih.gov

National Women's Health Information Center
Department of Health and Human Services
200 Independence Ave. SW, Room 730B
Washington, DC 20201
Toll-Free: 800-994-WOMAN
Phone: 202-690-7650
Fax: 202-205-2631
TDD: 888-220-5446
Website: http://www.4woman.gov

Office of Disease Prevention and Health Promotion (ODPHP)
1101 Wooton Parkway
Suite LL100
Rockville, MD 20852
Phone: 240-453-8280
Fax: 240-453-8282
Website: http://odphp.osophs.dhhs.gov

Office of Women's Health (OWH)
5600 Fishers Lane
Rockville, MD 20857-0001
Toll-Free: 888-463-6332
Phone: 301-827-0350
Website: http://www.fda.gov/womens

Texas Heart Institute
6770 Bertner Avenue
P.O. Box 20345
Houston, TX 77030
Phone: 823-355-4011
Website: http://www.tmc.edu/thi

U.S. Department of Health and Human Services (HHS)
200 Independence Ave. SW
Washington, DC 20201
Toll-Free: 877-696-6775
Phone: 202-619-0257
Website: http://www.hhs.gov

U.S. Food and Drug Administration (FDA)
5600 Fishers Lane
Rockville, MD 20857-0001
Toll-Free: 888-463-6332
Website: http://www.fda.gov

Vascular Disease Foundation
3333 South Wadsworth Blvd.,
Suite B104-37
Lakewood, CO 90227
Phone: 303-949-8337
Fax: 303-989-6522
Website: http://www.vdf.org
E-mail: info@vdf.org

WomenHeart: The National Coalition for Women with Heart Disease
818 18th Street, NW, Suite 230
Washington, DC 20006
Phone: 202-728-7199
Fax: 202-728-7238
Website: http://
www.womenheart.org
E-mail: mail@womenheart.org

Cardiovascular Rehabilitation

American Association of Cardiovascular and Pulmonary Rehabilitation
401 N. Michigan Ave., Suite 2200
Chicago, IL 60611
Phone: 312-321-5146
Fax: 312-527-6635
Website: http://www.aacvpr.org
E-mail: aacvpr@sba.com

Mended Hearts, Inc.
7272 Greenville Avenue
Dallas, TX 75231-4596
Phone: 214-706-1442
Fax: 214-706-5245
Website: http://
www.mendedhearts.org
E-mail: info@mendedhearts.org

Congenital Heart Defects

Congenital Heart Information Network
1561 Clark Drive
Yardley, PA 19067
Phone: 215-493-3068
Website: http://www.tchin.org

March of Dimes
1275 Mamaroneck Avenue
White Plains, NY 10605
Toll-Free: 800-367-6630
Website: http://
www.modimes.org

Diabetes

American Association of Diabetes Educators (AADE)
100 West Monroe, Suite 400
Chicago, IL 60603
Toll-Free 800-338-3633
Phone: 312-424-2426
Fax: 312-424-2427
Diabetes Educator Access Line:
800-TEAMUP4 (800-832-6874)
Website: http://www.aadenet.org
E-mail: aade@aadenet.org

American Diabetes Association (ADA)
1701 N. Beauregard St.
Alexandria, VA 22311
Toll-Free: 800-342-2383
Fax: 847-434-8000
Website: http://www.diabetes.org
E-mail: AskADA@diabetes.org

Centers for Disease Control and Prevention (CDC)

National Center for Chronic Disease Prevention and Health Promotion
Division of Diabetes Translation
Mail Stop K-10
4770 Buford Highway, N.E.
Atlanta, GA 30341-3717
Toll Free: 877-CDC-DIAB
Fax: 301-562-1050
E-mail: diabetes@cdc.gov
Website: http://www.cdc.gov/diabetes

Department of Veterans Affairs

Veterans Health Administration (VHA)
Program Chief, Diabetes
Veterans Health Affairs
810 Vermont Avenue, N.W.
Washington, DC 20420
Phone: 202-273-8490
Fax: 202-273-9142
Website: http://www.va.gov

Diabetes Action Research and Education Foundation

426 C Street, N.E.
Washington, DC 20002
Phone: 202-333-4520
Website: http://www.diabetesaction.org
E-mail: daref@diabetesaction.org

Diabetes Exercise and Sports Association (DESA)

8001 Montcastle Drive
Nashville, TN 37221
Toll Free: 800-898-4322
Fax: 615-673-2077
Website: http://www.diabetes-exercise.org
E-mail: desa@diabetes-exercise.org

Diabetes Endocrinology Research Centers (DERCs)

Joslin Diabetes Center DERC

One Joslin Place
Boston, MA 02215
Phone: 617-732-2400
Fax: 617-732-2487
Website: http://www.joslin.harvard.edu

Massachusetts General Hospital DERC

Diabetes Unit
Department of Molecular Biology
Wellman 8
50 Blossom Street
Boston, MA 02114
Phone: 617-726-6909
Website: http://www.mgh.harvard.edu/depts/diabetes/treatmentatMGH.htm

University of Colorado DERC

Barbara Davis Center for Childhood Diabetes
4200 East 9th Avenue
Box B-140
Denver, CO 80262
Phone: 303-315-8796
Fax: 303-315-4892
Website: http://www.uchsc.edu/misc/diabetes/index.html

University of Iowa DERC
Department of Internal
Medicine
200 Hawkins Drive
Iowa City, IA 52242
Phone: 319-338-0581, ext. 7625
Fax: 319-339-7025
Website: http://www.int-med
.uiowa.edu

*University of Massachusetts
Medical School DERC*
373 Plantation Street, Suite 218
Worcester, MA 01605
Phone: 508-856-3800
Fax: 508-856-4093
Website: http://
www.umassmed.edu/derc

*University of Pennsylvania
DERC*
Division of Endocrinology,
Diabetes and Metabolism
778 Clinical Research Building
415 Curie Boulevard
Philadelphia, PA 19104
Phone: 215-898-6893
Fax: 215-573-5809
Website: http://
www.med.upenn.edu/pdc

University of Washington DERC
Box 358285
DVA Puget Sound Health Care
System
1660 S. Columbian Way
Seattle, WA 98108
Phone: 206-764-2688
Fax: 206-764-2693
Website: http://depts.washington
.edu/diabetes/index.html

*Yale University School of
Medicine DERC*
Box 208020
333 Cedar Street, Fitikin 1
Section of Endocrinology
New Haven, CT 06520-8020
Phone: 203-785-6069
Fax: 203-785-6015
Website: http://
info.med.yale.edu/intmed/
endocrin/research_prog.html

Diabetes Research and Training Centers (DRTCs)

Albert Einstein DRTC
Belfer Building 701
1300 Morris Park Avenue
Bronx, NY 10461
Phone: 718-430-3345
Fax: 718-430-8634
Website: http://medicine.aecom.yu
.edu/endocrine/DiabetesCenter.htm

Indiana University DRTC
Indiana University School of
Medicine
250 University Blvd., Suite 122
Indianapolis, IN 46202
Phone: 317-630-6375
Fax: 317-278-0900
Website: http://www.indiana.edu/
~ovpr/ ctrdir/drtc.html

Michigan DRTC
University of Michigan Medical
School
1331 E. Ann Street, #5111
Ann Arbor, MI 48109-0580
Phone: 734-763-5730
Fax: 734-647-2307
Website: http://
www.med.umich.edu/mdrtc

University of Chicago DRTC
Howard Hughes Medical
Institute
University of Chicago
5841 S. Maryland Avenue
MC 1028, Room N-216
Chicago, IL 60637
Phone: 773-702-1334
Fax: 773-702-4292
Website: http://endocrinology
.uchicago.edu/clinicalpages/
drtc.html

Vanderbilt University DRTC
Vanderbilt University School of
Medicine
707 Light Hall
Nashville, TN 37232-0615
Phone: 615-322-4708
Fax: 615-322-7236
Website: http://www.mc.vanderbilt
.edu/vumc/centers/drtc

Washington University DRTC
Washington University School of
Medicine
660 S. Euclid Avenue, Box 8127
St. Louis, MO 63110
Phone: 314-362-8680
Fax: 314-747-2692
Website: http://
medicine.wustl.edu/~drtc

Indian Health Service (IHS)
Indian Health Service National
Diabetes Program
5300 Homestead Road, N.E.
Albuquerque, NM 87110
Phone: 505-248-4182 or
505-248-4236
Fax: 505-248-4188

Website: http://www.ihs.gov/Med
icalPrograms/Diabetes/index.asp
E-mail:
diabetesprogram@mail.ihs.gov

**Juvenile Diabetes Research
Foundation International
(JDRF)**
120 Wall Street
19th floor
New York, NY 10005-4001
Toll Free: 800-533-2873
Phone: 212-785-9500
Fax: 212-785-9595
E-mail: info@jdf.org
Website: http://www.jdf.org

**National Diabetes
Education Program**
1 Diabetes Way
Bethesda, MD 20802-3600
Toll-Free: 800-438-5383
Phone: 301-496-3583
Website: http://ndep.nih.gov
E-mail: ndep@info.nih.gov

**National Diabetes
Information Clearinghouse**
1 Information Way
Bethesda, MD 20892-3560
Toll-Free: 800-860-8747
Phone: 301-654-3327
Fax: 301-907-8906
Website: http://
diabetes.niddk.nih.gov
E-mail: ndic@info.niddk.nih.gov

National Eye Health Education Program (NEHEP)
National Eye Institute (NEI)
2020 Vision Place
Bethesda, MD 20892-3655
Toll Free: 800-869-2020 (for health professionals only)
Phone: 301-496-5248
Fax: 301-402-1065
Website: http://www.nei.nih.gov
E-mail: 2020@nei.nih.gov

National Institute of Diabetes and Digestive and Kidney Diseases
Building 31, Room 9A04 Center Drive, MCS 2560
Bethesda, MD 20892-2560
Website: http://www.niddk.nih.gov

National Kidney and Urologic Diseases Information Clearinghouse (NKUDIC)
3 Information Way
Bethesda, MD 20892-3580
Toll Free: 800-891-5390
Phone: 301-654-4415
Fax: 301-907-8906
Website: http://kidney.niddk.nih.gov
E-mail: nkudic@info.niddk.nih.gov

High Blood Pressure (Hypertension):

American Society of Hypertension, Inc.
148 Madison Ave., 5th Floor
New York, NY 10016
Phone: 212-696-9099
Fax: 212-696-0711
Website: http://www.ash-us.org
E-mail: ash@ash-us.org

BlackHealthCare.com
Website: http://www.blackhealthcare.com

Council for High Blood Pressure Research (CHBPR)
National Center
7272 Greenville Ave.
Dallas, TX 75231
Toll-Free: 800-242-8721
Website: http://www.americanheart.org/presenter.jhtml?identifier=1115

Hypertension Education Foundation
Box 651
Scarsdale, NY 10583
Website: http://www.hypertensionfoundation.org
E-mail: hyperedu@aol.com

Hypertension Online
Baylor College of Medicine
1 Baylor Plaza
Houston, TX 77030
Phone: 713-798-4951
Website: http://www.hypertensiononline.org
E-mail: www@bcm.tmc.edu

InteliHealth: High Blood Pressure

Website: http://www.intelihealth
.com/IH/ihtIH/WSIHW000/8315/
8315.html
E-mail:
comments@intelihealth.com

Inter-American Society of Hypertension (IASH)

University of Mississippi
Medical Center
Jackson, MS 39216-4505
Phone: 601-984-1820
Fax: 601-984-1817
Website: http://org.umc.edu/iash/
homepage.htm

International Society on Hypertension in Blacks, Inc. (ISHIB)

100 Auburn Ave., N.E.
Atlanta, GA 30303
Phone: 404-880-0343
Fax: 404-880-0347
Website: http://www.ishib.org
E-mail: inforequest@ishib.org

MayoClinic.com: High Blood Pressure Condition Center

200 1st St. SW
Rochester, MN 55905
Website: http://www.mayoclinic
.com/findinformation/condition
centers/centers.cfm?objectid
=0000C07D-38AE-1B32-82D
780C8D77A0000
E-mail:
comments@mayoclinic.com

National Hypertension Association

324 E. 30th St.
New York, NY 10016
Phone: 212-889-3557
Fax: 212-447-7031
Website: http://
www.nathypertension.org
E-mail:
nathypertension@aol.com

PHCentral–Pulmonary Hypertension: The Complete Resource

P.O. Box 477
Blue Bell, PA 19422
Website: http://www.phcentral.org
E-mail: info@PHCentral.org

Pulmonary Hypertension Association

850 Sligo Ave., Suite 800
Silver Spring, MD 20910
Toll-Free: 800-748-7274
Phone: 301-565-3004
Fax: 301-565-3994
Website: http://
www.phassociation.org

WebMD: Hypertension Health Center

Website: http://my.webmd.com/
medical_information/condition_
centers/hypertension/default
.htm

World Hypertension League

Website: http://www.mco.edu/whl
E-mail: whlsec@mco.edu
Visit the site to find a local
chapter.

Stroke

Administration on Aging
330 Independence Ave., S.W.
Washington, DC 20201
Toll-Free: 800-677-1116
Phone: 202-619-0725
Website: http://www.aoa.gov
E-mail: aoainfo@aoa.gov

American Stroke Association
American Heart Association
National Center
7272 Greenville Ave.
Dallas, TX 75231
Toll-Free: 800-242-7653
Website: http://
www.strokeassociation.org

Brain Resources and Information Network (BRAIN)
P.O. Box 5801
Bethesda, MD 20824
Toll-Free: 800-352-9424
Phone: 301-496-5751
Fax: 301-402-2186
Website: http://ninds.nih.gov

Children's Hemiplegia and Stroke Association (CHASA)
Suite 305, PMB 149
4101 West Green Oaks Blvd.
Arlington, TX 76016
Phone: 817-492-4325
Website: http://www.hemikids.org
E-mail: support@chasa.org

National Institute of Neurological Disorders and Stroke
P.O. Box 5801
Bethesda, MD 20824
Toll-Free: 800-352-9424
Phone: 301-496-5751
TTY: 301-468-5981
Website: http://
www.ninds.nih.gov

National Stroke Association
9707 East Easter Lane
Englewood, CO 80112-3747
Toll-Free: 800-STROKES (787-6537)
Phone: 303-649-9299
Fax: 303-649-1328
Website: http://www.stroke.org

Stroke Clubs International
805 12th Street
Galveston, TX 77550
Phone: 409-762-1022
E-mail: strokeclub@aol.com

Index

Index

Page numbers followed by 'n' indicate a footnote. Page numbers in *italics* indicate a table or illustration.

Health Reference Series
COMPLETE CATALOG

Adolescent Health Sourcebook

Basic Consumer Health Information about Common Medical, Mental, and Emotional Concerns in Adolescents, Including Facts about Acne, Body Piercing, Mononucleosis, Nutrition, Eating Disorders, Stress, Depression, Behavior Problems, Peer Pressure, Violence, Gangs, Drug Use, Puberty, Sexuality, Pregnancy, Learning Disabilities, and More

Along with a Glossary of Terms and Other Resources for Further Help and Information

Edited by Chad T. Kimball. 658 pages. 2002. 0-7808-0248-9. $78.

"It is written in clear, nontechnical language aimed at general readers. . . . Recommended for public libraries, community colleges, and other agencies serving health care consumers."
— *American Reference Books Annual, 2003*

"Recommended for school and public libraries. Parents and professionals dealing with teens will appreciate the easy-to-follow format and the clearly written text. This could become a 'must have' for every high school teacher." — *E-Streams, Jan '03*

"A good starting point for information related to common medical, mental, and emotional concerns of adolescents." — *School Library Journal, Nov '02*

"This book provides accurate information in an easy to access format. It addresses topics that parents and caregivers might not be aware of and provides practical, useable information." — *Doody's Health Sciences Book Review Journal, Sep-Oct '02*

"Recommended reference source."
— *Booklist, American Library Association, Sep '02*

▨

AIDS Sourcebook, 3rd Edition

Basic Consumer Health Information about Acquired Immune Deficiency Syndrome (AIDS) and Human Immunodeficiency Virus (HIV) Infection, Including Facts about Transmission, Prevention, Diagnosis, Treatment, Opportunistic Infections, and Other Complications, with a Section for Women and Children, Including Details about Associated Gynecological Concerns, Pregnancy, and Pediatric Care

Along with Updated Statistical Information, Reports on Current Research Initiatives, a Glossary, and Directories of Internet, Hotline, and Other Resources

Edited by Dawn D. Matthews. 664 pages. 2003. 0-7808-0631-X. $78.

ALSO AVAILABLE: AIDS Sourcebook, 1st Edition. Edited by Karen Bellenir and Peter D. Dresser. 831 pages. 1995. 0-7808-0031-1. $78.

AIDS Sourcebook, 2nd Edition. Edited by Karen Bellenir. 751 pages. 1999. 0-7808-0225-X. $78.

"The 3rd edition of the *AIDS Sourcebook,* part of Omnigraphics' *Health Reference Series,* is a welcome update. . . . This resource is highly recommended for academic and public libraries."
— *American Reference Books Annual, 2004*

"Excellent sourcebook. This continues to be a highly recommended book. There is no other book that provides as much information as this book provides."
— *AIDS Book Review Journal, Dec-Jan 2000*

"Recommended reference source."
— *Booklist, American Library Association, Dec '99*

"A solid text for college-level health libraries."
— *The Bookwatch, Aug '99*

Cited in *Reference Sources for Small and Medium-Sized Libraries, American Library Association, 1999*

▨

Alcoholism Sourcebook

Basic Consumer Health Information about the Physical and Mental Consequences of Alcohol Abuse, Including Liver Disease, Pancreatitis, Wernicke-Korsakoff Syndrome (Alcoholic Dementia), Fetal Alcohol Syndrome, Heart Disease, Kidney Disorders, Gastrointestinal Problems, and Immune System Compromise and Featuring Facts about Addiction, Detoxification, Alcohol Withdrawal, Recovery, and the Maintenance of Sobriety

Along with a Glossary and Directories of Resources for Further Help and Information

Edited by Karen Bellenir. 613 pages. 2000. 0-7808-0325-6. $78.

"This title is one of the few reference works on alcoholism for general readers. For some readers this will be a welcome complement to the many self-help books on the market. Recommended for collections serving general readers and consumer health collections."
— *E-Streams, Mar '01*

"This book is an excellent choice for public and academic libraries."
— *American Reference Books Annual, 2001*

"Recommended reference source."
— *Booklist, American Library Association, Dec '00*

"Presents a wealth of information on alcohol use and abuse and its effects on the body and mind, treatment, and prevention." — *SciTech Book News, Dec '00*

"Important new health guide which packs in the latest consumer information about the problems of alcoholism." — *Reviewer's Bookwatch, Nov '00*

SEE ALSO Drug Abuse Sourcebook, Substance Abuse Sourcebook

Allergies Sourcebook, 2nd Edition

Basic Consumer Health Information about Allergic Disorders, Triggers, Reactions, and Related Symptoms, Including Anaphylaxis, Rhinitis, Sinusitis, Asthma, Dermatitis, Conjunctivitis, and Multiple Chemical Sensitivity

Along with Tips on Diagnosis, Prevention, and Treatment, Statistical Data, a Glossary, and a Directory of Sources for Further Help and Information

Edited by Annemarie S. Muth. 598 pages. 2002. 0-7808-0376-0. $78.

ALSO AVAILABLE: *Allergies Sourcebook, 1st Edition.* Edited by Allan R. Cook. 611 pages. 1997. 0-7808-0036-2. $78.

"This book brings a great deal of useful material together. . . . This is an excellent addition to public and consumer health library collections."
— *American Reference Books Annual, 2003*

"This second edition would be useful to laypersons with little or advanced knowledge of the subject matter. This book would also serve as a resource for nursing and other health care professions students. It would be useful in public, academic, and hospital libraries with consumer health collections." — *E-Streams, Jul '02*

■

Alternative Medicine Sourcebook, 2nd Edition

Basic Consumer Health Information about Alternative and Complementary Medical Practices, Including Acupuncture, Chiropractic, Herbal Medicine, Homeopathy, Naturopathic Medicine, Mind-Body Interventions, Ayurveda, and Other Non-Western Medical Traditions

Along with Facts about such Specific Therapies as Massage Therapy, Aromatherapy, Qigong, Hypnosis, Prayer, Dance, and Art Therapies, a Glossary, and Resources for Further Information

Edited by Dawn D. Matthews. 618 pages. 2002. 0-7808-0605-0. $78.

ALSO AVAILABLE: *Alternative Medicine Sourcebook, 1st Edition.* Edited by Allan R. Cook. 737 pages. 1999. 0-7808-0200-4. $78.

"Recommended for public, high school, and academic libraries that have consumer health collections. Hospital libraries that also serve the public will find this to be a useful resource." — *E-Streams, Feb '03*

"Recommended reference source."
— *Booklist, American Library Association, Jan '03*

"An important alternate health reference."
— *MBR Bookwatch, Oct '02*

"A great addition to the reference collection of every type of library." — *American Reference Books Annual, 2000*

Alzheimer's Disease Sourcebook, 3rd Edition

Basic Consumer Health Information about Alzheimer's Disease, Other Dementias, and Related Disorders, Including Multi-Infarct Dementia, AIDS Dementia Complex, Dementia with Lewy Bodies, Huntington's Disease, Wernicke-Korsakoff Syndrome (Alcohol-Reated Dementia), Delirium, and Confusional States

Along with Information for People Newly Diagnosed with Alzheimer's Disease and Caregivers, Reports Detailing Current Research Efforts in Prevention, Diagnosis, and Treatment, Facts about Long-Term Care Issues, and Listings of Sources for Additional Information

Edited by Karen Bellenir. 645 pages. 2003. 0-7808-0666-2. $78.

ALSO AVAILABLE: *Alzheimer's, Stroke & 29 Other Neurological Disorders Sourcebook, 1st Edition.* Edited by Frank E. Bair. 579 pages. 1993. 1-55888-748-2. $78.

ALSO AVAILABLE: *Alzheimer's Disease Sourcebook, 2nd Edition.* Edited by Karen Bellenir. 524 pages. 1999. 0-7808-0223-3. $78.

"This very informative and valuable tool will be a great addition to any library serving consumers, students and health care workers."
— *American Reference Books Annual, 2004*

"This is a valuable resource for people affected by dementias such as Alzheimer's. It is easy to navigate and includes important information and resources."
— *Doody's Review Service, Feb. 2004*

"Recommended reference source."
— *Booklist, American Library Association, Oct '99*

SEE ALSO *Brain Disorders Sourcebook*

■

Arthritis Sourcebook, 2nd Edition

Basic Consumer Health Information about Osteoarthritis, Rheumatoid Arthritis, Other Rheumatic Disorders, Infectious Forms of Arthritis, and Diseases with Symptoms Linked to Arthritis, Featuring Facts about Diagnosis, Pain Management, and Surgical Therapies

Along with Coping Strategies, Research Updates, a Glossary, and Resources for Additional Help and Information

Edited by Amy L. Sutton. 593 pages. 2004. 0-7808-0667-0. $78.

ALSO AVAILABLE: *Arthritis Sourcebook, 1st Edition.* Edited by Allan R. Cook. 550 pages. 1998. 0-7808-0201-2. $78.

". . . accessible to the layperson."
— *Reference and Research Book News, Feb '99*

Asthma Sourcebook

Basic Consumer Health Information about Asthma, Including Symptoms, Traditional and Nontraditional Remedies, Treatment Advances, Quality-of-Life Aids, Medical Research Updates, and the Role of Allergies, Exercise, Age, the Environment, and Genetics in the Development of Asthma

Along with Statistical Data, a Glossary, and Directories of Support Groups, and Other Resources for Further Information

Edited by Annemarie S. Muth. 628 pages. 2000. 0-7808-0381-7. $78.

"A worthwhile reference acquisition for public libraries and academic medical libraries whose readers desire a quick introduction to the wide range of asthma information." — *Choice, Association of College & Research Libraries, Jun '01*

"Recommended reference source." — *Booklist, American Library Association, Feb '01*

"Highly recommended." — *The Bookwatch, Jan '01*

"There is much good information for patients and their families who deal with asthma daily." — *American Medical Writers Association Journal, Winter '01*

"This informative text is recommended for consumer health collections in public, secondary school, and community college libraries and the libraries of universities with a large undergraduate population." — *American Reference Books Annual, 2001*

Attention Deficit Disorder Sourcebook

Basic Consumer Health Information about Attention Deficit/Hyperactivity Disorder in Children and Adults, Including Facts about Causes, Symptoms, Diagnostic Criteria, and Treatment Options Such as Medications, Behavior Therapy, Coaching, and Homeopathy

Along with Reports on Current Research Initiatives, Legal Issues, and Government Regulations, and Featuring a Glossary of Related Terms, Internet Resources, and a List of Additional Reading Material

Edited by Dawn D. Matthews. 470 pages. 2002. 0-7808-0624-7. $78.

"Recommended reference source." — *Booklist, American Library Association, Jan '03*

"This book is recommended for all school libraries and the reference or consumer health sections of public libraries." — *American Reference Books Annual, 2003*

Back & Neck Sourcebook, 2nd Edition

Basic Consumer Health Information about Spinal Pain, Spinal Cord Injuries, and Related Disorders, Such as Degenerative Disk Disease, Osteoarthritis, Scoliosis, Sciatica, Spina Bifida, and Spinal Stenosis, and Featuring Facts about Maintaining Spinal Health, Self-Care, Pain Management, Rehabilitative Care, Chiropractic Care, Spinal Surgeries, and Complementary Therapies

Along with Suggestions for Preventing Back and Neck Pain, a Glossary of Related Terms, and a Directory of Resources

Edited by Amy L. Sutton. 633 pages. 2004. 0-7808-0738-3 $78.

ALSO AVAILABLE: *Back & Neck Disorders Sourcebook, 1st Edition.* Edited by Karen Bellenir. 548 pages. 1997. 0-7808-0202-0. $78.

"The strength of this work is its basic, easy-to-read format. Recommended." — *Reference and User Services Quarterly, American Library Association, Winter '97*

Blood & Circulatory Disorders Sourcebook

Basic Information about Blood and Its Components, Anemias, Leukemias, Bleeding Disorders, and Circulatory Disorders, Including Aplastic Anemia, Thalassemia, Sickle-Cell Disease, Hemochromatosis, Hemophilia, Von Willebrand Disease, and Vascular Diseases

Along with a Special Section on Blood Transfusions and Blood Supply Safety, a Glossary, and Source Listings for Further Help and Information

Edited by Karen Bellenir and Linda M. Shin. 554 pages. 1998. 0-7808-0203-9. $78.

"Recommended reference source." — *Booklist, American Library Association, Feb '99*

"An important reference sourcebook written in simple language for everyday, non-technical users. " — *Reviewer's Bookwatch, Jan '99*

Brain Disorders Sourcebook

Basic Consumer Health Information about Strokes, Epilepsy, Amyotrophic Lateral Sclerosis (ALS/Lou Gehrig's Disease), Parkinson's Disease, Brain Tumors, Cerebral Palsy, Headache, Tourette Syndrome, and More

Along with Statistical Data, Treatment and Rehabilitation Options, Coping Strategies, Reports on Current Research Initiatives, a Glossary, and Resource Listings for Additional Help and Information

Edited by Karen Bellenir. 481 pages. 1999. 0-7808-0229-2. $78.

"Belongs on the shelves of any library with a consumer health collection." — *E-Streams, Mar '00*

"Recommended reference source." — *Booklist, American Library Association, Oct '99*

SEE ALSO *Alzheimer's Disease Sourcebook*

Breast Cancer Sourcebook, 2nd Edition

Basic Consumer Health Information about Breast Cancer, Including Facts about Risk Factors, Prevention, Screening and Diagnostic Methods, Treatment Options, Complementary and Alternative Therapies, Post-Treatment Concerns, Clinical Trials, Special Risk Populations, and New Developments in Breast Cancer Research

Along with Breast Cancer Statistics, a Glossary of Related Terms, and a Directory of Resources for Additional Help and Information

Edited by Sandra J. Judd. 595 pages. 2004. 0-7808-0668-9. $78.

ALSO AVAILABLE: Breast Cancer Sourcebook, 1st Edition. Edited by Edward J. Prucha and Karen Bellenir. 580 pages. 2001. 0-7808-0244-6. $78.

"It would be a useful reference book in a library or on loan to women in a support group."
— *Cancer Forum, Mar '03*

"Recommended reference source."
— *Booklist, American Library Association, Jan '02*

"This reference source is highly recommended. It is quite informative, comprehensive and detailed in nature, and yet it offers practical advice in easy-to-read language. It could be thought of as the 'bible' of breast cancer for the consumer." — *E-Streams, Jan '02*

"The broad range of topics covered in lay language make the *Breast Cancer Sourcebook* an excellent addition to public and consumer health library collections."
— *American Reference Books Annual 2002*

"From the pros and cons of different screening methods and results to treatment options, *Breast Cancer Sourcebook* provides the latest information on the subject."
— *Library Bookwatch, Dec '01*

"This thoroughgoing, very readable reference covers all aspects of breast health and cancer. . . . Readers will find much to consider here. Recommended for all public and patient health collections."
— *Library Journal, Sep '01*

SEE ALSO Cancer Sourcebook for Women, Women's Health Concerns Sourcebook

Breastfeeding Sourcebook

Basic Consumer Health Information about the Benefits of Breastmilk, Preparing to Breastfeed, Breastfeeding as a Baby Grows, Nutrition, and More, Including Information on Special Situations and Concerns Such as Mastitis, Illness, Medications, Allergies, Multiple Births, Prematurity, Special Needs, and Adoption

Along with a Glossary and Resources for Additional Help and Information

Edited by Jenni Lynn Colson. 388 pages. 2002. 0-7808-0332-9. $78.

SEE ALSO Pregnancy & Birth Sourcebook

"Particularly useful is the information about professional lactation services and chapters on breastfeeding when returning to work. . . . *Breastfeeding Sourcebook* will be useful for public libraries, consumer health libraries, and technical schools offering nurse assistant training, especially in areas where Internet access is problematic."
— *American Reference Books Annual, 2003*

Burns Sourcebook

Basic Consumer Health Information about Various Types of Burns and Scalds, Including Flame, Heat, Cold, Electrical, Chemical, and Sun Burns

Along with Information on Short-Term and Long-Term Treatments, Tissue Reconstruction, Plastic Surgery, Prevention Suggestions, and First Aid

Edited by Allan R. Cook. 604 pages. 1999. 0-7808-0204-7. $78.

"This is an exceptional addition to the series and is highly recommended for all consumer health collections, hospital libraries, and academic medical centers."
— *E-Streams, Mar '00*

"This key reference guide is an invaluable addition to all health care and public libraries in confronting this ongoing health issue."
— *American Reference Books Annual, 2000*

"Recommended reference source."
— *Booklist, American Library Association, Dec '99*

SEE ALSO Skin Disorders Sourcebook

Cancer Sourcebook, 4th Edition

Basic Consumer Health Information about Major Forms and Stages of Cancer, Featuring Facts about Head and Neck Cancers, Lung Cancers, Gastrointestinal Cancers, Genitourinary Cancers, Lymphomas, Blood Cell Cancers, Endocrine Cancers, Skin Cancers, Bone Cancers, Sarcomas, and Others, and Including Information about Cancer Treatments and Therapies, Identifying and Reducing Cancer Risks, and Strategies for Coping with Cancer and the Side Effects of Treatment

Along with a Cancer Glossary, Statistical and Demographic Data, and a Directory of Sources for Additional Help and Information

Edited by Karen Bellenir. 1,119 pages. 2003. 0-7808-0633-6. $78.

ALSO AVAILABLE: Cancer Sourcebook, 1st Edition. Edited by Frank E. Bair. 932 pages. 1990. 1-55888-888-8. $78.

New Cancer Sourcebook, 2nd Edition. Edited by Allan R. Cook. 1,313 pages. 1996. 0-7808-0041-9. $78.

Cancer Sourcebook, 3rd Edition. Edited by Edward J. Prucha. 1,069 pages. 2000. 0-7808-0227-6. $78.

"With cancer being the second leading cause of death for Americans, a prodigious work such as this one, which locates centrally so much cancer-related information, is clearly an asset to this nation's citizens and others." — *Journal of the National Medical Association, 2004*

"This title is recommended for health sciences and public libraries with consumer health collections."
— *E-Streams, Feb '01*

". . . can be effectively used by cancer patients and their families who are looking for answers in a language they can understand. Public and hospital libraries should have it on their shelves."
— *American Reference Books Annual, 2001*

"Recommended reference source."
— *Booklist, American Library Association, Dec '00*

Cited in *Reference Sources for Small and Medium-Sized Libraries, American Library Association, 1999*

"The amount of factual and useful information is extensive. The writing is very clear, geared to general readers. Recommended for all levels."   — *Choice, Association of College & Research Libraries, Jan '97*

SEE ALSO Breast Cancer Sourcebook, Cancer Sourcebook for Women, Pediatric Cancer Sourcebook, Prostate Cancer Sourcebook

Cancer Sourcebook for Women, 2nd Edition

Basic Consumer Health Information about Gynecologic Cancers and Related Concerns, Including Cervical Cancer, Endometrial Cancer, Gestational Trophoblastic Tumor, Ovarian Cancer, Uterine Cancer, Vaginal Cancer, Vulvar Cancer, Breast Cancer, and Common Non-Cancerous Uterine Conditions, with Facts about Cancer Risk Factors, Screening and Prevention, Treatment Options, and Reports on Current Research Initiatives

Along with a Glossary of Cancer Terms and a Directory of Resources for Additional Help and Information

Edited by Karen Bellenir. 604 pages. 2002. 0-7808-0226-8. $78.

ALSO AVAILABLE: Cancer Sourcebook for Women, 1st Edition. Edited by Allan R. Cook and Peter D. Dresser. 524 pages. 1996. 0-7808-0076-1. $78.

"An excellent addition to collections in public, consumer health, and women's health libraries."
— *American Reference Books Annual, 2003*

"Overall, the information is excellent, and complex topics are clearly explained. As a reference book for the consumer it is a valuable resource to assist them to make informed decisions about cancer and its treatments."   — *Cancer Forum, Nov '02*

"Highly recommended for academic and medical reference collections."   — *Library Bookwatch, Sep '02*

"This is a highly recommended book for any public or consumer library, being reader friendly and containing accurate and helpful information."
— *E-Streams, Aug '02*

"Recommended reference source."
— *Booklist, American Library Association, Jul '02*

SEE ALSO Breast Cancer Sourcebook, Women's Health Concerns Sourcebook

Cardiovascular Diseases & Disorders Sourcebook, 3rd Edition

Basic Consumer Health Information about Heart and Vascular Diseases and Disorders, Such as Angina, Heart Attacks, Arrhythmias, Cardiomyopathy, Valve Disease, Atherosclerosis, and Aneurysms, with Information about Managing Cardiovascular Risk Factors and Maintaining Heart Health, Medications and Procedures Used to Treat Cardiovascular Disorders, and Concerns of Special Significance to Women

long with Reports on Current Research Initiatives, a Glossary of Related Medical Terms, and a Directory of Sources for Further Help and Information

Edited by Sandra J. Judd. 713 pages. 2005. 0-7808-0739-1. $78.

ALSO AVAILABLE: Heart Diseases & Disorders Sourcebook, 2nd Edition. Edited by Karen Bellenir. 612 pages. 2000. 0-7808-0238-1. $78.

Cardiovascular Diseases & Disorders Sourcebook, 1st Edition. Edited by Karen Bellenir and Peter D. Dresser. 683 pages. 1995. 0-7808-0032-X. $78.

"This work stands out as an imminently accessible resource for the general public. It is recommended for the reference and circulating shelves of school, public, and academic libraries."
— *American Reference Books Annual, 2001*

"Recommended reference source."
— *Booklist, American Library Association, Dec '00*

"Provides comprehensive coverage of matters related to the heart. This title is recommended for health sciences and public libraries with consumer health collections."
— *E-Streams, Oct '00*

SEE ALSO Healthy Heart Sourcebook for Women

Caregiving Sourcebook

Basic Consumer Health Information for Caregivers, Including a Profile of Caregivers, Caregiving Responsibilities and Concerns, Tips for Specific Conditions, Care Environments, and the Effects of Caregiving

Along with Facts about Legal Issues, Financial Information, and Future Planning, a Glossary, and a Listing of Additional Resources

Edited by Joyce Brennfleck Shannon. 600 pages. 2001. 0-7808-0331-0. $78.

"Essential for most collections."
— *Library Journal, Apr 1, 2002*

"An ideal addition to the reference collection of any public library. Health sciences information professionals may also want to acquire the *Caregiving Sourcebook* for their hospital or academic library for use as a ready reference tool by health care workers interested in aging and caregiving."   — *E-Streams, Jan '02*

"Recommended reference source."
— *Booklist, American Library Association, Oct '01*

Child Abuse Sourcebook

Basic Consumer Health Information about the Physical, Sexual, and Emotional Abuse of Children, with Additional Facts about Neglect, Munchausen Syndrome by Proxy (MSBP), Shaken Baby Syndrome, and Controversial Issues Related to Child Abuse, Such as Withholding Medical Care, Corporal Punishment, and Child Maltreatment in Youth Sports, and Featuring Facts about Child Protective Services, Foster Care, Adoption, Parenting Challenges, and Other Abuse Prevention Efforts

Along with a Glossary of Related Terms and Resources for Additional Help and Information

Edited by Dawn D. Matthews. 620 pages. 2004. 0-7808-0705-7. $78.

Childhood Diseases & Disorders Sourcebook

Basic Consumer Health Information about Medical Problems Often Encountered in Pre-Adolescent Children, Including Respiratory Tract Ailments, Ear Infections, Sore Throats, Disorders of the Skin and Scalp, Digestive and Genitourinary Diseases, Infectious Diseases, Inflammatory Disorders, Chronic Physical and Developmental Disorders, Allergies, and More

Along with Information about Diagnostic Tests, Common Childhood Surgeries, and Frequently Used Medications, with a Glossary of Important Terms and Resource Directory

Edited by Chad T. Kimball. 662 pages. 2003. 0-7808-0458-9. $78.

"This is an excellent book for new parents and should be included in all health care and public libraries."
— *American Reference Books Annual, 2004*

Colds, Flu & Other Common Ailments Sourcebook

Basic Consumer Health Information about Common Ailments and Injuries, Including Colds, Coughs, the Flu, Sinus Problems, Headaches, Fever, Nausea and Vomiting, Menstrual Cramps, Diarrhea, Constipation, Hemorrhoids, Back Pain, Dandruff, Dry and Itchy Skin, Cuts, Scrapes, Sprains, Bruises, and More

Along with Information about Prevention, Self-Care, Choosing a Doctor, Over-the-Counter Medications, Folk Remedies, and Alternative Therapies, and Including a Glossary of Important Terms and a Directory of Resources for Further Help and Information

Edited by Chad T. Kimball. 638 pages. 2001. 0-7808-0435-X. $78.

"A good starting point for research on common illnesses. It will be a useful addition to public and consumer health library collections."
— *American Reference Books Annual 2002*

"Will prove valuable to any library seeking to maintain a current, comprehensive reference collection of health resources. . . . Excellent reference."
— *The Bookwatch, Aug '01*

"Recommended reference source."
— *Booklist, American Library Association, July '01*

Communication Disorders Sourcebook

Basic Information about Deafness and Hearing Loss, Speech and Language Disorders, Voice Disorders, Balance and Vestibular Disorders, and Disorders of Smell, Taste, and Touch

Edited by Linda M. Ross. 533 pages. 1996. 0-7808-0077-X. $78.

"This is skillfully edited and is a welcome resource for the layperson. It should be found in every public and medical library." — *Booklist Health Sciences Supplement, American Library Association, Oct '97*

Congenital Disorders Sourcebook

Basic Information about Disorders Acquired during Gestation, Including Spina Bifida, Hydrocephalus, Cerebral Palsy, Heart Defects, Craniofacial Abnormalities, Fetal Alcohol Syndrome, and More

Along with Current Treatment Options and Statistical Data

Edited by Karen Bellenir. 607 pages. 1997. 0-7808-0205-5. $78.

"Recommended reference source."
— *Booklist, American Library Association, Oct '97*

SEE ALSO *Pregnancy & Birth Sourcebook*

Consumer Issues in Health Care Sourcebook

Basic Information about Health Care Fundamentals and Related Consumer Issues, Including Exams and Screening Tests, Physician Specialties, Choosing a Doctor, Using Prescription and Over-the-Counter Medications Safely, Avoiding Health Scams, Managing Common Health Risks in the Home, Care Options for Chronically or Terminally Ill Patients, and a List of Resources for Obtaining Help and Further Information

Edited by Karen Bellenir. 618 pages. 1998. 0-7808-0221-7. $78.

"Both public and academic libraries will want to have a copy in their collection for readers who are interested in self-education on health issues."
— *American Reference Books Annual, 2000*

"The editor has researched the literature from government agencies and others, saving readers the time and effort of having to do the research themselves. Recommended for public libraries."
— *Reference and User Services Quarterly, American Library Association, Spring '99*

"Recommended reference source."
— *Booklist, American Library Association, Dec '98*

694

Contagious Diseases Sourcebook

Basic Consumer Health Information about Infectious Diseases Spread by Person-to-Person Contact through Direct Touch, Airborne Transmission, Sexual Contact, or Contact with Blood or Other Body Fluids, Including Hepatitis, Herpes, Influenza, Lice, Measles, Mumps, Pinworm, Ringworm, Severe Acute Respiratory Syndrome (SARS), Streptococcal Infections, Tuberculosis, and Others

Along with Facts about Disease Transmission, Antimicrobial Resistance, and Vaccines, with a Glossary and Directories of Resources for More Information

Edited by Karen Bellenir. 643 pages. 2004. 0-7808-0736-7. $78.

Contagious & Non-Contagious Infectious Diseases Sourcebook

Basic Information about Contagious Diseases like Measles, Polio, Hepatitis B, and Infectious Mononucleosis, and Non-Contagious Infectious Diseases like Tetanus and Toxic Shock Syndrome, and Diseases Occurring as Secondary Infections Such as Shingles and Reye Syndrome

Along with Vaccination, Prevention, and Treatment Information, and a Section Describing Emerging Infectious Disease Threats

Edited by Karen Bellenir and Peter D. Dresser. 566 pages. 1996. 0-7808-0075-3. $78.

Death & Dying Sourcebook

Basic Consumer Health Information for the Layperson about End-of-Life Care and Related Ethical and Legal Issues, Including Chief Causes of Death, Autopsies, Pain Management for the Terminally Ill, Life Support Systems, Insurance, Euthanasia, Assisted Suicide, Hospice Programs, Living Wills, Funeral Planning, Counseling, Mourning, Organ Donation, and Physician Training

Along with Statistical Data, a Glossary, and Listings of Sources for Further Help and Information

Edited by Annemarie S. Muth. 641 pages. 1999. 0-7808-0230-6. $78.

"Public libraries, medical libraries, and academic libraries will all find this sourcebook a useful addition to their collections."
— *American Reference Books Annual, 2001*

"An extremely useful resource for those concerned with death and dying in the United States."
— *Respiratory Care, Nov '00*

"Recommended reference source."
—*Booklist, American Library Association, Aug '00*

"This book is a definite must for all those involved in end-of-life care." — *Doody's Review Service, 2000*

Dental Care & Oral Health Sourcebook, 2nd Edition

Basic Consumer Health Information about Dental Care, Including Oral Hygiene, Dental Visits, Pain Management, Cavities, Crowns, Bridges, Dental Implants, and Fillings, and Other Oral Health Concerns, Such as Gum Disease, Bad Breath, Dry Mouth, Genetic and Developmental Abnormalities, Oral Cancers, Orthodontics, and Temporomandibular Disorders

Along with Updates on Current Research in Oral Health, a Glossary, a Directory of Dental and Oral Health Organizations, and Resources for People with Dental and Oral Health Disorders

Edited by Amy L. Sutton. 609 pages. 2003. 0-7808-0634-4. $78.

ALSO AVAILABLE: *Oral Health Sourcebook, 1st Edition.* Edited by Allan R. Cook. 558 pages. 1997. 0-7808-0082-6. $78.

"This book could serve as a turning point in the battle to educate consumers in issues concerning oral health."
— *American Reference Books Annual, 2004*

"Unique source which will fill a gap in dental sources for patients and the lay public. A valuable reference tool even in a library with thousands of books on dentistry. Comprehensive, clear, inexpensive, and easy to read and use. It fills an enormous gap in the health care literature." — *Reference and User Services Quarterly, American Library Association, Summer '98*

"Recommended reference source."
— *Booklist, American Library Association, Dec '97*

Depression Sourcebook

Basic Consumer Health Information about Unipolar Depression, Bipolar Disorder, Postpartum Depression, Seasonal Affective Disorder, and Other Types of Depression in Children, Adolescents, Women, Men, the Elderly, and Other Selected Populations

Along with Facts about Causes, Risk Factors, Diagnostic Criteria, Treatment Options, Coping Strategies, Suicide Prevention, a Glossary, and a Directory of Sources for Additional Help and Information

Edited by Karen Belleni. 602 pages. 2002. 0-7808-0611-5. $78.

"*Depression Sourcebook* is of a very high standard. Its purpose, which is to serve as a reference source to the lay reader, is very well served."
— *Journal of the National Medical Association, 2004*

"Invaluable reference for public and school library collections alike." — *Library Bookwatch, Apr '03*

"Recommended for purchase."
— *American Reference Books Annual, 2003*

Diabetes Sourcebook, 3rd Edition

Basic Consumer Health Information about Type 1 Diabetes (Insulin-Dependent or Juvenile-Onset Diabetes), Type 2 Diabetes (Noninsulin-Dependent or Adult-Onset

Diabetes), Gestational Diabetes, Impaired Glucose Tolerance (IGT), and Related Complications, Such as Amputation, Eye Disease, Gum Disease, Nerve Damage, and End-Stage Renal Disease, Including Facts about Insulin, Oral Diabetes Medications, Blood Sugar Testing, and the Role of Exercise and Nutrition in the Control of Diabetes

Along with a Glossary and Resources for Further Help and Information

Edited by Dawn D. Matthews. 622 pages. 2003. 0-7808-0629-8. $78.

ALSO AVAILABLE: Diabetes Sourcebook, 1st Edition. Edited by Karen Bellenir and Peter D. Dresser. 827 pages. 1994. 1-55888-751-2. $78.

Diabetes Sourcebook, 2nd Edition. Edited by Karen Bellenir. 688 pages. 1998. 0-7808-0224-1. $78.

"This edition is even more helpful than earlier versions. . . . It is a truly valuable tool for anyone seeking readable and authoritative information on diabetes."
— American Reference Books Annual, 2004

"An invaluable reference." *— Library Journal, May '00*

Selected as one of the 250 "Best Health Sciences Books of 1999." *— Doody's Rating Service, Mar-Apr 2000*

"Provides useful information for the general public."
— Healthlines, University of Michigan Health Management Research Center, Sep/Oct '99

". . . provides reliable mainstream medical information . . . belongs on the shelves of any library with a consumer health collection." *— E-Streams, Sep '99*

"Recommended reference source."
— Booklist, American Library Association, Feb '99

■

Diet & Nutrition Sourcebook, 2nd Edition

Basic Consumer Health Information about Dietary Guidelines, Recommended Daily Intake Values, Vitamins, Minerals, Fiber, Fat, Weight Control, Dietary Supplements, and Food Additives

Along with Special Sections on Nutrition Needs throughout Life and Nutrition for People with Such Specific Medical Concerns as Allergies, High Blood Cholesterol, Hypertension, Diabetes, Celiac Disease, Seizure Disorders, Phenylketonuria (PKU), Cancer, and Eating Disorders, and Including Reports on Current Nutrition Research and Source Listings for Additional Help and Information

Edited by Karen Bellenir. 650 pages. 1999. 0-7808-0228-4. $78.

ALSO AVAILABLE: Diet & Nutrition Sourcebook, 1st Edition. Edited by Dan R. Harris. 662 pages. 1996. 0-7808-0084-2. $78.

"This book is an excellent source of basic diet and nutrition information." *— Booklist Health Sciences Supplement, American Library Association, Dec '00*

"This reference document should be in any public library, but it would be a very good guide for beginning students in the health sciences. If the other books in this publisher's series are as good as this, they should all be in the health sciences collections."
— American Reference Books Annual, 2000

"This book is an excellent general nutrition reference for consumers who desire to take an active role in their health care for prevention. Consumers of all ages who select this book can feel confident they are receiving current and accurate information." *— Journal of Nutrition for the Elderly, Vol. 19, No. 4, '00*

"Recommended reference source."
— Booklist, American Library Association, Dec '99

SEE ALSO Digestive Diseases & Disorders Sourcebook, Eating Disorders Sourcebook, Gastrointestinal Diseases & Disorders Sourcebook, Vegetarian Sourcebook

■

Digestive Diseases & Disorders Sourcebook

Basic Consumer Health Information about Diseases and Disorders that Impact the Upper and Lower Digestive System, Including Celiac Disease, Constipation, Crohn's Disease, Cyclic Vomiting Syndrome, Diarrhea, Diverticulosis and Diverticulitis, Gallstones, Heartburn, Hemorrhoids, Hernias, Indigestion (Dyspepsia), Irritable Bowel Syndrome, Lactose Intolerance, Ulcers, and More

Along with Information about Medications and Other Treatments, Tips for Maintaining a Healthy Digestive Tract, a Glossary, and Directory of Digestive Diseases Organizations

Edited by Karen Bellenir. 335 pages. 2000. 0-7808-0327-2. $78.

"This title would be an excellent addition to all public or patient-research libraries."
— American Reference Books Annual, 2001

"This title is recommended for public, hospital, and health sciences libraries with consumer health collections." *— E-Streams, Jul-Aug '00*

"Recommended reference source."
— Booklist, American Library Association, May '00

SEE ALSO Diet & Nutrition Sourcebook, Eating Disorders Sourcebook, Gastrointestinal Diseases & Disorders Sourcebook

■

Disabilities Sourcebook

Basic Consumer Health Information about Physical and Psychiatric Disabilities, Including Descriptions of Major Causes of Disability, Assistive and Adaptive Aids, Workplace Issues, and Accessibility Concerns

Along with Information about the Americans with Disabilities Act, a Glossary, and Resources for Additional Help and Information

Edited by Dawn D. Matthews. 616 pages. 2000. 0-7808-0389-2. $78.

"It is a must for libraries with a consumer health section." *— American Reference Books Annual 2002*

"A much needed addition to the Omnigraphics *Health Reference Series*. A current reference work to provide people with disabilities, their families, caregivers or those who work with them, a broad range of information in one volume, has not been available until now.... It is recommended for all public and academic library reference collections." — *E-Streams, May '01*

"An excellent source book in easy-to-read format covering many current topics; highly recommended for all libraries." — *Choice, Association of College and Research Libraries, Jan '01*

"Recommended reference source."
—*Booklist, American Library Association, Jul '00*

Domestic Violence Sourcebook, 2nd Edition

Basic Consumer Health Information about the Causes and Consequences of Abusive Relationships, Including Physical Violence, Sexual Assault, Battery, Stalking, and Emotional Abuse, and Facts about the Effects of Violence on Women, Men, Young Adults, and the Elderly, with Reports about Domestic Violence in Selected Populations, and Featuring Facts about Medical Care, Victim Assistance and Protection, Prevention Strategies, Mental Health Services, and Legal Issues

Along with a Glossary of Related Terms and Resources for Additional Help and Information

Edited by Dawn D. Matthews. 628 pages. 2004. 0-7808-0669-7. $78.

ALSO AVAILABLE: *Domestic Violence & Child Abuse Sourcebook, 1st Edition.* Edited by Helene Henderson. 1,064 pages. 2001. 0-7808-0235-7. $78.

"Interested lay persons should find the book extremely beneficial.... A copy of *Domestic Violence and Child Abuse Sourcebook* should be in every public library in the United States."
— *Social Science & Medicine, No. 56, 2003*

"This is important information. The Web has many resources but this sourcebook fills an important societal need. I am not aware of any other resources of this type." — *Doody's Review Service, Sep '01*

"Recommended for all libraries, scholars, and practitioners." — *Choice, Association of College & Research Libraries, Jul '01*

"Recommended reference source."
— *Booklist, American Library Association, Apr '01*

"Important pick for college-level health reference libraries." — *The Bookwatch, Mar '01*

"Because this problem is so widespread and because this book includes a lot of issues within one volume, this work is recommended for all public libraries."
— *American Reference Books Annual, 2001*

Drug Abuse Sourcebook, 2nd Edition

Basic Consumer Health Information about Illicit Substances of Abuse and the Misuse of Prescription and Over-the-Counter Medications, Including Depressants, Hallucinogens, Inhalants, Marijuana, Stimulants, and Anabolic Steroids

Along with Facts about Related Health Risks, Treatment Programs, Prevention Programs, a Glossary of Abuse and Addiction Terms, a Glossary of Drug-Related Street Terms, and a Directory of Resources for More Information

Edited by Catherine Ginther. 607 pages. 2004. 0-7808-0740-5. $78.

ALSO AVAILABLE: Drug Abuse Sourcebook, 1st Edition. Edited by Karen Bellenir. 629 pages. 2000. 0-7808-0242-X. $78.

"Containing a wealth of information.... This resource belongs in libraries that serve a lower-division undergraduate or community college clientele as well as the general public." — *Choice, Association of College and Research Libraries, Jun '01*

"Recommended reference source."
— *Booklist, American Library Association, Feb '01*

"Highly recommended." — *The Bookwatch, Jan '01*

"Even though there is a plethora of books on drug abuse, this volume is recommended for school, public, and college libraries."
—*American Reference Books Annual, 2001*

SEE ALSO Alcoholism Sourcebook, Substance Abuse Sourcebook

Ear, Nose & Throat Disorders Sourcebook

Basic Information about Disorders of the Ears, Nose, Sinus Cavities, Pharynx, and Larynx, Including Ear Infections, Tinnitus, Vestibular Disorders, Allergic and Non-Allergic Rhinitis, Sore Throats, Tonsillitis, and Cancers That Affect the Ears, Nose, Sinuses, and Throat

Along with Reports on Current Research Initiatives, a Glossary of Related Medical Terms, and a Directory of Sources for Further Help and Information

Edited by Karen Bellenir and Linda M. Shin. 576 pages. 1998. 0-7808-0206-3. $78.

"Overall, this sourcebook is helpful for the consumer seeking information on ENT issues. It is recommended for public libraries."
—*American Reference Books Annual, 1999*

"Recommended reference source."
—*Booklist, American Library Association, Dec '98*

Eating Disorders Sourcebook

Basic Consumer Health Information about Eating Disorders, Including Information about Anorexia Nervosa, Bulimia Nervosa, Binge Eating, Body Dysmorphic

Disorder, Pica, Laxative Abuse, and Night Eating Syndrome

Along with Information about Causes, Adverse Effects, and Treatment and Prevention Issues, and Featuring a Section on Concerns Specific to Children and Adolescents, a Glossary, and Resources for Further Help and Information

Edited by Dawn D. Matthews. 322 pages. 2001. 0-7808-0335-3. $78.

"Recommended for health science libraries that are open to the public, as well as hospital libraries. This book is a good resource for the consumer who is concerned about eating disorders." — *E-Streams, Mar '02*

"This volume is another convenient collection of excerpted articles. Recommended for school and public library patrons; lower-division undergraduates; and two-year technical program students." — *Choice, Association of College & Research Libraries, Jan '02*

"Recommended reference source." — *Booklist, American Library Association, Oct '01*

SEE ALSO Diet & Nutrition Sourcebook, Digestive Diseases & Disorders Sourcebook, Gastrointestinal Diseases & Disorders Sourcebook

Emergency Medical Services Sourcebook

Basic Consumer Health Information about Preventing, Preparing for, and Managing Emergency Situations, When and Who to Call for Help, What to Expect in the Emergency Room, the Emergency Medical Team, Patient Issues, and Current Topics in Emergency Medicine

Along with Statistical Data, a Glossary, and Sources of Additional Help and Information

Edited by Jenni Lynn Colson. 494 pages. 2002. 0-7808-0420-1. $78.

"Handy and convenient for home, public, school, and college libraries. Recommended."
— *Choice, Association of College and Research Libraries, Apr '03*

"This reference can provide the consumer with answers to most questions about emergency care in the United States, or it will direct them to a resource where the answer can be found."
— *American Reference Books Annual, 2003*

"Recommended reference source."
— *Booklist, American Library Association, Feb '03*

Endocrine & Metabolic Disorders Sourcebook

Basic Information for the Layperson about Pancreatic and Insulin-Related Disorders Such as Pancreatitis, Diabetes, and Hypoglycemia; Adrenal Gland Disorders Such as Cushing's Syndrome, Addison's Disease, and Congenital Adrenal Hyperplasia; Pituitary Gland Disorders Such as Growth Hormone Deficiency, Acromegaly, and Pituitary Tumors; Thyroid Disorders Such

as Hypothyroidism, Graves' Disease, Hashimoto's Disease, and Goiter; Hyperparathyroidism; and Other Diseases and Syndromes of Hormone Imbalance or Metabolic Dysfunction

Along with Reports on Current Research Initiatives

Edited by Linda M. Shin. 574 pages. 1998. 0-7808-0207-1. $78.

"Omnigraphics has produced another needed resource for health information consumers."
— *American Reference Books Annual, 2000*

"Recommended reference source."
— *Booklist, American Library Association, Dec '98*

Environmental Health Sourcebook, 2nd Edition

Basic Consumer Health Information about the Environment and Its Effect on Human Health, Including the Effects of Air Pollution, Water Pollution, Hazardous Chemicals, Food Hazards, Radiation Hazards, Biological Agents, Household Hazards, Such as Radon, Asbestos, Carbon Monoxide, and Mold, and Information about Associated Diseases and Disorders, Including Cancer, Allergies, Respiratory Problems, and Skin Disorders

Along with Information about Environmental Concerns for Specific Populations, a Glossary of Related Terms, and Resources for Further Help and Information

Edited by Dawn D. Matthews. 673 pages. 2003. 0-7808-0632-8. $78.

ALSO AVAILABLE: Environmentally Induced Disorders Sourcebook, 1st Edition. Edited by Allan R. Cook. 620 pages. 1997. 0-7808-0083-4. $78.

"This recently updated edition continues the level of quality and the reputation of the numerous other volumes in Omnigraphics' *Health Reference Series.*"
— *American Reference Books Annual, 2004*

"Recommended reference source."
— *Booklist, American Library Association, Sep '98*

"This book will be a useful addition to anyone's library." — *Choice Health Sciences Supplement, Association of College and Research Libraries, May '98*

". . . a good survey of numerous environmentally induced physical disorders . . . a useful addition to anyone's library."
— *Doody's Health Sciences Book Reviews, Jan '98*

". . . provide[s] introductory information from the best authorities around. Since this volume covers topics that potentially affect everyone, it will surely be one of the most frequently consulted volumes in the *Health Reference Series.*" — *Rettig on Reference, Nov '97*

Environmentally Induced Disorders Sourcebook, 1st Edition

SEE Environmental Health Sourcebook, 2nd Edition

Ethnic Diseases Sourcebook

Basic Consumer Health Information for Ethnic and Racial Minority Groups in the United States, Including General Health Indicators and Behaviors, Ethnic Diseases, Genetic Testing, the Impact of Chronic Diseases, Women's Health, Mental Health Issues, and Preventive Health Care Services

Along with a Glossary and a Listing of Additional Resources

Edited by Joyce Brennfleck Shannon. 664 pages. 2001. 0-7808-0336-1. $78.

"Recommended for health sciences libraries where public health programs are a priority."
— *E-Streams, Jan '02*

"Not many books have been written on this topic to date, and the *Ethnic Diseases Sourcebook* is a strong addition to the list. It will be an important introductory resource for health consumers, students, health care personnel, and social scientists. It is recommended for public, academic, and large hospital libraries."
— *American Reference Books Annual 2002*

"Recommended reference source."
— *Booklist, American Library Association, Oct '01*

"Will prove valuable to any library seeking to maintain a current, comprehensive reference collection of health resources.... An excellent source of health information about genetic disorders which affect particular ethnic and racial minorities in the U.S."
— *The Bookwatch, Aug '01*

∎

Eye Care Sourcebook, 2nd Edition

Basic Consumer Health Information about Eye Care and Eye Disorders, Including Facts about the Diagnosis, Prevention, and Treatment of Common Refractive Problems Such as Myopia, Hyperopia, Astigmatism, and Presbyopia, and Eye Diseases, Including Glaucoma, Cataract, Age-Related Macular Degeneration, and Diabetic Retinopathy

Along with a Section on Vision Correction and Refractive Surgeries, Including LASIK and LASEK, a Glossary, and Directories of Resources for Additional Help and Information

Edited by Amy L. Sutton. 543 pages. 2003. 0-7808-0635-2. $78.

ALSO AVAILABLE: Ophthalmic Disorders Sourcebook, 1st Edition. Edited by Linda M. Ross. 631 pages. 1996. 0-7808-0081-8. $78.

". . . a solid reference tool for eye care and a valuable addition to a collection."
— *American Reference Books Annual, 2004*

∎

Family Planning Sourcebook

Basic Consumer Health Information about Planning for Pregnancy and Contraception, Including Traditional Methods, Barrier Methods, Hormonal Methods, Permanent Methods, Future Methods, Emergency Contraception, and Birth Control Choices for Women at Each Stage of Life

Along with Statistics, a Glossary, and Sources of Additional Information

Edited by Amy Marcaccio Keyzer. 520 pages. 2001. 0-7808-0379-5. $78.

"Recommended for public, health, and undergraduate libraries as part of the circulating collection."
— *E-Streams, Mar '02*

"Information is presented in an unbiased, readable manner, and the sourcebook will certainly be a necessary addition to those public and high school libraries where Internet access is restricted or otherwise problematic." — *American Reference Books Annual 2002*

"Recommended reference source."
— *Booklist, American Library Association, Oct '01*

"Will prove valuable to any library seeking to maintain a current, comprehensive reference collection of health resources.... Excellent reference."
— *The Bookwatch, Aug '01*

SEE ALSO Pregnancy & Birth Sourcebook

∎

Fitness & Exercise Sourcebook, 2nd Edition

Basic Consumer Health Information about the Fundamentals of Fitness and Exercise, Including How to Begin and Maintain a Fitness Program, Fitness as a Lifestyle, the Link between Fitness and Diet, Advice for Specific Groups of People, Exercise as It Relates to Specific Medical Conditions, and Recent Research in Fitness and Exercise

Along with a Glossary of Important Terms and Resources for Additional Help and Information

Edited by Kristen M. Gledhill. 646 pages. 2001. 0-7808-0334-5. $78.

ALSO AVAILABLE: Fitness & Exercise Sourcebook, 1st Edition. Edited by Dan R. Harris. 663 pages. 1996. 0-7808-0186-5. $78.

"This work is recommended for all general reference collections."
— *American Reference Books Annual 2002*

"Highly recommended for public, consumer, and school grades fourth through college."
— *E-Streams, Nov '01*

"Recommended reference source." — *Booklist, American Library Association, Oct '01*

"The information appears quite comprehensive and is considered reliable. . . . This second edition is a welcomed addition to the series."
— *Doody's Review Service, Sep '01*

"This reference is a valuable choice for those who desire a broad source of information on exercise, fitness, and chronic-disease prevention through a healthy lifestyle." — *American Medical Writers Association Journal, Fall '01*

"Will prove valuable to any library seeking to maintain a current, comprehensive reference collection of health resources. . . . Excellent reference."
— The Bookwatch, Aug '01

Food & Animal Borne Diseases Sourcebook

Basic Information about Diseases That Can Be Spread to Humans through the Ingestion of Contaminated Food or Water or by Contact with Infected Animals and Insects, Such as Botulism, E. Coli, Hepatitis A, Trichinosis, Lyme Disease, and Rabies

Along with Information Regarding Prevention and Treatment Methods, and Including a Special Section for International Travelers Describing Diseases Such as Cholera, Malaria, Travelers' Diarrhea, and Yellow Fever, and Offering Recommendations for Avoiding Illness

Edited by Karen Bellenir and Peter D. Dresser. 535 pages. 1995. 0-7808-0033-8. $78.

"Targeting general readers and providing them with a single, comprehensive source of information on selected topics, this book continues, with the excellent caliber of its predecessors, to catalog topical information on health matters of general interest. Readable and thorough, this valuable resource is highly recommended for all libraries."
— Academic Library Book Review, Summer '96

"A comprehensive collection of authoritative information."
— Emergency Medical Services, Oct '95

Food Safety Sourcebook

Basic Consumer Health Information about the Safe Handling of Meat, Poultry, Seafood, Eggs, Fruit Juices, and Other Food Items, and Facts about Pesticides, Drinking Water, Food Safety Overseas, and the Onset, Duration, and Symptoms of Foodborne Illnesses, Including Types of Pathogenic Bacteria, Parasitic Protozoa, Worms, Viruses, and Natural Toxins

Along with the Role of the Consumer, the Food Handler, and the Government in Food Safety; a Glossary, and Resources for Additional Help and Information

Edited by Dawn D. Matthews. 339 pages. 1999. 0-7808-0326-4. $78.

"This book is recommended for public libraries and universities with home economic and food science programs."
— E-Streams, Nov '00

"Recommended reference source."
— Booklist, American Library Association, May '00

"This book takes the complex issues of food safety and foodborne pathogens and presents them in an easily understood manner. [It does] an excellent job of covering a large and often confusing topic."
— American Reference Books Annual, 2000

Forensic Medicine Sourcebook

Basic Consumer Information for the Layperson about Forensic Medicine, Including Crime Scene Investigation, Evidence Collection and Analysis, Expert Testimony, Computer-Aided Criminal Identification, Digital Imaging in the Courtroom, DNA Profiling, Accident Reconstruction, Autopsies, Ballistics, Drugs and Explosives Detection, Latent Fingerprints, Product Tampering, and Questioned Document Examination

Along with Statistical Data, a Glossary of Forensics Terminology, and Listings of Sources for Further Help and Information

Edited by Annemarie S. Muth. 574 pages. 1999. 0-7808-0232-2. $78.

"Given the expected widespread interest in its content and its easy to read style, this book is recommended for most public and all college and university libraries."
— E-Streams, Feb '01

"Recommended for public libraries."
— Reference & User Services Quarterly, American Library Association, Spring 2000

"Recommended reference source."
— Booklist, American Library Association, Feb '00

"A wealth of information, useful statistics, references are up-to-date and extremely complete. This wonderful collection of data will help students who are interested in a career in any type of forensic field. It is a great resource for attorneys who need information about types of expert witnesses needed in a particular case. It also offers useful information for fiction and nonfiction writers whose work involves a crime. A fascinating compilation. All levels." — Choice, Association of College and Research Libraries, Jan 2000

"There are several items that make this book attractive to consumers who are seeking certain forensic data. . . . This is a useful current source for those seeking general forensic medical answers."
— American Reference Books Annual, 2000

Gastrointestinal Diseases & Disorders Sourcebook

Basic Information about Gastroesophageal Reflux Disease (Heartburn), Ulcers, Diverticulosis, Irritable Bowel Syndrome, Crohn's Disease, Ulcerative Colitis, Diarrhea, Constipation, Lactose Intolerance, Hemorrhoids, Hepatitis, Cirrhosis, and Other Digestive Problems, Featuring Statistics, Descriptions of Symptoms, and Current Treatment Methods of Interest for Persons Living with Upper and Lower Gastrointestinal Maladies

Edited by Linda M. Ross. 413 pages. 1996. 0-7808-0078-8. $78.

". . . very readable form. The successful editorial work that brought this material together into a useful and understandable reference makes accessible to all readers information that can help them more effectively understand and obtain help for digestive tract problems."
— Choice, Association of College & Research Libraries, Feb '97

■

Genetic Disorders Sourcebook, 3rd Edition

Basic Consumer Health Information about Hereditary Diseases and Disorders, Including Facts about the Human Genome, Genetic Inheritance Patterns, Disorders Associated with Specific Genes, Such as Sickle Cell Disease, Hemophilia, and Cystic Fibrosis, Chromosome Disorders, Such as Down Syndrome, Fragile X Syndrome, and Turner Syndrome, and Complex Diseases and Disorders Resulting from the Interaction of Environmental and Genetic Factors, Such as Allergies, Cancer, and Obesity

Along with Facts about Genetic Testing, Suggestions for Parents of Children with Special Needs, Reports on Current Research Initiatives, a Glossary of Genetic Terminology, and Resources for Additional Help and Information

Edited by Karen Bellenir. 777 pages. 2004. 0-7808-0742-1. $78.

ALSO AVAILABLE: Genetic Disorders Sourcebook, 1st Edition. Edited by Karen Bellenir. 642 pages. 1996. 0-7808-0034-6. $78.

Genetic Disorders Sourcebook, 2nd Edition. Edited by Kathy Massimini. 768 pages. 2001. 0-7808-0241-1. $78.

"Recommended for public libraries and medical and hospital libraries with consumer health collections."
— E-Streams, May '01

"Recommended reference source."
— Booklist, American Library Association, Apr '01

"Important pick for college-level health reference libraries." — The Bookwatch, Mar '01

"Provides essential medical information to both the general public and those diagnosed with a serious or fatal genetic disease or disorder." —Choice, Association of College and Research Libraries, Jan '97

■

Head Trauma Sourcebook

Basic Information for the Layperson about Open-Head and Closed-Head Injuries, Treatment Advances, Recovery, and Rehabilitation

Along with Reports on Current Research Initiatives

Edited by Karen Bellenir. 414 pages. 1997. 0-7808-0208-X. $78.

■

Headache Sourcebook

Basic Consumer Health Information about Migraine, Tension, Cluster, Rebound and Other Types of Headaches, with Facts about the Cause and Prevention of Headaches, the Effects of Stress and the Environment, Headaches during Pregnancy and Menopause, and Childhood Headaches

Along with a Glossary and Other Resources for Additional Help and Information

Edited by Dawn D. Matthews. 362 pages. 2002. 0-7808-0337-X. $78.

"Highly recommended for academic and medical reference collections." — Library Bookwatch, Sep '02

■

Health Insurance Sourcebook

Basic Information about Managed Care Organizations, Traditional Fee-for-Service Insurance, Insurance Portability and Pre-Existing Conditions Clauses, Medicare, Medicaid, Social Security, and Military Health Care

Along with Information about Insurance Fraud

Edited by Wendy Wilcox. 530 pages. 1997. 0-7808-0222-5. $78.

"Particularly useful because it brings much of this information together in one volume. This book will be a handy reference source in the health sciences library, hospital library, college and university library, and medium to large public library."
— Medical Reference Services Quarterly, Fall '98

Awarded "Books of the Year Award"
— American Journal of Nursing, 1997

"The layout of the book is particularly helpful as it provides easy access to reference material. A most useful addition to the vast amount of information about health insurance. The use of data from U.S. government agencies is most commendable. Useful in a library or learning center for healthcare professional students."
— Doody's Health Sciences Book Reviews, Nov '97

■

Health Reference Series Cumulative Index 1999

A Comprehensive Index to the Individual Volumes of the Health Reference Series, Including a Subject Index, Name Index, Organization Index, and Publication Index

Along with a Master List of Acronyms and Abbreviations

Edited by Edward J. Prucha, Anne Holmes, and Robert Rudnick. 990 pages. 2000. 0-7808-0382-5. $78.

"This volume will be most helpful in libraries that have a relatively complete collection of the Health Reference Series." — American Reference Books Annual, 2001

"Essential for collections that hold any of the numerous Health Reference Series titles."
— Choice, Association of College and Research Libraries, Nov '00

■

Healthy Aging Sourcebook

Basic Consumer Health Information about Maintaining Health through the Aging Process, Including Advice on Nutrition, Exercise, and Sleep, Help in Making Decisions about Midlife Issues and Retirement, and

Guidance Concerning Practical and Informed Choices in Health Consumerism

Along with Data Concerning the Theories of Aging, Different Experiences in Aging by Minority Groups, and Facts about Aging Now and Aging in the Future; and Featuring a Glossary, a Guide to Consumer Help, Additional Suggested Reading, and Practical Resource Directory

Edited by Jenifer Swanson. 536 pages. 1999. 0-7808-0390-6. $78.

"Recommended reference source."
—Booklist, American Library Association, Feb '00

SEE ALSO Physical & Mental Issues in Aging Sourcebook

■

Healthy Children Sourcebook

Basic Consumer Health Information about the Physical and Mental Development of Children between the Ages of 3 and 12, Including Routine Health Care, Preventative Health Services, Safety and First Aid, Healthy Sleep, Dental Care, Nutrition, and Fitness, and Featuring Parenting Tips on Such Topics as Bedwetting, Choosing Day Care, Monitoring TV and Other Media, and Establishing a Foundation for Substance Abuse Prevention

Along with a Glossary of Commonly Used Pediatric Terms and Resources for Additional Help and Information.

Edited by Chad T. Kimball. 647 pages. 2003. 0-7808-0247-0. $78.

"It is hard to imagine that any other single resource exists that would provide such a comprehensive guide of timely information on health promotion and disease prevention for children aged 3 to 12."
—American Reference Books Annual, 2004

"The strengths of this book are many. It is clearly written, presented and structured."
—Journal of the National Medical Association, 2004

■

Healthy Heart Sourcebook for Women

Basic Consumer Health Information about Cardiac Issues Specific to Women, Including Facts about Major Risk Factors and Prevention, Treatment and Control Strategies, and Important Dietary Issues

Along with a Special Section Regarding the Pros and Cons of Hormone Replacement Therapy and Its Impact on Heart Health, and Additional Help, Including Recipes, a Glossary, and a Directory of Resources

Edited by Dawn D. Matthews. 336 pages. 2000. 0-7808-0329-9. $78.

"A good reference source and recommended for all public, academic, medical, and hospital libraries."
—Medical Reference Services Quarterly, Summer '01

"Because of the lack of information specific to women on this topic, this book is recommended for public libraries and consumer libraries."
—American Reference Books Annual, 2001

"Contains very important information about coronary artery disease that all women should know. The information is current and presented in an easy-to-read format. The book will make a good addition to any library."
—American Medical Writers Association Journal, Summer '00

"Important, basic reference."
—Reviewer's Bookwatch, Jul '00

SEE ALSO Heart Diseases & Disorders Sourcebook, Women's Health Concerns Sourcebook

■

Heart Diseases & Disorders Sourcebook, 2nd Edition

SEE Cardiovascular Diseases & Disorders Sourcebook, 3rd Edition

■

Household Safety Sourcebook

Basic Consumer Health Information about Household Safety, Including Information about Poisons, Chemicals, Fire, and Water Hazards in the Home

Along with Advice about the Safe Use of Home Maintenance Equipment, Choosing Toys and Nursery Furniture, Holiday and Recreation Safety, a Glossary, and Resources for Further Help and Information

Edited by Dawn D. Matthews. 606 pages. 2002. 0-7808-0338-8. $78.

"This work will be useful in public libraries with large consumer health and wellness departments."
—American Reference Books Annual, 2003

"As a sourcebook on household safety this book meets its mark. It is encyclopedic in scope and covers a wide range of safety issues that are commonly seen in the home."
—E-Streams, Jul '02

■

Hypertension Sourcebook

Basic Consumer Health Information about the Causes, Diagnosis, and Treatment of High Blood Pressure, with Facts about Consequences, Complications, and Co-Occurring Disorders, Such as Coronary Heart Disease, Diabetes, Stroke, Kidney Disease, and Hypertensive Retinopathy, and Issues in Blood Pressure Control, Including Dietary Choices, Stress Management, and Medications

Along with Reports on Current Research Initiatives and Clinical Trials, a Glossary, and Resources for Additional Help and Information

Edited by Dawn D. Matthews and Karen Bellenir. 613 pages. 2004. 0-7808-0674-3. $78.

Immune System Disorders Sourcebook

Basic Information about Lupus, Multiple Sclerosis, Guillain-Barré Syndrome, Chronic Granulomatous Disease, and More

Along with Statistical and Demographic Data and Reports on Current Research Initiatives

Edited by Allan R. Cook. 608 pages. 1997. 0-7808-0209-8. $78.

■

Infant & Toddler Health Sourcebook

Basic Consumer Health Information about the Physical and Mental Development of Newborns, Infants, and Toddlers, Including Neonatal Concerns, Nutrition Recommendations, Immunization Schedules, Common Pediatric Disorders, Assessments and Milestones, Safety Tips, and Advice for Parents and Other Caregivers

Along with a Glossary of Terms and Resource Listings for Additional Help

Edited by Jenifer Swanson. 585 pages. 2000. 0-7808-0246-2. $78.

"As a reference for the general public, this would be useful in any library." —*E-Streams, May '01*

"Recommended reference source."
—*Booklist, American Library Association, Feb '01*

"This is a good source for general use."
—*American Reference Books Annual, 2001*

■

Infectious Diseases Sourcebook

Basic Consumer Health Information about Non-Contagious Bacterial, Viral, Prion, Fungal, and Parasitic Diseases Spread by Food and Water, Insects and Animals, or Environmental Contact, Including Botulism, E. Coli, Encephalitis, Legionnaires' Disease, Lyme Disease, Malaria, Plague, Rabies, Salmonella, Tetanus, and Others, and Facts about Newly Emerging Diseases, Such as Hantavirus, Mad Cow Disease, Monkeypox, and West Nile Virus

Along with Information about Preventing Disease Transmission, the Threat of Bioterrorism, and Current Research Initiatives, with a Glossary and Directory of Resources for More Information

Edited by Karen Bellenir. 634 pages. 2004. 0-7808-0675-1. $78.

■

Injury & Trauma Sourcebook

Basic Consumer Health Information about the Impact of Injury, the Diagnosis and Treatment of Common and Traumatic Injuries, Emergency Care, and Specific Injuries Related to Home, Community, Workplace, Transportation, and Recreation

Along with Guidelines for Injury Prevention, a Glossary, and a Directory of Additional Resources

Edited by Joyce Brennfleck Shannon. 696 pages. 2002. 0-7808-0421-X. $78.

"This publication is the most comprehensive work of its kind about injury and trauma."
—*American Reference Books Annual, 2003*

"This sourcebook provides concise, easily readable, basic health information about injuries. . . . This book is well organized and an easy to use reference resource suitable for hospital, health sciences and public libraries with consumer health collections."
—*E-Streams, Nov '02*

"Practitioners should be aware of guides such as this in order to facilitate their use by patients and their families." —*Doody's Health Sciences Book Review Journal, Sep-Oct '02*

"Recommended reference source."
—*Booklist, American Library Association, Sep '02*

"Highly recommended for academic and medical reference collections." —*Library Bookwatch, Sep '02*

■

Kidney & Urinary Tract Diseases & Disorders Sourcebook

Basic Information about Kidney Stones, Urinary Incontinence, Bladder Disease, End Stage Renal Disease, Dialysis, and More

Along with Statistical and Demographic Data and Reports on Current Research Initiatives

Edited by Linda M. Ross. 602 pages. 1997. 0-7808-0079-6. $78.

■

Learning Disabilities Sourcebook, 2nd Edition

Basic Consumer Health Information about Learning Disabilities, Including Dyslexia, Developmental Speech and Language Disabilities, Non-Verbal Learning Disorders, Developmental Arithmetic Disorder, Developmental Writing Disorder, and Other Conditions That Impede Learning Such as Attention Deficit/ Hyperactivity Disorder, Brain Injury, Hearing Impairment, Klinefelter Syndrome, Dyspraxia, and Tourette Syndrome

Along with Facts about Educational Issues and Assistive Technology, Coping Strategies, a Glossary of Related Terms, and Resources for Further Help and Information

Edited by Dawn D. Matthews. 621 pages. 2003. 0-7808-0626-3. $78.

ALSO AVAILABLE: Learning Disabilities Sourcebook, 1st Edition. Edited by Linda M. Shin. 579 pages. 1998. 0-7808-0210-1. $78.

"The second edition of *Learning Disabilities Sourcebook* far surpasses the earlier edition in that it is more focused on information that will be useful as a consumer health resource."
—*American Reference Books Annual, 2004*

"Teachers as well as consumers will find this an essential guide to understanding various syndromes and their latest treatments. [An] invaluable reference for public and school library collections."
— *Library Bookwatch, Apr '03*

Named "Outstanding Reference Book of 1999."
— *New York Public Library, Feb 2000*

"An excellent candidate for inclusion in a public library reference section. It's a great source of information. Teachers will also find the book useful. Definitely worth reading."
— *Journal of Adolescent & Adult Literacy, Feb 2000*

"Readable . . . provides a solid base of information regarding successful techniques used with individuals who have learning disabilities, as well as practical suggestions for educators and family members. Clear language, concise descriptions, and pertinent information for contacting multiple resources add to the strength of this book as a useful tool."
— *Choice, Association of College and Research Libraries, Feb '99*

"Recommended reference source."
— *Booklist, American Library Association, Sep '98*

"A useful resource for libraries and for those who don't have the time to identify and locate the individual publications."
— *Disability Resources Monthly, Sep '98*

■

Leukemia Sourcebook

Basic Consumer Health Information about Adult and Childhood Leukemias, Including Acute Lymphocytic Leukemia (ALL), Chronic Lymphocytic Leukemia (CLL), Acute Myelogenous Leukemia (AML), Chronic Myelogenous Leukemia (CML), and Hairy Cell Leukemia, and Treatments Such as Chemotherapy, Radiation Therapy, Peripheral Blood Stem Cell and Marrow Transplantation, and Immunotherapy

Along with Tips for Life During and After Treatment, a Glossary, and Directories of Additional Resources

Edited by Joyce Brennfleck Shannon. 587 pages. 2003. 0-7808-0627-1. $78.

"Unlike other medical books for the layperson, . . . the language does not talk down to the reader. . . . This volume is highly recommended for all libraries."
— *American Reference Books Annual, 2004*

■

Liver Disorders Sourcebook

Basic Consumer Health Information about the Liver and How It Works; Liver Diseases, Including Cancer, Cirrhosis, Hepatitis, and Toxic and Drug Related Diseases; Tips for Maintaining a Healthy Liver; Laboratory Tests, Radiology Tests, and Facts about Liver Transplantation

Along with a Section on Support Groups, a Glossary, and Resource Listings

Edited by Joyce Brennfleck Shannon. 591 pages. 2000. 0-7808-0383-3. $78.

"A valuable resource."
— *American Reference Books Annual, 2001*

"This title is recommended for health sciences and public libraries with consumer health collections."
— *E-Streams, Oct '00*

"Recommended reference source."
— *Booklist, American Library Association, Jun '00*

■

Lung Disorders Sourcebook

Basic Consumer Health Information about Emphysema, Pneumonia, Tuberculosis, Asthma, Cystic Fibrosis, and Other Lung Disorders, Including Facts about Diagnostic Procedures, Treatment Strategies, Disease Prevention Efforts, and Such Risk Factors as Smoking, Air Pollution, and Exposure to Asbestos, Radon, and Other Agents

Along with a Glossary and Resources for Additional Help and Information

Edited by Dawn D. Matthews. 678 pages. 2002. 0-7808-0339-6. $78.

"This title is a great addition for public and school libraries because it provides concise health information on the lungs."
— *American Reference Books Annual, 2003*

"Highly recommended for academic and medical reference collections." — *Library Bookwatch, Sep '02*

■

Medical Tests Sourcebook, 2nd Edition

Basic Consumer Health Information about Medical Tests, Including Age-Specific Health Tests, Important Health Screenings and Exams, Home-Use Tests, Blood and Specimen Tests, Electrical Tests, Scope Tests, Genetic Testing, and Imaging Tests, Such as X-Rays, Ultrasound, Computed Tomography, Magnetic Resonance Imaging, Angiography, and Nuclear Medicine

Along with a Glossary and Directory of Additional Resources

Edited by Joyce Brennfleck Shannon. 654 pages. 2004. 0-7808-0670-0. $78.

ALSO AVAILABLE: Medical Tests, 1st Edition. Edited by Joyce Brennfleck Shannon. 691 pages. 1999. 0-7808-0243-8. $78.

"Recommended for hospital and health sciences libraries with consumer health collections."
— *E-Streams, Mar '00*

"This is an overall excellent reference with a wealth of general knowledge that may aid those who are reluctant to get vital tests performed."
— *Today's Librarian, Jan 2000*

"A valuable reference guide."
— *American Reference Books Annual, 2000*

Men's Health Concerns Sourcebook, 2nd Edition

Basic Consumer Health Information about the Medical and Mental Concerns of Men, Including Theories about the Shorter Male Lifespan, the Leading Causes of Death and Disability, Physical Concerns of Special Significance to Men, Reproductive and Sexual Concerns, Sexually Transmitted Diseases, Men's Mental and Emotional Health, and Lifestyle Choices That Affect Wellness, Such as Nutrition, Fitness, and Substance Use

Along with a Glossary of Related Terms and a Directory of Organizational Resources in Men's Health

Edited by Robert Aquinas McNally. 644 pages. 2004. 0-7808-0671-9. $78.

ALSO AVAILABLE: *Men's Health Concerns Sourcebook, 1st Edition.* Edited by Allan R. Cook. 738 pages. 1998. 0-7808-0212-8. $78.

"This comprehensive resource and the series are highly recommended."
— *American Reference Books Annual, 2000*

"Recommended reference source."
— *Booklist, American Library Association, Dec '98*

■

Mental Health Disorders Sourcebook, 2nd Edition

Basic Consumer Health Information about Anxiety Disorders, Depression and Other Mood Disorders, Eating Disorders, Personality Disorders, Schizophrenia, and More, Including Disease Descriptions, Treatment Options, and Reports on Current Research Initiatives

Along with Statistical Data, Tips for Maintaining Mental Health, a Glossary, and Directory of Sources for Additional Help and Information

Edited by Karen Bellenir. 605 pages. 2000. 0-7808-0240-3. $78.

ALSO AVAILABLE: *Mental Health Disorders Sourcebook, 1st Edition.* Edited by Karen Bellenir. 548 pages. 1995. 0-7808-0040-0. $78.

"Well organized and well written."
— *American Reference Books Annual, 2001*

"Recommended reference source."
— *Booklist, American Library Association, Jun '00*

■

Mental Retardation Sourcebook

Basic Consumer Health Information about Mental Retardation and Its Causes, Including Down Syndrome, Fetal Alcohol Syndrome, Fragile X Syndrome, Genetic Conditions, Injury, and Environmental Sources

Along with Preventive Strategies, Parenting Issues, Educational Implications, Health Care Needs, Employment and Economic Matters, Legal Issues, a Glossary, and a Resource Listing for Additional Help and Information

Edited by Joyce Brennfleck Shannon. 642 pages. 2000. 0-7808-0377-9. $78.

"Public libraries will find the book useful for reference and as a beginning research point for students, parents, and caregivers."
— *American Reference Books Annual, 2001*

"The strength of this work is that it compiles many basic fact sheets and addresses for further information in one volume. It is intended and suitable for the general public. This sourcebook is relevant to any collection providing health information to the general public."
— *E-Streams, Nov '00*

"From preventing retardation to parenting and family challenges, this covers health, social and legal issues and will prove an invaluable overview."
— *Reviewer's Bookwatch, Jul '00*

■

Movement Disorders Sourcebook

Basic Consumer Health Information about Neurological Movement Disorders, Including Essential Tremor, Parkinson's Disease, Dystonia, Cerebral Palsy, Huntington's Disease, Myasthenia Gravis, Multiple Sclerosis, and Other Early-Onset and Adult-Onset Movement Disorders, Their Symptoms and Causes, Diagnostic Tests, and Treatments

Along with Mobility and Assistive Technology Information, a Glossary, and a Directory of Additional Resources

Edited by Joyce Brennfleck Shannon. 655 pages. 2003. 0-7808-0628-X. $78.

". . . a good resource for consumers and recommended for public, community college and undergraduate libraries."
— *American Reference Books Annual, 2004*

■

Muscular Dystrophy Sourcebook

Basic Consumer Health Information about Congenital, Childhood-Onset, and Adult-Onset Forms of Muscular Dystrophy, Such as Duchenne, Becker, Emery-Dreifuss, Distal, Limb-Girdle, Facioscapulohumeral (FSHD), Myotonic, and Ophthalmoplegic Muscular Dystrophies, Including Facts about Diagnostic Tests, Medical and Physical Therapies, Management of Co-Occurring Conditions, and Parenting Guidelines

Along with Practical Tips for Home Care, a Glossary, and Directories of Additional Resources

Edited by Joyce Brennfleck Shannon. 577 pages. 2004. 0-7808-0676-X. $78.

■

Obesity Sourcebook

Basic Consumer Health Information about Diseases and Other Problems Associated with Obesity, and Including Facts about Risk Factors, Prevention Issues, and Management Approaches

Along with Statistical and Demographic Data, Information about Special Populations, Research Updates, a Glossary, and Source Listings for Further Help and Information

Edited by Wilma Caldwell and Chad T. Kimball. 376 pages. 2001. 0-7808-0333-7. $78.

"The book synthesizes the reliable medical literature on obesity into one easy-to-read and useful resource for the general public."
— *American Reference Books Annual 2002*

"This is a very useful resource book for the lay public."
—*Doody's Review Service, Nov '01*

"Well suited for the health reference collection of a public library or an academic health science library that serves the general population." —*E-Streams, Sep '01*

"Recommended reference source."
—*Booklist, American Library Association, Apr '01*

" Recommended pick both for specialty health library collections and any general consumer health reference collection." — *The Bookwatch, Apr '01*

■

Ophthalmic Disorders Sourcebook, 1st Edition
SEE *Eye Care Sourcebook, 2nd Edition*

■

Oral Health Sourcebook
SEE *Dental Care & Oral Health Sourcebook, 2nd Ed.*

■

Osteoporosis Sourcebook
Basic Consumer Health Information about Primary and Secondary Osteoporosis and Juvenile Osteoporosis and Related Conditions, Including Fibrous Dysplasia, Gaucher Disease, Hyperthyroidism, Hypophosphatasia, Myeloma, Osteopetrosis, Osteogenesis Imperfecta, and Paget's Disease

Along with Information about Risk Factors, Treatments, Traditional and Non-Traditional Pain Management, a Glossary of Related Terms, and a Directory of Resources

Edited by Allan R. Cook. 584 pages. 2001. 0-7808-0239-X. $78.

"This would be a book to be kept in a staff or patient library. The targeted audience is the layperson, but the therapist who needs a quick bit of information on a particular topic will also find the book useful."
—*Physical Therapy, Jan '02*

"This resource is recommended as a great reference source for public, health, and academic libraries, and is another triumph for the editors of Omnigraphics."
—*American Reference Books Annual 2002*

"Recommended for all public libraries and general health collections, especially those supporting patient education or consumer health programs."
—*E-Streams, Nov '01*

"Will prove valuable to any library seeking to maintain a current, comprehensive reference collection of health resources. . . . From prevention to treatment and associated conditions, this provides an excellent survey."
—*The Bookwatch, Aug '01*

"Recommended reference source."
—*Booklist, American Library Association, July '01*

SEE ALSO *Women's Health Concerns Sourcebook*

■

Pain Sourcebook, 2nd Edition
Basic Consumer Health Information about Specific Forms of Acute and Chronic Pain, Including Muscle and Skeletal Pain, Nerve Pain, Cancer Pain, and Disorders Characterized by Pain, Such as Fibromyalgia, Shingles, Angina, Arthritis, and Headaches

Along with Information about Pain Medications and Management Techniques, Complementary and Alternative Pain Relief Options, Tips for People Living with Chronic Pain, a Glossary, and a Directory of Sources for Further Information

Edited by Karen Bellenir. 670 pages. 2002. 0-7808-0612-3. $78.

ALSO AVAILABLE: *Pain Sourcebook, 1st Edition.* Edited by Allan R. Cook. 667 pages. 1997. 0-7808-0213-6. $78.

"A source of valuable information. . . . This book offers help to nonmedical people who need information about pain and pain management. It is also an excellent reference for those who participate in patient education."
—*Doody's Review Service, Sep '02*

"The text is readable, easily understood, and well indexed. This excellent volume belongs in all patient education libraries, consumer health sections of public libraries, and many personal collections."
—*American Reference Books Annual, 1999*

"A beneficial reference." —*Booklist Health Sciences Supplement, American Library Association, Oct '98*

"The information is basic in terms of scholarship and is appropriate for general readers. Written in journalistic style . . . intended for non-professionals. Quite thorough in its coverage of different pain conditions and summarizes the latest clinical information regarding pain treatment." — *Choice, Association of College and Research Libraries, Jun '98*

"Recommended reference source."
—*Booklist, American Library Association, Mar '98*

■

Pediatric Cancer Sourcebook
Basic Consumer Health Information about Leukemias, Brain Tumors, Sarcomas, Lymphomas, and Other Cancers in Infants, Children, and Adolescents, Including Descriptions of Cancers, Treatments, and Coping Strategies

Along with Suggestions for Parents, Caregivers, and Concerned Relatives, a Glossary of Cancer Terms, and Resource Listings

Edited by Edward J. Prucha. 587 pages. 1999. 0-7808-0245-4. $78.

"An excellent source of information. Recommended for public, hospital, and health science libraries with consumer health collections." —*E-Streams, Jun '00*

"Recommended reference source."
—*Booklist, American Library Association, Feb '00*

Physical & Mental Issues in Aging Sourcebook

Basic Consumer Health Information on Physical and Mental Disorders Associated with the Aging Process, Including Concerns about Cardiovascular Disease, Pulmonary Disease, Oral Health, Digestive Disorders, Musculoskeletal and Skin Disorders, Metabolic Changes, Sexual and Reproductive Issues, and Changes in Vision, Hearing, and Other Senses

Along with Data about Longevity and Causes of Death, Information on Acute and Chronic Pain, Descriptions of Mental Concerns, a Glossary of Terms, and Resource Listings for Additional Help

Edited by Jenifer Swanson. 660 pages. 1999. 0-7808-0233-0. $78.

SEE ALSO Healthy Aging Sourcebook

Podiatry Sourcebook

Basic Consumer Health Information about Foot Conditions, Diseases, and Injuries, Including Bunions, Corns, Calluses, Athlete's Foot, Plantar Warts, Hammertoes and Clawtoes, Clubfoot, Heel Pain, Gout, and More

Along with Facts about Foot Care, Disease Prevention, Foot Safety, Choosing a Foot Care Specialist, a Glossary of Terms, and Resource Listings for Additional Information

Edited by M. Lisa Weatherford. 380 pages. 2001. 0-7808-0215-2. $78.

Pregnancy & Birth Sourcebook, 2nd Edition

Basic Consumer Health Information about Conception and Pregnancy, Including Facts about Fertility, Infertility, Pregnancy Symptoms and Complications, Fetal Growth and Development, Labor, Delivery, and the Postpartum Period, as Well as Information about Maintaining Health and Wellness during Pregnancy and Caring for a Newborn

Along with Information about Public Health Assistance for Low-Income Pregnant Women, a Glossary, and Directories of Agencies and Organizations Providing Help and Support

Edited by Amy L. Sutton. 626 pages. 2004. 0-7808-0672-7. $78.

ALSO AVAILABLE: Pregnancy & Birth Sourcebook, 1st Edition. Edited by Heather E. Aldred. 737 pages. 1997. 0-7808-0216-0. $78.

SEE ALSO Congenital Disorders Sourcebook, Family Planning Sourcebook

Prostate Cancer Sourcebook

Basic Consumer Health Information about Prostate Cancer, Including Information about the Associated Risk Factors, Detection, Diagnosis, and Treatment of Prostate Cancer

Along with Information on Non-Malignant Prostate Conditions, and Featuring a Section Listing Support and Treatment Centers and a Glossary of Related Terms

Edited by Dawn D. Matthews. 358 pages. 2001. 0-7808-0324-8. $78.

Public Health Sourcebook

Basic Information about Government Health Agencies, Including National Health Statistics and Trends, Healthy People 2000 Program Goals and Objectives, the Centers for Disease Control and Prevention, the Food and Drug Administration, and the National Institutes of Health

Along with Full Contact Information for Each Agency

Edited by Wendy Wilcox. 698 pages. 1998. 0-7808-0220-9. $78.

Reconstructive & Cosmetic Surgery Sourcebook

Basic Consumer Health Information on Cosmetic and Reconstructive Plastic Surgery, Including Statistical Information about Different Surgical Procedures, Things to Consider Prior to Surgery, Plastic Surgery Techniques and Tools, Emotional and Psychological Considerations, and Procedure-Specific Information

Along with a Glossary of Terms and a Listing of Resources for Additional Help and Information

Edited by M. Lisa Weatherford. 374 pages. 2001. 0-7808-0214-4. $78.

"An excellent reference that addresses cosmetic and medically necessary reconstructive surgeries. . . . The style of the prose is calm and reassuring, discussing the many positive outcomes now available due to advances in surgical techniques."
— *American Reference Books Annual 2002*

"Recommended for health science libraries that are open to the public, as well as hospital libraries that are open to the patients. This book is a good resource for the consumer interested in plastic surgery."
— *E-Streams, Dec '01*

"Recommended reference source."
— *Booklist, American Library Association, July '01*

■

Rehabilitation Sourcebook

Basic Consumer Health Information about Rehabilitation for People Recovering from Heart Surgery, Spinal Cord Injury, Stroke, Orthopedic Impairments, Amputation, Pulmonary Impairments, Traumatic Injury, and More, Including Physical Therapy, Occupational Therapy, Speech/ Language Therapy, Massage Therapy, Dance Therapy, Art Therapy, and Recreational Therapy

Along with Information on Assistive and Adaptive Devices, a Glossary, and Resources for Additional Help and Information

Edited by Dawn D. Matthews. 531 pages. 1999. 0-7808-0236-5. $78.

"This is an excellent resource for public library reference and health collections."
— *American Reference Books Annual, 2001*

"Recommended reference source."
— *Booklist, American Library Association, May '00*

■

Respiratory Diseases & Disorders Sourcebook

Basic Information about Respiratory Diseases and Disorders, Including Asthma, Cystic Fibrosis, Pneumonia, the Common Cold, Influenza, and Others, Featuring Facts about the Respiratory System, Statistical and Demographic Data, Treatments, Self-Help Management Suggestions, and Current Research Initiatives

Edited by Allan R. Cook and Peter D. Dresser. 771 pages. 1995. 0-7808-0037-0. $78.

"Designed for the layperson and for patients and their families coping with respiratory illness. . . . an extensive array of information on diagnosis, treatment, management, and prevention of respiratory illnesses for the general reader."
— *Choice, Association of College and Research Libraries, Jun '96*

"A highly recommended text for all collections. It is a comforting reminder of the power of knowledge that good books carry between their covers."
— *Academic Library Book Review, Spring '96*

"A comprehensive collection of authoritative information presented in a nontechnical, humanitarian style for patients, families, and caregivers." — *Association of Operating Room Nurses, Sep/Oct '95*

SEE ALSO Lung Disorders Sourcebook

■

Sexually Transmitted Diseases Sourcebook, 2nd Edition

Basic Consumer Health Information about Sexually Transmitted Diseases, Including Information on the Diagnosis and Treatment of Chlamydia, Gonorrhea, Hepatitis, Herpes, HIV, Mononucleosis, Syphilis, and Others

Along with Information on Prevention, Such as Condom Use, Vaccines, and STD Education; And Featuring a Section on Issues Related to Youth and Adolescents, a Glossary, and Resources for Additional Help and Information

Edited by Dawn D. Matthews. 538 pages. 2001. 0-7808-0249-7. $78.

ALSO AVAILABLE: Sexually Transmitted Diseases Sourcebook, 1st Edition. Edited by Linda M. Ross. 550 pages. 1997. 0-7808-0217-9. $78.

"Recommended for consumer health collections in public libraries, and secondary school and community college libraries."
— *American Reference Books Annual 2002*

"Every school and public library should have a copy of this comprehensive and user-friendly reference book."
— *Choice, Association of College & Research Libraries, Sep '01*

"This is a highly recommended book. This is an especially important book for all school and public libraries." — *AIDS Book Review Journal, Jul-Aug '01*

"Recommended reference source."
— *Booklist, American Library Association, Apr '01*

"Recommended pick both for specialty health library collections and any general consumer health reference collection." — *The Bookwatch, Apr '01*

■

Skin Disorders Sourcebook

Basic Information about Common Skin and Scalp Conditions Caused by Aging, Allergies, Immune Reactions, Sun Exposure, Infectious Organisms, Parasites, Cosmetics, and Skin Traumas, Including Abrasions, Cuts, and Pressure Sores

Along with Information on Prevention and Treatment

Edited by Allan R. Cook. 647 pages. 1997. 0-7808-0080-X. $78.

"... comprehensive, easily read reference book."
— *Doody's Health Sciences Book Reviews, Oct '97*

SEE ALSO Burns Sourcebook

Sleep Disorders Sourcebook, 2nd Edition

Basic Consumer Health Information about Sleep and Sleep Disorders, Including Insomnia, Sleep Apnea, Restless Legs Syndrome, Narcolepsy, Parasomnias, and Other Health Problems That Affect Sleep, Plus Facts about Diagnostic Procedures, Treatment Strategies, Sleep Medications, and Tips for Improving Sleep Quality

Along with a Glossary of Related Terms and Resources for Additional Help and Information

Edited by Amy L. Sutton. 575 pages. 2005. 0-7808-0745-6. $78.

ALSO AVAILABLE: Sleep Disorders Sourcebook, 1st Edition. Edited by Jenifer Swanson. 439 pages. 1998. 0-7808-0234-9. $78.

"This text will complement any home or medical library. It is user-friendly and ideal for the adult reader."
— *American Reference Books Annual, 2000*

"A useful resource that provides accurate, relevant, and accessible information on sleep to the general public. Health care providers who deal with sleep disorders patients may also find it helpful in being prepared to answer some of the questions patients ask."
— *Respiratory Care, Jul '99*

"Recommended reference source."
— *Booklist, American Library Association, Feb '99*

Smoking Concerns Sourcebook

Basic Consumer Health Information about Nicotine Addiction and Smoking Cessation, Featuring Facts about the Health Effects of Tobacco Use, Including Lung and Other Cancers, Heart Disease, Stroke, and Respiratory Disorders, Such as Emphysema and Chronic Bronchitis

Along with Information about Smoking Prevention Programs, Suggestions for Achieving and Maintaining a Smoke-Free Lifestyle, Statistics about Tobacco Use, Reports on Current Research Initiatives, a Glossary of Related Terms, and Directories of Resources for Additional Help and Information

Edited by Karen Bellenir. 621 pages. 2004. 0-7808-0323-X. $78.

Sports Injuries Sourcebook, 2nd Edition

Basic Consumer Health Information about the Diagnosis, Treatment, and Rehabilitation of Common Sports-Related Injuries in Children and Adults

Along with Suggestions for Conditioning and Training, Information and Prevention Tips for Injuries Frequently Associated with Specific Sports and Special Populations, a Glossary, and a Directory of Additional Resources

Edited by Joyce Brennfleck Shannon. 614 pages. 2002. 0-7808-0604-2. $78.

ALSO AVAILABLE: Sports Injuries Sourcebook, 1st Edition. Edited by Heather E. Aldred. 624 pages. 1999. 0-7808-0218-7. $78.

"This is an excellent reference for consumers and it is recommended for public, community college, and undergraduate libraries."
— *American Reference Books Annual, 2003*

"Recommended reference source."
— *Booklist, American Library Association, Feb '03*

Stress-Related Disorders Sourcebook

Basic Consumer Health Information about Stress and Stress-Related Disorders, Including Stress Origins and Signals, Environmental Stress at Work and Home, Mental and Emotional Stress Associated with Depression, Post-Traumatic Stress Disorder, Panic Disorder, Suicide, and the Physical Effects of Stress on the Cardiovascular, Immune, and Nervous Systems

Along with Stress Management Techniques, a Glossary, and a Listing of Additional Resources

Edited by Joyce Brennfleck Shannon. 610 pages. 2002. 0-7808-0560-7. $78.

"Well written for a general readership, the *Stress-Related Disorders Sourcebook* is a useful addition to the health reference literature."
— *American Reference Books Annual, 2003*

"I am impressed by the amount of information. It offers a thorough overview of the causes and consequences of stress for the layperson.... A well-done and thorough reference guide for professionals and nonprofessionals alike."
— *Doody's Review Service, Dec '02*

Stroke Sourcebook

Basic Consumer Health Information about Stroke, Including Ischemic, Hemorrhagic, Transient Ischemic Attack (TIA), and Pediatric Stroke, Stroke Triggers and Risks, Diagnostic Tests, Treatments, and Rehabilitation Information

Along with Stroke Prevention Guidelines, Legal and Financial Information, a Glossary, and a Directory of Additional Resources

Edited by Joyce Brennfleck Shannon. 606 pages. 2003. 0-7808-0630-1. $78.

"This volume is highly recommended and should be in every medical, hospital, and public library."
— *American Reference Books Annual, 2004*

Substance Abuse Sourcebook

Basic Health-Related Information about the Abuse of Legal and Illegal Substances Such as Alcohol, Tobacco, Prescription Drugs, Marijuana, Cocaine, and Heroin; and Including Facts about Substance Abuse Prevention Strategies, Intervention Methods, Treatment and Recovery Programs, and a Section Addressing the Special Problems Related to Substance Abuse during Pregnancy

Edited by Karen Bellenir. 573 pages. 1996. 0-7808-0038-9. $78.

"A valuable addition to any health reference section. Highly recommended."
— *The Book Report, Mar/Apr '97*

". . . a comprehensive collection of substance abuse information that's both highly readable and compact. Families and caregivers of substance abusers will find the information enlightening and helpful, while teachers, social workers and journalists should benefit from the concise format. Recommended."
— *Drug Abuse Update, Winter '96/'97*

SEE ALSO Alcoholism Sourcebook, Drug Abuse Sourcebook

■

Surgery Sourcebook

Basic Consumer Health Information about Inpatient and Outpatient Surgeries, Including Cardiac, Vascular, Orthopedic, Ocular, Reconstructive, Cosmetic, Gynecologic, and Ear, Nose, and Throat Procedures and More

Along with Information about Operating Room Policies and Instruments, Laser Surgery Techniques, Hospital Errors, Statistical Data, a Glossary, and Listings of Sources for Further Help and Information

Edited by Annemarie S. Muth and Karen Bellenir. 596 pages. 2002. 0-7808-0380-9. $78.

"Large public libraries and medical libraries would benefit from this material in their reference collections."
— *American Reference Books Annual, 2004*

"Invaluable reference for public and school library collections alike."   — *Library Bookwatch, Apr '03*

■

Transplantation Sourcebook

Basic Consumer Health Information about Organ and Tissue Transplantation, Including Physical and Financial Preparations, Procedures and Issues Relating to Specific Solid Organ and Tissue Transplants, Rehabilitation, Pediatric Transplant Information, the Future of Transplantation, and Organ and Tissue Donation

Along with a Glossary and Listings of Additional Resources

Edited by Joyce Brennfleck Shannon. 628 pages. 2002. 0-7808-0322-1. $78.

"Along with these advances [in transplantation technology] have come a number of daunting questions for potential transplant patients, their families, and their health care providers. This reference text is the best single tool to address many of these questions. . . . It will be a much-needed addition to the reference collections in health care, academic, and large public libraries."
— *American Reference Books Annual, 2003*

"Recommended for libraries with an interest in offering consumer health information."   — *E-Streams, Jul '02*

"This is a unique and valuable resource for patients facing transplantation and their families."
— *Doody's Review Service, Jun '02*

■

Traveler's Health Sourcebook

Basic Consumer Health Information for Travelers, Including Physical and Medical Preparations, Transportation Health and Safety, Essential Information about Food and Water, Sun Exposure, Insect and Snake Bites, Camping and Wilderness Medicine, and Travel with Physical or Medical Disabilities

Along with International Travel Tips, Vaccination Recommendations, Geographical Health Issues, Disease Risks, a Glossary, and a Listing of Additional Resources

Edited by Joyce Brennfleck Shannon. 613 pages. 2000. 0-7808-0384-1. $78.

"Recommended reference source."
— *Booklist, American Library Association, Feb '01*

"This book is recommended for any public library, any travel collection, and especially any collection for the physically disabled."
— *American Reference Books Annual, 2001*

■

Vegetarian Sourcebook

Basic Consumer Health Information about Vegetarian Diets, Lifestyle, and Philosophy, Including Definitions of Vegetarianism and Veganism, Tips about Adopting Vegetarianism, Creating a Vegetarian Pantry, and Meeting Nutritional Needs of Vegetarians, with Facts Regarding Vegetarianism's Effect on Pregnant and Lactating Women, Children, Athletes, and Senior Citizens

Along with a Glossary of Commonly Used Vegetarian Terms and Resources for Additional Help and Information

Edited by Chad T. Kimball. 360 pages. 2002. 0-7808-0439-2. $78.

"Organizes into one concise volume the answers to the most common questions concerning vegetarian diets and lifestyles. This title is recommended for public and secondary school libraries."   — *E-Streams, Apr '03*

"Invaluable reference for public and school library collections alike."   — *Library Bookwatch, Apr '03*

"The articles in this volume are easy to read and come from authoritative sources. The book does not necessarily support the vegetarian diet but instead provides the pros and cons of this important decision. The *Vegetarian Sourcebook* is recommended for public libraries and consumer health libraries."
— *American Reference Books Annual, 2003*

Women's Health Concerns Sourcebook, 2nd Edition

Basic Consumer Health Information about the Medical and Mental Concerns of Women, Including Maintaining Health and Wellness, Gynecological Concerns, Breast Health, Sexuality and Reproductive Issues, Menopause, Cancer in Women, the Leading Causes of Death and Disability among Women, Physical Concerns of Special Significance to Women, and Women's Mental and Emotional Health

Along with a Glossary of Related Terms and Directories of Resources for Additional Help and Information

Edited by Amy L. Sutton. 748 pages. 2004. 0-7808-0673-5. $78.

ALSO AVAILABLE: *Women's Health Concerns Sourcebook, 1st Edition.* Edited by Heather E. Aldred. 567 pages. 1997. 0-7808-0219-5. $78.

"Handy compilation. There is an impressive range of diseases, devices, disorders, procedures, and other physical and emotional issues covered . . . well organized, illustrated, and indexed." *— Choice, Association of College and Research Libraries, Jan '98*

SEE ALSO *Breast Cancer Sourcebook, Cancer Sourcebook for Women, Healthy Heart Sourcebook for Women, Osteoporosis Sourcebook*

■

Workplace Health & Safety Sourcebook

Basic Consumer Health Information about Workplace Health and Safety, Including the Effect of Workplace Hazards on the Lungs, Skin, Heart, Ears, Eyes, Brain, Reproductive Organs, Musculoskeletal System, and Other Organs and Body Parts

Along with Information about Occupational Cancer, Personal Protective Equipment, Toxic and Hazardous Chemicals, Child Labor, Stress, and Workplace Violence

Edited by Chad T. Kimball. 626 pages. 2000. 0-7808-0231-4. $78.

"As a reference for the general public, this would be useful in any library." *—E-Streams, Jun '01*

"Provides helpful information for primary care physicians and other caregivers interested in occupational medicine. . . . General readers; professionals." *— Choice, Association of College & Research Libraries, May '01*

"Recommended reference source." *— Booklist, American Library Association, Feb '01*

"Highly recommended." *— The Bookwatch, Jan '01*

■

Worldwide Health Sourcebook

Basic Information about Global Health Issues, Including Malnutrition, Reproductive Health, Disease Dispersion and Prevention, Emerging Diseases, Risky Health Behaviors, and the Leading Causes of Death

Along with Global Health Concerns for Children, Women, and the Elderly, Mental Health Issues, Research and Technology Advancements, and Economic, Environmental, and Political Health Implications, a Glossary, and a Resource Listing for Additional Help and Information

Edited by Joyce Brennfleck Shannon. 614 pages. 2001. 0-7808-0330-2. $78.

"Named an Outstanding Academic Title." *—Choice, Association of College & Research Libraries, Jan '02*

"Yet another handy but also unique compilation in the extensive Health Reference Series, this is a useful work because many of the international publications reprinted or excerpted are not readily available. Highly recommended." *—Choice, Association of College & Research Libraries, Nov '01*

"Recommended reference source." *—Booklist, American Library Association, Oct '01*

711

Teen Health Series

Helping Young Adults Understand, Manage, and Avoid Serious Illness

Alcohol Information For Teens

Health Tips About Alcohol And Alcoholism

Including Facts about Underage Drinking, Preventing Teen Alcohol Use, Alcohol's Effects on the Brain and the Body, Alcohol Abuse Treatment, Help for Children of Alcoholics, and More

Edited by Joyce Brennfleck Shannon. 370 pages. 2005. 0-7808-0741-3. $58.

Cancer Information for Teens

Health Tips about Cancer Awareness, Prevention, Diagnosis, and Treatment

Including Facts about Frequently Occurring Cancers, Cancer Risk Factors, and Coping Strategies for Teens Fighting Cancer or Dealing with Cancer in Friends or Family Members

Edited by Wilma R. Caldwell. 428 pages. 2004. 0-7808-0678-6. $58.

Diet Information for Teens

Health Tips about Diet and Nutrition

Including Facts about Nutrients, Dietary Guidelines, Breakfasts, School Lunches, Snacks, Party Food, Weight Control, Eating Disorders, and More

Edited by Karen Bellenir. 399 pages. 2001. 0-7808-0441-4. $58.

"Full of helpful insights and facts throughout the book. ... An excellent resource to be placed in public libraries or even in personal collections."
—*American Reference Books Annual 2002*

"Recommended for middle and high school libraries and media centers as well as academic libraries that educate future teachers of teenagers. It is also a suitable addition to health science libraries that serve patrons who are interested in teen health promotion and education."
—*E-Streams, Oct '01*

"This comprehensive book would be beneficial to collections that need information about nutrition, dietary guidelines, meal planning, and weight control. ... This reference is so easy to use that its purchase is recommended."
—*The Book Report, Sep-Oct '01*

"This book is written in an easy to understand format describing issues that many teens face every day, and then provides thoughtful explanations so that teens can make informed decisions. This is an interesting book that provides important facts and information for today's teens."
—*Doody's Health Sciences Book Review Journal, Jul-Aug '01*

"A comprehensive compendium of diet and nutrition. The information is presented in a straightforward, plain-spoken manner. This title will be useful to those working on reports on a variety of topics, as well as to general readers concerned about their dietary health."
—*School Library Journal, Jun '01*

Drug Information for Teens

Health Tips about the Physical and Mental Effects of Substance Abuse

Including Facts about Alcohol, Anabolic Steroids, Club Drugs, Cocaine, Depressants, Hallucinogens, Herbal Products, Inhalants, Marijuana, Narcotics, Stimulants, Tobacco, and More

Edited by Karen Bellenir. 452 pages. 2002. 0-7808-0444-9. $58.

"A clearly written resource for general readers and researchers alike."
—*School Library Journal*

"The chapters are quick to make a connection to their teenage reading audience. The prose is straightforward and the book lends itself to spot reading. It should be useful both for practical information and for research, and it is suitable for public and school libraries."
—*American Reference Books Annual, 2003*

"Recommended reference source."
—*Booklist, American Library Association, Feb '03*

"This is an excellent resource for teens and their parents. Education about drugs and substances is key to discouraging teen drug abuse and this book provides this much needed information in a way that is interesting and factual."
—*Doody's Review Service, Dec '02*

Fitness Information for Teens

Health Tips about Exercise, Physical Well-Being, and Health Maintenance

Including Facts about Aerobic and Anaerobic Conditioning, Stretching, Body Shape and Body Image, Sports Training, Nutrition, and Activities for Non-Athletes

Edited by Karen Bellenir. 425 pages. 2004. 0-7808-0679-4. $58.

Mental Health Information for Teens

Health Tips about Mental Health and Mental Illness

Including Facts about Anxiety, Depression, Suicide, Eating Disorders, Obsessive-Compulsive Disorders, Panic Attacks, Phobias, Schizophrenia, and More

Edited by Karen Bellenir. 406 pages. 2001. 0-7808-0442-2. $58.

"In both language and approach, this user-friendly entry in the *Teen Health Series* is on target for teens needing information on mental health concerns." — *Booklist, American Library Association, Jan '02*

"Readers will find the material accessible and informative, with the shaded notes, facts, and embedded glossary insets adding appropriately to the already interesting and succinct presentation."
— *School Library Journal, Jan '02*

"This title is highly recommended for any library that serves adolescents and parents/caregivers of adolescents." — *E-Streams, Jan '02*

"Recommended for high school libraries and young adult collections in public libraries. Both health professionals and teenagers will find this book useful."
— *American Reference Books Annual 2002*

"This is a nice book written to enlighten the society, primarily teenagers, about common teen mental health issues. It is highly recommended to teachers and parents as well as adolescents."
— *Doody's Review Service, Dec '01*

Sexual Health Information for Teens

Health Tips about Sexual Development, Human Reproduction, and Sexually Transmitted Diseases

Including Facts about Puberty, Reproductive Health, Chlamydia, Human Papillomavirus, Pelvic Inflammatory Disease, Herpes, AIDS, Contraception, Pregnancy, and More

Edited by Deborah A. Stanley. 391 pages. 2003. 0-7808-0445-7. $58.

"This work should be included in all high school libraries and many larger public libraries. . . . highly recommended."
— *American Reference Books Annual 2004*

"Sexual Health approaches its subject with appropriate seriousness and offers easily accessible advice and information." — *School Library Journal, Feb. 2004*

Skin Health Information For Teens

Health Tips about Dermatological Concerns and Skin Cancer Risks

Including Facts about Acne, Warts, Hives, and Other Conditions and Lifestyle Choices, Such as Tanning, Tattooing, and Piercing, That Affect the Skin, Nails, Scalp, and Hair

Edited by Robert Aquinas McNally. 429 pages. 2003. 0-7808-0446-5. $58.

"This volume, as with others in the series, will be a useful addition to school and public library collections."
— *American Reference Books Annual 2004*

"This volume serves as a one-stop source and should be a necessity for any health collection."
— *Library Media Connection*

Sports Injuries Information For Teens

Health Tips about Sports Injuries and Injury Protection

Including Facts about Specific Injuries, Emergency Treatment, Rehabilitation, Sports Safety, Competition Stress, Fitness, Sports Nutrition, Steroid Risks, and More

Edited by Joyce Brennfleck Shannon. 405 pages. 2003. 0-7808-0447-3. $58.

"This work will be useful in the young adult collections of public libraries as well as high school libraries."
— *American Reference Books Annual 2004*

Suicide Information for Teens

Health Tips about Suicide Causes and Prevention

Including Facts about Depression, Risk Factors, Getting Help, Survivor Support, and More

Edited by Joyce Brennfleck Shannon. 375 pages. 2005. 0-7808-0737-5. $58.

Health Reference Series